Overcoming Resistance in Cognitive Therapy

ROBERT L. LEAHY

THE GUILFORD PRESS
New York London

© 2001 Robert L. Leahy
Published by The Guilford Press
A Division of Guilford Publications, Inc.
72 Spring Street, New York, NY 10012
www.guilford.com

Paperback edition 2003

Printed in the United States of America

This book is printed on acid-free paper.

Last digit is print number: 9   8   7   6   5   4   3   2

Library of Congress Cataloging-in-Publication Data

Leahy, Robert L.
   Overcoming resistance in cognitive therapy / Robert L. Leahy.
      p. cm.
   Includes bibliographical references and index.
   ISBN 1-57230-684-X (hardcover) ISBN 1-57230-936-9 (paper)
      1. Cognitive therapy. 2. Resistance (Psychoanalysis) I. Title.

   RC489.C63 L384 2001
   616.89′142—dc21

                        2001033291

*To those patients who have
taught me about their struggles*

Open your eyes.
Why open my eyes when the form
of Krishna resides within?
        —RUSKHAN, 16th century

About the Author

Robert L. Leahy, PhD, is President-Elect of the International Association of Cognitive Psychotherapy and Editor of the *Journal of Cognitive Psychotherapy: An International Quarterly*. The author or editor of nine books, including *Treatment Plans and Interventions for Depression and Anxiety Disorders* (with Stephen J. Holland) and *Bipolar Disorder: A Cognitive Therapy Approach* (with Cory Newman, Aaron T. Beck, Noreen Reilly-Harrington, and Laszylo Gyulai), Dr. Leahy is also the Founder and Director of the American Institute for Cognitive Therapy in New York (*www.CognitiveTherapyNYC.com*) and Clinical Associate Professor in the Department of Psychiatry at Weill–Cornell Medical College.

Acknowledgments

I would like to begin by thanking Seymour Weingarten of The Guilford Press, who had the patience to recognize that a book on "resistance" was bound to come in past the deadline. Jim Nageotte of Guilford was very helpful in providing me with editorial feedback to tighten the manuscript. Tony Papa and Lisa Wu of Columbia University tirelessly reviewed the manuscript and assisted with its production.

My ideas about an integrative cognitive model of resistance have benefited over several years from discussions with members of the American Institute for Cognitive Therapy in New York. I would like to thank Mudita Buhadur, Christiane Humke, Lynn Marcinko, Laura Oliff, and Elizabeth Winkelman. My friend and colleague Stephen Holland has been an invaluable source of knowledge and support over the years and has given me many insights into the understanding of personality and resistance. David Clark made numerous helpful comments on the manuscript. Needless to say, any errors and oversights are mine.

Of course, I wish to thank my wife, Helen, who often had the ironic humor to comment on my resistance to completing a book on resistance. And my gratitude is especially extended to the many patients whom I have seen who have taught me about the reasons and the "logic" of resistance, and have helped me understand that it is much easier to change what you say than to change how you feel.

Contents

PART III. COGNITIVE THERAPY
AND COUNTERTRANSFERENCE

1

Introduction

He who saves a single life saves the world entire.
—TALMUD, SANHEDRIN

*D*espite the efforts of therapists and patients, many patients in cognitive-behavioral therapy—or any therapy—do not improve. For example, perhaps one out of three patients treated for depression in cognitive therapy shows clinically significant change. Moreover, some studies indicate that about 40% of patients terminate prematurely. These results pertain to *cognitive therapy*, a modality often praised as a treatment with proven efficacy. Why do so many patients drop out? Of those remaining, why do one-third not improve? What could account for these less-than-spectacular results?

A common view of cognitive-behavioral therapy is that it relies on structured treatment packages and specific intervention techniques, often applied in what appears to some as a manner that does not take into account the individuality of the patient. Unlike psychodynamic therapists, who emphasize the patient's earlier developmental history and current transference as impediments to current change, the cognitive therapist is often viewed as driven by naive optimism while ignoring the fundamental resistance that the patient displays.

As cognitive therapy has matured as a therapeutic model, there has been an increased awareness of the need to adapt the model to overcome impediments to individual change. In the last decade there has been considerable interest among cognitive therapists in individualizing treatment by utilizing *case conceptualization* (Beck, Freeman, & Associates, 1990; J. Beck, 1996; Leahy, 1991; 1996a, 1999a; Needleman, 1999; Persons, 1989; Tompkins, 1999). Case conceptualization includes an analysis of the patient's current cognitive schemas, interpersonal problems and

1

behavioral deficits, and excesses as related to early childhood experiences. But case conceptualization may take a form different from these standard guidelines—a point that will be illustrated in my discussions of varieties of resistance. Throughout this book, I rely on case conceptualizations as a guide in dealing with resistance and countertransference.

DIMENSIONS OF RESISTANCE

My purpose is to outline *several* causes or dimensions of resistance to change and to indicate how these may be addressed within a cognitive therapy model. Before individual change can occur, the therapist must first learn what the patient's view of this change is and what the patient sees he is giving up in abandoning his current position. For example, consider the woman who has been married for 15 years to an abusive, withholding, passive–aggressive, alcoholic husband who refuses to have sex with her. She is having problems in her career. From the therapist's point of view, almost anything that gets the patient out of the marriage would be a positive change. The therapist is bewildered that the patient stays in the relationship, even after her practical problems—such as where to live and how to support herself—are resolved. Why does she "resist" change? The naive therapist might assume that the patient does not want to change or suffers from psychological masochism. But the patient feels trapped and complains of her suffering. How does the patient see change?

Contrary to the beliefs of the naive therapist, who views personal change *only* from the perspective of solving practical problems, the therapist who addresses the patient's resistance learns that change is often about *solving psychological problems, not just solving practical problems.* Solving practical problems may help address psychological problems, but it is seldom enough in the case of patients presenting with longer term personality problems.

Several dimensions must be addressed to help the resistant patient. First, she may need *validation* for her feelings and for her perspective. If the therapist says, in a cavalier manner, "Just move out and get divorced," he may be viewed by the patient as unable to understand how badly she feels and how difficult she sees her future to be. Validating her suffering and her sense of hopelessness may be a necessary component of helping her to change. His recommendations may be viewed as condescending and may add to the patient's sense of hopelessness. The patient may think, "How can he help me if he doesn't understand me?"

A patient's resistance to change may be related to her inability to handle her emotional intensity. When she experiences anxiety, she focuses on bodily sensations and describes how "bad" she feels in general. These complaints appear diffuse and vague to the therapist, but their very ambiguity contributes to her feeling of being overwhelmed. After all, if she cannot specifically identify the complaint, it is difficult for her to develop a strategy to cope with it. She claims that "feelings come over her" and has trouble identifying the thoughts that give rise to these feelings or the specific problems that need to be addressed. She turns plaintively toward the therapist, hoping he will find a solution to her distress. She states her problems in terms of their pain, not in terms of their solutions. The first dimension of resistance may be her demands for validation.

A second impediment to change may be *self-consistency*. She may resist change because of her belief that she has already committed a great deal of time, effort, and self-esteem to the relationship and she is reluctant to walk away from it. She may be trapped by the "sunk-cost" that holds her to a decision she made in the past that has proven to be a failure. From her perspective, walking away from the relationship may be evidence that she is incompetent in making any decisions, thereby making the future even more problematic.

Thus, the woman in the 15-year marriage has to make "sense" of why she has stayed. She is committed to justifying her past behavior. In the absence of clear, positive reasons for staying now, she is even more motivated to come up with stronger reasons for staying in the future. She may think, "If leaving makes so much sense and would be so easy, then why did I not leave a long time ago?" She has several choices in explaining this consistency—that is, she may think she is an idiot for staying, she may think she has a moral obligation, or she may view herself as helpless (unable to change).

A third impediment is her habitual pattern of viewing herself as unlovable and helpless—that is, her *personal schemas*. We generally like to see our past behavior as consistent with our view of ourselves—that is, as consistent with our identity. Once we form a concept of who we are, we tend to seek or to remember information that is consistent with this personal concept or *schema*. Having a personal schema allows us to predict how we will act in the future and enables us to make sense of our behavior. In the case of the unhappy wife, her personal schema is one of helplessness. Thus, change for her may activate her belief that she cannot take care of herself: that she will not be able to manage the home, continue at work, or raise the children. Ironically, by staying with her demeaning, passive–aggressive husband, she increases her sense of personal helplessness, making it even more difficult to leave. Thus, the psychological abuse that the therapist sees as the very reason for her to leave may be the psychological glue that keeps her in the marriage.

A fourth impediment for the patient may be *moral resistance*. She may believe in a "just world," in which bad things happen to bad people. Thus, she may conclude from her experience that she does not deserve positives, since her distress is evidence of her unworthiness. Or she may believe she has an obligation to make the marriage work out.

A fifth dimension may be her view that she is a *victim*. She may feel entitled to her complaints and her suffering: "I have a right to feel bad— look how he's treating me!" She may feel she has a right to stay in the house and that he should move out. She may feel obligated to change his drinking habits and may view his alcoholism as evidence of her own character defects. She may derive some satisfaction in proving she is right and he is wrong.

A sixth dimension is that she views change as too *risky*. Since her self-esteem has been lowered by the relationship, and since the abusive husband tells her daily that she cannot take care of herself, she believes she has little room for error. If she leaves, she may not be able to take care of herself. She fears her financial assets will be depleted, she will get sick and have no one to take care of her, or she will leave and recognize that she has made a mistake, only to face the public humiliation of going home again. As she anticipates "how things will not work out if I leave," she looks for any sign of possible failure. She fears getting her hopes up too high, lest she get too far ahead of herself and risk too much. In fact, she finds herself getting angry with the therapist who, naively, believes his encouragement will help her feel better. What he sees as an opportunity, she sees as a test of her incompetence.

A seventh dimension of resistance is that she may be using the marital problem as a *self-handicapping strategy*. As long as she focuses on her personal relationship as "the problem," she may be able to utilize it as an excuse for why she is not making progress in her career. She may tell herself and her friends, "What do you expect of me? I have a problem in my marriage." The problems about which she complains—which may include somatic as well as relationship problems—can be viewed as "sufficient" explanations for a lack of success in other areas of her life. Perhaps she actually has fears of being evaluated in her true potential at work, but uses her relationship preoccupations as a distraction from those challenges.

The example of the woman "trapped" in her marriage is not untypical of the long-term problems the experienced therapist may confront. The patient may receive some abatement of symptoms from medication and therapy, but the core problems remain. Many therapists who have been practicing for more than 10 years can attest that their practices appear to be focused on patients whose problems continue. Nor is resistance confined to the longer term patient. Patients entering therapy may present their resistance in the first two sessions: some patients refuse to fill out intake forms, some cancel even before they come to their first session. One patient told me in her first session, "I am not going to do any self-help homework. If you are going to help me, it is going to have to be in here—in the session."

COUNTERTRANSFERENCE

Needless to say, these patients activate a strong countertransference in the therapist. Cognitive therapists may wonder why I—a cognitive therapist—have chosen to use the term "countertransference"—a term so closely associated with the psychodynamic approach. There are several reasons I am willing to borrow—if not steal—from our dynamic colleagues. First, the countertransference exists, no matter how objective or technique-driven you are as a therapist. We all know that certain patients or issues "push our buttons" more than others. Second, none of us has a monopoly on the truth. Psychodynamic concepts of transference, countertransference, and even ego defenses may be useful in helping us understand and change our patients' problems. Indeed, a recent review of some of the major components of psychodynamic theory indicates substantial empirical support for several of the main tenets of this model, including unconscious motivation, developmental precursors, and various personality types (Weston, 1998). Third, my use of "transference" and "countertransference" does not imply that I have abandoned the cognitive model. Quite the contrary—I will attempt to assimilate these concepts *into* the cognitive model, by indicating how we can understand the patient's relationship to the therapist and the therapist's response to this relationship by utilizing the cognitive constructs outlined above, such as affective dysregulation, moral resistance, schematic processes, and risk aversion. When we, as therapists, consider ourselves "our own patient" (as we should do in examining the countertransference), we come to recognize that just as it is difficult for the patient to abandon old patterns, it is difficult for ourselves, as therapists, to modify our habitual patterns of responding. In the therapeutic relationship, both patient and therapist are *patients*.

ORGANIZATION OF THE BOOK

I begin with a very brief discussion of the importance of resistance in psychotherapy. In Part I, I describe how resistance is explained in psychoanalytic, behavioral, and (traditional) cognitive models. One conclusion we can draw from this review is that the meaning of "resistance" can best be understood in the context of the theoretical or clinical model. What appears to be "resistance" in behavioral therapy is called "regression" in the dynamic model—and regression may be the goal of treatment. Also in Part I, I describe "procedural resistance"—that is, the specific elements of resistance related to the cognitive model.

In Part II, I describe seven dimensions of resistance: validation, self-consistency, schematic resistance, moral resistance, victim resistance, risk aversion, and self-handicapping. These constitute the core dimensions of resistance in the cognitive model I am proposing. This model is not meant to be a comprehensive model of all resistance. For example, attachment issues and family-systems issues, so central to the nature of resistance, are not included in this model. These issues are better addressed by other models and should be considered by the clinician in modifying resistance.

In Part III, I discuss countertransference issues. I examine the various schematic issues that give rise to our countertransference and how it interacts with the different kinds of patients we encounter. I also examine how the therapist can use cognitive therapy to help him- or herself modify the countertransference and, in the process, assist the patient. I propose that the countertransference is an excellent window into the interpersonal world of the patient. By utilizing the countertransference, the clinician gains insight into the "real" world of the patient and may learn from the patient how his or her early maladaptive schemas were formed.

This book is directed toward clinicians familiar with the cognitive therapy approach. However, it is not necessary that the reader even practice this approach. I have found that discussions of the issues outlined in this book are relevant to clinicians from almost any approach. Perhaps because I have attempted to bridge the theoretical gap between cognitive therapy and other models, readers may find that the content and the suggestions that are offered here clash less with their theoretical preconceptions and conform more with their own clinical experience.

PART I
Theoretical and Conceptual Foundations

2

Models of Resistance

The idea that patients may resist change has been a central theme in psychotherapy for over a century. During the 19th century, many neurologists (the precursors of psychiatrists) viewed psychopathology precisely in terms of resistance. These early observers of neurosis claimed that much of psychopathology was due to malingering—that is, patients simply faked their symptoms in order to derive social benefits, such as claims of disability, freedom from responsibility, and attention and sympathy from others (Shorter, 1997). Indeed, the advance made by Breuer and Freud (1895/1955) was to suggest that mental illness was due to internal conflicts in the patient's psyche, many of which the patient was presumed to be unaware of.

WHAT IS RESISTANCE?

Before we can develop a model of resistance, we need to determine what resistance is. This is not such an easy task. Resistance is a contextual construct in that it refers to how a patient does not comply with a specific role defined by the therapist. If the patient is resisting in therapy, we must first understand what is expected of him or her in therapy. For example, depending on the particular therapy, resistance could take the form of overfocusing or underfocusing on emotions, of talking too much or too little about the past, of asking the therapist for advice or not asking the therapist for advice. Psychoanalytic models of therapy might stress the importance of catharsis of emotions, whereas cognitive-behavioral models might stress problem-solving strategies. What is regarded as resistance in one treatment might be viewed as appropriate in another treatment.

But certain behaviors are generally considered "resistance" or "noncompliance" regardless of the treatment modality. For example, not coming to sessions, coming late, not paying for treatment, devaluing the therapist or the treatment, or dissociating in sessions all qualify as resistance. In cognitive-behavioral treatment, patient resistance or noncompliance might take the form of not setting an agenda, changing the topic frequently, refusing to answer questions, trivializing the sessions, and not carrying out homework assignments. These are examples of "procedural resistance," which I discuss later. In psychodynamically oriented treatment, resistance might take the form of appearing cut off from feelings, not recalling important events, idealizing or devaluing the therapist, or acting out between sessions. In the cognitive-behavioral model, resistance is understood as noncompliance, or noncollaboration, with a here-and-now problem-solving role (Beck et al., 1990), whereas in psychoanalytic treatment resistance is conceptualized in terms of the patient's inability to maintain awareness of relevant unpleasant thoughts and the tendency to "act out" in the transference (Strean, 1990).

Resistance is not simply the failure to improve in treatment. Patients may not get better for many reasons: because of biological impediments in refractory cases, because of misdiagnosis, or because the appropriate treatment has not been administered. But theoretical models might look differently at improvement and resistance. Psychoanalytic models seek "structural" changes, primarily through insight and working through a long process in the transference in treatment. Consistent with the view that the process of change is essential, some analysts might view rapid improvement in the patient's mood as a "flight into health" or a "transference cure," and therefore as a resistance on the part of the patient to directly address underlying neurotic conflicts.

It is rare for cognitive therapists to view rapid improvement as resistance. We tend to pride ourselves (perhaps too much) on quick results. But it is consistent with a cognitive model to view rapid improvement, followed by termination of treatment, as avoidance of the need to address underlying cognitive vulnerabilities, such as maladaptive assumptions and maladaptive schemas (Ingram, Miranda, & Segal, 1998; Young, 1990). We can make a legitimate distinction between "feeling better" and "getting better," where the latter involves modification of the assumptions and schemas that make one vulnerable to depression. We can also argue that the patient's therapy is incomplete if he or she has not acquired the self-help skills that will assist him or her in the future, should a crisis arise. Thus, we would not conclude that therapy has been successful or completed if a narcissistic patient feels better because, in the course of treatment, he has acquired a new admirer. Nor would we claim that a patient who attempted suicide last week has completed treatment simply because she is not suicidal today.

Psychoanalytic models and cognitive-behavioral models (as advanced in recent years) share some common ground in viewing therapy as incomplete unless it has addressed the underlying vulnerabilities of the patient. Perhaps the psychoanalytic therapist views these vulnerabilities as more profound, complicated, and difficult to access in treatment, whereas the cognitive therapist may believe these vulnerabilities can be specified in terms of maladaptive schemas and assumptions and the acquisition of self-help skills. But incomplete treatment may be one marker of resistance. It may be that many cognitive-behavioral therapists wish to view treatment as completed before it really is—perhaps because of the therapist's desire to feel competent—whereas psychoanalytic therapists may view therapy almost as interminable—perhaps because of their desire to be complete. With cognitive therapy, the patient may leave therapy prematurely because of the "illusion of functionality"—that is, the patient appears to feel better and to function better. Yet the patient's underlying vulnerabilities may not have been resolved. With psychoanalytic treatment, the goals of therapy may have been so unclear that the patient and therapist may never agree regarding the criteria for completion of treatment.

There is no generally shared definition of resistance. Therefore, at the risk of appearing arbitrary, I shall offer a definition for cognitive-behavioral resistance. *Resistance* is anything in the patient's behavior, thinking, affective response, and interpersonal style that interferes with the ability of that patient to utilize the treatment and to acquire the ability to handle problems outside of therapy and after therapy has been terminated. The "demand characteristics" of cognitive therapy include the following: emphasis on the here-and-now, structured sessions, continuity across sessions, problem-solving orientation, rational thinking, collaboration with the therapist, psychoeducation and information sharing, an active role for both patient and therapist, accountability as evidenced by identifying and measuring goals and attainment of goals, and compliance with self-help assignments (see Beck, Rush, Shaw, & Emery, 1979; J. Beck, 1996; Leahy, 1996a). According to the definition of resistance I offered above, resistance is anything that interferes with these demand characteristics. Moreover, my definition of resistance suggests that resistance can occur with premature termination, even if the patient is feeling better. This is because the goal of treatment is to help the patient acquire self-help skills and to modify those assumptions and schemas that confer vulnerability. It may be that many cognitive-behavioral therapists will argue that I am expecting too much from therapy. Perhaps. But I believe patients who do have these cognitive vulnerabilities or who lack the ability to utilize self-help have a substantial risk of reoccurrence of their problem.

In the remaining sections of this chapter, I offer a brief overview of psychoanalytic, behavioral, and cognitive models of resistance. In Chapter 3, I begin the discussion of procedural resistance in cognitive-behavioral treatment, in order to identify some specific interventions that have quite general applicability. Part II, "Dimensions of Resistance," follows, in which I outline seven different dimensions of resistance and how the therapist can address them. In Part III, I address countertransference—which I view as the therapist resisting the patient—especially how the therapist's resistance can be understood as a response to the patient's resistance.

PSYCHOANALYTIC MODELS OF RESISTANCE

Freud's model of resistance is based on the view that the patient is confronted with unresolvable conflicts (Breuer & Freud, 1895/1955; Freud, 1923/1961). Freud advanced a structural theory in which he proposed that the psyche could be divided into id, ego, and superego. The id corresponded to strong instinctual energies, such as sexuality and aggression, which sought immediate gratification regardless of consequences. At the other extreme, the superego reflected the internalization of standards, customs, and morality learned from parents and other socializing agents. The ego moderated the conflicts between the id and the superego, by providing reality testing, by controlling the impulsive and primitive id, and by moderating the excessive demands of the superego. Thus, id impulses of sexual gratification demanding immediate satisfaction would be confronted by the superego, which might "demand" the suppression of all sexual desire as "evil." The ego, serving its moderating function, might turn this sexual gratification into socially acceptable behavior, such as affection toward one's spouse, or it might redirect these sexual energies into sports or some other physical outlet.

The redirection of the id impulses by the ego constitutes the foundation of Freud's model of the ego defenses. According to the psychoanalytic model, these ego defenses, which suppress and redirect id impulses, are an economic, or efficient, solution to the demands of both id and superego. Sigmund Freud (1912/1958, 1923/1961) and Anna Freud (1946) identified numerous ego defenses (or defenses in the "service of the ego"). These include repression, denial, sublimation, isolation, intellectualization, displacement, regression, projection, and reaction formation. The ego defenses are said to provide the most efficient means of moderating id impulses, implying that the removal of these ego defenses, without the acquisition of corresponding adaptive functions, will result in an increase in psychopathology.

The psychoanalytic model of therapy stresses the importance of resistance. Patients, according to this model, are usually unaware of the true problem precisely because their defenses keep them from developing awareness of their real conflicts. The "symptom" that is presented in treatment is seldom the true problem, but is rather a symbolic representation of inner conflicts. According to this ego defense model, the patient holds onto the symptom because it protects him or her from the emergence of this inner conflict, which is viewed as overwhelming and primitive. If the symptom is removed, other neurotic symptoms would arise to take the defensive position of the original symptom. Thus, according to the ego psychology model within psychoanalytic theory, resistance is viewed in terms of specific mechanisms of defense, such as projection, denial, intellectualization, isolation, displacement, repression, and sublimation. The ego psychologist focuses her attention on analyzing these specific defense mechanisms and how they operate to impede improvement in therapy. We shall see, in my later discussion of schematic processes, that schema-focused cognitive therapy of personality disorders also emphasizes cognitive mechanisms of avoidance and compensation—mechanisms that appear quite similar to ego defenses (see Beck et al., 1990; Young, 1990).

The goal of psychoanalytic therapy is to analyze the patient's unconscious conflicts in an attempt to replace the primitive id–ego–superego conflicts with more adaptive functioning. As Freud indicated, "Where id is, ego shall be"—the goal of therapy is the repair of the ego structure. The emphasis in therapy is to assist the patient in regression toward the earlier conflicts and to lead the patient back through the restorative nature of interpretation and the importance of the therapeutic relationship.

Freud began with a strong emphasis on directing patients to change their thinking and behavior (not unlike many cognitive therapists!). But he abandoned this approach because he believed patients would revert to their original problems or, in some cases, develop new and different symptoms. Freud's therapeutic model as it developed focused more on the therapeutic relationship itself—which he called the "transference" because of his belief that this relationship reflected the patient's transfer, or generalization, of original conflicts with the parents onto the therapist. Thus, according to Freud, the transference relationship provided a unique opportunity for the patient to "regress," and thereby to relive his original conflicts, but this time in the context of the neutral, interpretative analyst.

The psychoanalytic model views resistance as an essential component of treatment. According to the model, the patient and the therapist are entangled in a long process of transference and countertransference, such that therapy entails working through the resistances in the transference and the regression of the patient to earlier conflicts. Since psycho-pathology is viewed as a dysfunction in ego defenses (which maintain the conflict), therapy involves confronting these ego defenses. Depending on the specific analytic model, the therapist may directly interpret defenses, focus on how the patient's transference interferes with treatment, provide a corrective emotional experience through empathic reflection and relating, or engage in corrective "reparenting" (see Kernberg, 1975, 1978; Kohut, 1971, 1977; Masterson, 1976; Winnicott, 1986).

Cognitive-behavioral therapists are generally unfriendly toward the psychoanalytic models. This theoretical antipathy results from a number of factors. First, it may simply be that cognitive-behavioral therapists wish to establish their theoretical "turf" by excluding all other therapeutic modalities. Quite frankly, I have found this theoretical "purity" to be more common among novices or among people who do not see many patients in clinical practice. Many experienced clinicians—regardless of their orientation—are willing to borrow or steal from any modality simply to be more effective as a clinician. Second, psychoanalytic thinking is rejected because cognitive and behavioral therapy initially emphasized either observable behaviors or conscious here-and-now thinking. Indeed, Beck's early work in cognitive therapy was a response to the apparent limitations of psychoanalytic treatment. However, cognitive therapy has a long history of development since the early 1980s, beginning with Guidano and Liotti's (1983) integration of Bowlby's attachment theory with Beck's theory; followed by Beck et al.'s (1990) analysis of personality disorders, which stressed the importance of compensatory styles and the continued influence of early maladaptive schemas; and resulting most recently in the integrative models proposed by Safran (1998) and Young (1990). Third, cognitive-behavioral therapists emphasize the manualization of treatment, stressing the uniformity of technique, independent of the patient's specific characteristics. This emphasis on manualization and short-term approaches has led to an interesting controversy, contrasting an emphasis on treatment plans, on the one hand, and case conceptualization, on the other hand (see Persons, 1989).

This theoretical polarization offers a false dichotomy. Experienced cognitive therapists whom I know address the transference, consider the importance of defense mechanisms, stress the influence of early developmental issues, and—indeed—talk about resistance. The cognitive-behavioral therapist may use different jargon—referring to resistance as "treatment non-compliance" or "motivation," calling defense mechanisms "compensation for a schema," and referring to developmental issues or regressive functioning as "the influence of early maladaptive schemas"—but he or she is addressing the same issues.

Throughout this book I utilize whatever theoretical ideas I think are important in helping us to understand resistance. I have borrowed from psychoanalytic thinking, Bowlby, Piaget, moral philosophy, microeconomic models, cognitive psychology, behavioral models, and—most importantly, for me—from my own experience in treating patients.

BEHAVIORAL MODELS
OF NONCOMPLIANCE AND RESISTANCE

Although behaviorists traditionally avoid the term "resistance," they are well aware that many patients do not follow therapeutic instructions. Preferring to refer to these patients as "noncompliant," rather than "resistant" (since the latter term assigns a motivational component to the patient's behavior), behaviorists have addressed this issue in terms of the learning and reinforcement model.

According to the behavioral model, the failure of the patient to comply with therapy may be the result of inappropriate reinforcers or reinforcement contingencies. Inappropriate reinforcers include reinforcements, or consequences, that are not relevant to the patient, that are not salient, or that are applied when the patient is satiated. An *irrelevant* reinforcement would be a consequence that is not highly desired by the patient—for example, an oppositional adolescent is not reinforced by praise from his teacher since such public praise is viewed by him as conflicting with his macho role with his peers. Reinforcements that are not *salient* would include weak reinforcers that the patient does not notice—such as nodding one's head when the patient complies. Reinforcements will not be effective if the patient is *satiated* in that domain: for example, opportunities to interact with others will not be reinforcing if the patient already has a lot of social contacts.

Noncontingency—or the perception of noncontingency—will affect reinforcement. If the reinforcement occurs independent of the frequency of the behavior, then it will fail to maintain or increase the desired behavior. Other reasons for noncompliance include reinforcement for behaviors that conflict with the goals of therapy. For example, the alcoholic patient may be reinforced for drinking by his drinking friends; indeed, he may be ridiculed or excluded for abstaining.

Frequently, resistant patients have a short duration in terms of delay of gratification. They often expect reinforcement immediately at a 100% schedule. Resistance to weight control or modification of addictive behavior often involves increased frustration. Removing the rewarding consequences of overeating, drinking, or smoking only increases the patient's frustration and makes delay of gratification even more difficult. Delay of gratification may be enhanced by addressing this issue directly:

"You may have to wait longer than you want for the result you desire." During the time in which the patient is practicing the delay, intermediate steps in reinforcement may be introduced. These include keeping track of desirable behaviors, such as calorie restriction and abstinence, with self-monitoring.

In addition, the patient and therapist may employ *mediating reinforcers,* reinforcers with symbolic value or those that can be used in exchange for other reinforcers—for example, symbolic tokens. Furthermore, the patient's delay of gratification may be improved by focusing on behaviors, rather than on outcomes: rather than count pounds lost, the patient may self-monitor positive behaviors in the process of change. Self-statements also dramatically enhance the ability to tolerate delay. The value of self-statements, or self-reinforcers, is that they are potentially always available and within the control of the patient. External support, from peers, group members (especially 12-step groups for addicts), family members, the therapist, and others (e.g., personal trainers), can also moderate delays of gratification.

Behavioral approaches also stress the importance of "shaping" behavior in dealing with noncompliance. Too often the therapist and the patient may have set the baseline and the goal too high. The patient who does not comply with self-help assignments may need to have the units of the behavior identified in the simplest steps. These steps can then be rehearsed in the session and practiced outside the session. The therapist may also model these behaviors in the session, including modeling the self-reward statements that may enhance patient compliance and behavioral maintenance. Behavioral chains may be established, such that the noncompliant patient may perform one link in the chain, obtain a prescheduled reward, and then perform subsequent links in the chain. "Bridging the gap" with reinforcements is useful in establishing and maintaining behavior the patient may be avoiding.

Modeling is important not only in sessions, but also outside of sessions. The patient may be asked to identify individuals who exhibit the desired behaviors, and then to identify the other person's behavioral repertoire. These individual behaviors may then be self-assigned and self-monitored. The patient who has difficulty initiating the desired behavior on his own may be asked to write out a behavioral description of a successful model he observes. For example, a patient who has difficulty getting along with his boss may identify a coworker who is successful with his boss and then write out a behavioral description of the coworker's effective behavior. This can then be employed as a list of target behaviors for the patient, with the patient self-monitoring his performance of these behaviors.

Therapy failures may be due to the fact that the patient simply does not know what to do to achieve a reinforcement. For example, sending a chronically shy and awkward individual to social gatherings with the instruction to "meet some people" will backfire if the patient does not know how or when to engage in appropriate social behaviors. Similarly, some patients may "resist" change because they simply do not know how to engage in effective problem solving—or if they do, they do not think it is appropriate in a given context (Nezu & Nezu, 1989). These examples point to the importance of skill acquisition in treating noncompliance, where the therapist assists the patient in acquiring appropriate social behaviors and problem-solving skills.

Noncompliance can also be addressed through punishment techniques, more euphemistically described as "response cost." These techniques involve the use of negative or to-be-avoided consequences for noncompliance with homework. Examples of response cost include simply reassigning the homework, carrying out the homework in the session, increasing the amount of homework to be done due to noncompliance, or attaching a "fine" that the patient pays in advance of the next homework assignment. Take the case of a patient who continually failed to do her exercise program for weight loss. She agreed to write a check to her least favored organization, which would then be mailed to it by the therapist if she failed to comply with the next self-assigned homework. This proved to be highly motivating, and so she complied.

The cognitive approach suggests that individuals differ considerably in their tendency to "process" reinforcements. Depressed individuals are often *negative trackers*, that is, they focus on their past mistakes and the frustrations associated with these mistakes. They fail to see the reinforcers available. Furthermore, they may discount reinforcements when they do see them, claiming that these reinforcements do not really matter because they are so mundane or so weak. Some noncompliant individuals, especially in couple therapy, have *perfectionistic reciprocity demands* for reinforcements: they expect to obtain a reinforcement for every positive behavior they demonstrate. Others have expectations that their spouse should reinforce them before they change. Still others will not reinforce their spouse unless the other spouse has demonstrated a stable and lasting change. These "rules for reinforcements" are the target of the cognitive interventions that I discuss throughout this book.

COGNITIVE MODELS OF RESISTANCE

Ellis's Model

Albert Ellis's model of resistance places considerable emphasis on the role of current dysfunctional thinking. Ellis (1985) proposes that resistance is often the result of "shoulds," low frustration tolerance, unrealistic expectations, absolutistic thinking, and other "irrational beliefs." Ellis's model of resistance—and the treatment that follows from this model—does not differ from Ellis's general rational-emotive approach. Ellis's approach stresses a direct confrontation with the patient's irrational thinking, such that the patient "must" recognize that she must relinquish or "surrender" her irrational beliefs before she can improve.

Ellis stresses that many irrational beliefs, such as "I am a worthless person," are meaningless statements. He indicates that concepts such as "worthlessness" are not empirically verifiable. Therefore, they are meaningless. In addition to the usual cognitive disputations in rational-emotive therapy (RET), Ellis recommends encouraging resistant patients to proselytize others, use thought stopping, and sing rational songs that challenge irrational thinking. Furthermore, Ellis recognizes the value of behavioral and experiential techniques in addressing resistance.

Although some of the RET techniques (such as evaluating the costs and benefits of a belief) are incorporated in the model that I will advance here, Ellis's approach to resistance does not stress anything that is not already part of the typical RET approach. Furthermore, although Ellis stresses "vigor" and "forcefulness" in challenging resistance, many therapists may find that a confrontational approach will only result in greater resistance from their patients. As I attempt to demonstrate later, confrontational approaches may actually confirm many of the underlying resistant thoughts that patients have—especially those patients who resist because of their need for validation or because of their moral and ethical beliefs.

Burns's Model

Similar to Ellis's model of resistance, Burns's (1989) model targets the role of cognitive distortions that determine the patient's participation in therapy. Burns focuses on noncompliance with self-help assignments, although there is greater generality to his approach. In *The Feeling Good Handbook*, Burns identifies 25 "reasons not to do homework." Some examples of these reasons include perfectionism, the need for approval, adherence to the belief that all problems are medical, "coercion sensitivity" (reactance), labeling, entitlement, and emotional reasoning. Each of these beliefs may be challenged by the therapist using cognitive therapy techniques, including examining the costs and benefits, evaluating the evidence, considering alternatives, and setting up experiments to test these beliefs.

Many of the automatic thoughts that depressed patients have are examples of resistance to change. These include fortune telling ("It won't work out"), all-or-nothing thinking ("I don't succeed at anything"), discounting the positives ("Even if it does get better here, it doesn't count"), or labeling ("I'm a loser, so why bother?"). Many of these traditional cognitive therapy approaches are incorporated in the next chapter and in each of the chapters on resistance.

Beck's Schema Model

Beck et al. (1990) extended Beck's (Beck, 1967; Beck et al., 1979) schema model of depression and anxiety to create a schema model of personality disorders. According to this model, individuals with chronic or reoccurring problems, often coexisting with personality disorders, have established early maladaptive schemas in childhood. These schemas direct attention to and increase recall of information consistent with the schema. Depressive schemas focus on loss, deprivation, and failure, while anxious schemas focus on threat, such as danger to valued aspects of the self (Beck, Emery, & Greenberg, 1985). *Personality schemas* are general themes of interpersonal and self-functioning, which correspond to vulnerabilities that may be activated by current life events. For example, a dependent individual with the schema of helplessness and abandonment may function reasonably well while she is in a relationship. However, should the relationship disintegrate, she will become depressed because of her concerns over helplessness and abandonment. Indeed, even within the relationship, she may be sensitized to issues of abandonment, since independent functioning seems impossible for her due to her schema of helplessness.

Beck et al. (1990) model stresses avoidance and compensation as two general coping styles for these personality schemas. *Avoidance* is the tendency either not to enter into or to escape from situations where the schema might be activated. For example, the dependent individual might avoid situations that require independent functioning: taking on new tasks, moving to a new city, or changing a job. *Compensation* is the tendency to overcome the threat of schema exposure by engaging in "extra-adaptive" behavior. For example, the dependent individual may be nonassertive, overly pleasing, and deferential, simply to maintain the relationship.

Resistance to change for these individuals would involve both avoidance and compensation. These individuals may view therapy as threatening the schema. Change may imply that the coping styles of avoidance and compensation will be abandoned and that there will be a direct threat that will overwhelm the individual (Beck et al., 1990;

Guidano & Liotti, 1983). In therapy, avoidance may take the form of poor attendance, dissociative responses, trivialization of the agenda, and premature termination. Compensation, for the dependent individual, may be reflected in becoming overly attached to the therapist, idealizing and eroticizing the therapist, and attempts to be overly pleasing to the therapist.

According to the Beck–Freeman model of personality disorders, we would expect that schemas would be activated in therapy and would result in individual differences in resistance. For example, the narcissistic patient with a schema of being a special and unique individual might resist the role of being a patient because he sees it as humiliating. His compensation for his "inferior" status could be to distance himself from and devalue the therapist. A schizoid patient who views relationships as intrusive could view therapy as threatening his identity and his boundaries. His adaptation would be to restrict emotional expression or to limit the areas of discussion in sessions. In Chapter 6 I examine in greater detail the importance of schemas in understanding and treating resistance.

AN INTEGRATIVE SOCIAL-COGNITIVE MODEL OF RESISTANCE

The Value of Other Models of Resistance

Each of the previous models of resistance provides a foundation for the model I propose in this book. The psychoanalytic models stress the importance of the self-protective mechanisms of defense, many of which may lie outside the patient's conscious awareness. The integrated social-cognitive model of resistance recognizes that resistance is often the result of emotional dysregulation (or overregulation), early (and later) childhood experiences, and unconscious processes. Ego defense mechanisms—such as projection, repression, denial, isolation, and intellectualization—are viewed as important tactics that maintain a resistant position. Moreover, this model emphasizes both the transference and the countertransference in the manifestation and modification of resistance. However, the model I propose is not derived from the psychoanalytic model of psychosexual determinism, nor does the model stress the nondirective and neutral position of the therapist, nor do I endorse a hydraulic energy model.

As I indicated above, the behavioral model is useful in addressing some issues in noncompliance, where noncompliance is the result of reinforcement contingencies, quality of reinforcement, relevance of reinforcement, and ability to produce reinforcements. The behavioral approach addresses the simplest aspect of "motivation" in noncompliance, but does not adequately address the intrapsychic qualities of resistance, which are my focus in this book. The behavioral therapist might argue that the patient needs to perceive reinforcement possibilities, thereby appearing to introduce the relevance of cognitive processes. However, this is a quite limited view of cognition, as I hope to make clear later in this volume. Behavioral interventions are often used to test or challenge dysfunctional thoughts and assumptions (Wells, 1997). However, to adequately test a thought or hypothesis, the patient may need assistance in stating predictions in a manner in which they can be made falsifiable. Indeed, as I illustrate later, cognitive consistency and risk-aversion processes in resistance often include discounting mechanisms, such that the nonoccurrence of an event is viewed not as evidence of disconfirmation, but as either irrelevant or as evidence that greater hypervigilance is required. The probable limitations of a simple behavioral model in understanding resistance will be addressed in several forthcoming chapters.

Dimensions of Resistance

The integrated social-cognitive model is really a collection of separate models of resistance. Resistance is expressed in different dimensions, where each dimension is a relatively self-contained style of thinking. Each of these self-contained dimensions needs to be understood and addressed in therapy within its own rules and logic. The dimensions of resistance that I identify and discuss in this volume include validation, self-consistency, schematic resistance, moral resistance, victim roles, risk aversion, and self-handicapping. Each has a distinctive "psycho-logic." Some individuals may utilize more than one dimension of resistance— for example, a patient may express resistance through validation demands, schematic resistance, and victim roles. However, the therapist and patient can separate these modes and address the dimensions separately.

Each dimension of resistance reflects a potentially healthy or adaptive way to function. Thus, as therapists, we would not want to say to the patient that being validated or maintaining self-consistency (or reliability) is trivial. Nor would we want to claim that the goal of therapy is to eliminate all moral considerations or to say that no one is a legitimate victim. To use Beck and Freeman's nonpejorative language in describing schematic processes, the dimension may simply be an "overdeveloped" style of coping. The general approach advocated throughout this book is to find the "truth" that exists in the dimension, but also to examine how overextension and rigidity may be modified in therapy.

SUMMARY

The topic of resistance is a central one in psychodynamic psychotherapy. Perhaps because of the analytic emphasis on unconscious motivation, the protective functions of the ego defenses, and the importance of the transference neurosis, "resistance" gained center stage in psychodynamic models. One assumption that analytic models share is that much of resistance may appear to function as an unconscious strategy to keep threatening material from overwhelming the patient. The function of the therapist, depending on the analytic approach utilized, is to interpret the resistance, to encourage regression within treatment, to assist the patient in relinquishing the defenses, and to rebuild a healthier or more adaptive ego.

Cognitive and behavioral approaches to resistance have been less articulated. Perhaps because of their emphasis on here-and-now functioning, their use of interventions that can be readily implemented, and their apparent rejection of the importance of the unconscious and its concomitant defenses, cognitive and behavioral approaches have generally eschewed discussion of resistance. Even when resistance, noncollaboration, or noncompliance have been discussed, the conceptualization has seldom strayed much from the more conventional plan and thinking of cognitive-behavioral therapy.

In the next chapter, I turn to more conventional cognitive-behavioral approaches to "procedural resistance"—that is, the patient's noncompliance with the typical approach that cognitive-behavioral therapists use. In subsequent chapters, I elaborate a more differentiated social-cognitive model of resistance that incorporates many of the ideas of traditional cognitive therapy, but takes us in new directions.

3

Resistance to Procedure

Cognitive therapy involves a set of procedures or expectations regarding patient behavior. Each procedural guideline, if not followed, represents a possibility of a clear departure from the task of collaboration in psychotherapy. Beck et al. (1979) and Leahy (1996a) have outlined a number of these "expectations," or guidelines, for cognitive therapy. The specific guidelines that apply directly to the patient include the following: the patient sets the agenda; the patient and the therapist will work together collaboratively; the agenda or current topic will define what is "on-task"; the goal will be to modify thoughts, feelings, and behavior; the focus is on the here-and-now; the emphasis will be on solving problems; the patient and therapist reject the idea of "readiness to change"; and the patient will conduct self-help homework outside the session. In addition to these guidelines, which are more relevant to cognitive-behavioral therapy than to traditional psychodynamic therapy, there are general expectations regarding patients in psychotherapy. These would include the patient's commitment to show up for a series of appointments, the patient's responsibility to pay for appointments, the importance of controlling self-destructive behavior, the necessity of honesty, and the patient's responsibility to refrain from abusive or seductive behavior toward the therapist.

Cognitive therapy presents a "demand" for rational, here-and-now, active problem solving. Rather than viewing therapy as a chance for the patient to regress to more primitive modes of functioning or to engage in "free association," the cognitive therapist presents a social demand that calls for patient responsibility. This is not a judgmental position on the part of the therapist, but rather a *procedural guideline*. The purpose of these procedural guidelines is to enhance efficiency, productivity, and the patient's development of independence and competence in solving his or her own problems. The therapist hopes that the collaborative problem solving set within sessions will generalize to the patient's life outside of therapy and that the therapist will serve as a role model of rational, effective problem solving.

Of course, the reason many people are in treatment is that they do not approach their problems with this procedural set. Rather than setting agendas and focusing on how they can solve their problems, many patients focus on changing topics, complaining, or even demonstrating that their problems are unsolvable. Rather than focus on the here-and-now of making progress, many patients focus on the injuries they experienced as children. In fact, the very nature of procedural guidelines lends itself to uncovering the schemas and resistance that beset the patient. Let us examine some of these procedural issues and how individual resistance arises and can be resolved.

BEHAVIORAL INTERVENTIONS

Psychoeducation

Some patients are under the misconception that getting better involves a long-term psychoanalytic process. Some believe that the effects of early (often unknown) childhood events cannot be overcome in later life. The behavioral component of cognitive-behavioral therapy requires the socialization of the patient to the intervention model. For example, the patient who complains about loneliness and indicates that he spends much of his time isolated in his apartment can be informed of the behavioral model of avoidance:

> "Let's examine the effects of your avoiding going out and trying to meet people. Whenever you think of leaving your apartment, you begin to feel anxious. As you go out the door your anxiety increases even more. What if you decide to turn around and go back into your apartment and spend the rest of the night watching television? Well, your anxiety decreases—you feel less anxious. This drop in your anxiety acts as a reward for you to avoid—every time you decide to avoid you are rewarded by a decrease in your anxiety.
>
> "For example, let's imagine that every time that you felt anxious you decided to have a drink. What would happen? Over time you would learn to drink when you feel anxious. You would start drinking more and more during the week until you became an alcoholic. So, in order to overcome your loneliness, you will have to learn to do things that make you anxious."

Evaluating Homework Instructions

Simply assigning self-help homework is not enough to get a patient to change. For example, telling the lonely patient, "I want you to go out more this week and try to meet people," may seem clear enough to the therapist, but may be remarkably vague and threatening to the patient. There are several guidelines to use in assigning homework:

1. *Practice the homework in session.* The therapist and the patient can engage in modeling and behavioral rehearsal in session. For example, the therapist can illustrate in session what he would do in terms of going out and planning an evening, while the patient can indicate to the therapist how he would apply this example to his own behavior—in this case, the patient might indicate that he would go out shopping, then later go to a museum and try to start a conversation with someone. The therapist and the patient could rehearse such a conversation. These sessions can be tape-recorded and the patient can listen to the tape over the next week (increasing the likelihood of imitating the behavior).

2. *Explain the rationale for the homework to the patient.* Just because the homework makes sense to the therapist, it does not follow that it makes sense to the patient. The patient might think, "How will going out shopping or going to a museum help me find a relationship?" The clinician needs to explain the rationale for all homework assignments, keeping in mind that the patient may not be familiar with concepts such as shaping or response generalization.

3. *Have the patient explain the rationale for the homework.* After the therapist explains the rationale for the homework and assigns specific behavior to be self-monitored, he should ask the patient what he understands the rationale to be: "Can you tell me in your own words what the reason would be for this homework?"

4. *Assign specific behaviors—that is, make clear what behavior should occur, how frequently (or with what intensity) it should occur, and in what situations.* Homework needs to be specific. Do not say, "Write down your negative thoughts and bring them in." The patient may have no idea when and how often he should do this. It is more effective to say, "Write down two negative thoughts each day and list three rational responses to these thoughts. Use the Daily Record of Dysfunctional Thoughts that we just used here in the session. Here are three copies of that form." Activity schedules may be useful in assigning specific times or situations in which the patient will engage in the assigned behavior. You must be specific about homework because patients vary: some patients may believe that simply thinking about a rational response

is sufficient, while perfectionistic and self-critical patients may think that they must write an extensive treatise to comply with the assignment.

5. *Illustrate and practice in session how the behavior will be monitored by the patient.* It is valuable for patients to keep track of their self-help by writing down what they said, did, or thought. Self-monitoring forms, including the Activity Schedule, Self-Monitoring Form, or Daily Record of Dysfunctional Thoughts, should be given to the patient. Self-monitoring can be practiced in the session—for example, the therapist can ask the patient to fill out the Activity Schedule in session and examine any problems that may ensue.

6. *Elicit feedback from the patient regarding ambivalence about doing the homework or uncertainty about what the homework is.* Since many patients feel hopeless or may have ambivalence about therapy in general, it is common for the patient to doubt whether self-help assignments will be useful. Some may not understand what is expected of them. It is helpful for the clinician to be direct about this: "Let's examine some of the reasons you might have for not doing this" or "Sometimes I don't make myself completely clear about homework that I assign. Perhaps you have some questions that you'd like to ask so I can clarify what you will be doing."

Shaping

A common problem in therapy is that the therapist assigns too much too quickly. When this occurs, it adds to the patient's sense of helplessness, hopelessness, and self-criticism and leads the patient to conclude that the therapist does not really understand what the patient is experiencing. For example, the lonely patient described above, who may have been isolated for years and who has never started a conversation with a stranger in a public place, might well find the assignment of going out and starting a conversation in a museum to be overwhelming. The therapist needs to be mindful of precisely where the patient is in the behavioral repertoire and the behavioral hierarchy. Social skills training may be broken down into smaller units—for example, collecting information by observing people who seem to be successful, practicing smiling behavior in the privacy of one's own apartment, evaluating proper grooming behavior, establishing proximity with others by being in the same place that they are in, and so on. The best place to begin is with simple assignments that are less threatening—for example, "Write out descriptions of people who you think are successful at meeting people," "What are some ways in which other people are rewarding or pleasurable to others? Make a list," or "What are some places that you can list where people come in contact with other people?"

Take the case of a woman who was shy when meeting men. She was asked to list a series of positive social behaviors that people could direct *toward her.* These included looking in her direction, standing closer to her in a public place, smiling, making eye contact, starting a conversation, and the like. She was then given a list of these behaviors to monitor while observing others. She viewed focusing on monitoring others' behaviors as much less threatening than engaging in these behaviors herself. It also allowed her to recognize that many of these positive social behaviors were already directed toward her. This led her therapist to ask her, "What is the consequence of your not noticing and rewarding people for these behaviors?" The patient was able to recognize that her nonreward of these behaviors may have led others to stop engaging in these positive behaviors toward her (i.e., extinction).

The next items in the assignment hierarchy included facing in the general direction of others in public places (e.g., elevators, train stations, parties) and noticing what clothing others wore. Partly as a consequence of her prior monitoring of others' positive behaviors and partly as a function of her own increasingly positive behavior, she began to receive some positive social rewards—that is, others looked back at her, smiled, and started conversations. As we moved up the hierarchy—toward initiating smiling, asking questions, or complimenting others—she was encouraged to reinforce positive behaviors in others.

Modification of Rewards

In order for rewards to be effective, they need to be related to some motivational system that is valued by the patient. The therapist and the patient may have very different ideas of what is rewarding. For practical purposes, we can simply define a *reward* or *reinforcement* as any event that increases the probability of a reoccurence of a desired behavior. The therapist may think that praise will be rewarding, but the patient may view praise as artificial or as leading to too much attention directed to himself. For example, shy individuals may find praise to be unpleasant; thus, the therapist's reward of praise may, inadvertently, serve as a punishment.

The therapist and the patient can collaborate on establishing a "reward menu"—that is, a list of different events that the patient identifies as pleasurable. Lewinsohn, Breckenridge, Antonuccio, and Teri's (1987) reward menu is a useful place to begin. It is important that rewards come from a variety of motivational systems—for example, you would not want all rewards to be food rewards, since the patient can easily become satiated. Moreover, the therapist should identify rewards of various intensities, durations, and costs, since obtaining or consuming a reward should not be viewed as an added burden. The therapist may use the "Premack principle" in defining a reward—that is, behaviors that the patient generally chooses to engage in at high frequencies are then specified as rewarding consequences for behaviors that the patient wishes to increase in frequency (Premack, 1965). For example, if the patient reads frequently, this behavior can serve as a reward for a lower frequency behavior, such as exercising. One problem with using the Premack principle with chronically depressed or anxious patients is that many of their high-frequency behaviors are negative—for example, ruminating, complaining, or viewing television by themselves.

The therapist and the patient can use the Activity Schedule to determine which current behaviors are associated with relatively high levels of mastery or pleasure. This information can then be used to construct a reward menu of current behaviors that can be used as contingent rewards. Family members or significant individuals in the patient's life can also be used as sources of information concerning what the patient does find rewarding or used to find rewarding. Since many severely depressed or anxious patients do not recall pleasurable experiences, others in the patient's life may be a more accurate source of this information. This information may then be added to the reward menu, and the patient's automatic thoughts about these previously rewarding behaviors may be examined. For example, the depressed patient may claim that what used to be rewarding will not be at all rewarding now, or that it will remind him of how bad off he is, or that he is too exhausted to engage in this behavior now. These thoughts can then be examined using the cognitive techniques described later in this book.

Increasing Contingency

Many patients do not reinforce themselves on a contingent basis. In order for a reward to be *contingent*, the individual must recognize a clear predictability of getting the reward as a consequence of the specified behavior. For example, a patient who was trying to lose weight was urged to specify a list of "healthy behaviors." His list included planning meals, reducing fattening food items in his house, eating slowly, exercising for 20 minutes, and so on. However, his prior "contingency" of reward was as follows: "If I didn't lose weight this week, I'll criticize myself." Consequently, all of the positive healthy behaviors specified would have no predictable relationship to a reward. Contingency can be increased by monitoring the behavior, checking off every instance of the behavior over the day, listing specific self-praising statements to the specific behaviors, and setting up larger rewards that follow after a specified number of positive behaviors are performed.

Related to increasing contingency is *changing reinforcement schedules*. Many people do not have a clear predictability (or contingency), but rather rely on variable schedules of reinforcement, such as variable ratio or variable time schedules. Thus, the individual does not know how many behaviors he needs to perform in order to obtain a reinforcement. The patient should be encouraged to follow a *fixed ratio* schedule of reinforcement, such that a specific number of behaviors lead to a fixed amount of reward. Not all schedules of reinforcement need to be *continuous*—that is, the individual need not be rewarded on a 100% reward schedule. This is generally impractical and may lead to satiation of reward. Once the behavior is established—which may initially require a continuous schedule of reward—the therapist may encourage the patient to modify the schedule to a fixed ratio. For example, rewards may follow on the average of 50% of behaviors, eventually dropping to 30% or lower. This increases resistance to extinction.

Response Cost

Once the patient has evaluated the costs and benefits of changing behavior, but has been unable to modify his behavior using the techniques proposed by the therapist, the therapist may change the focus of treatment to attaching a negative consequence to the negative behavior or the absence of the positive behavior. For example, if the patient does not engage in the behavior he has agreed to pursue—such as initiating three conversations per day—the therapist and patient may contract on a negative consequence. The negative consequence may include either the withdrawal of a positive (e.g., "You cannot watch television tonight") or the introduction of a negative ("You will walk around the block three times").

Some patients observe that if they are unwilling to engage in the positive behavior that they have contracted to do, then it is unlikely that they will engage in the negative behavior. The therapist may avoid this problem by getting the patient to agree to a response cost that can be initiated by the therapist. For example, the patient might agree to give the therapist a check (for a small amount of money) made out to an organization that the patient does not like, with the stipulation that this check will be mailed by the therapist only if the patient does not engage in the desired behavior. Alternatively, the patient and the therapist might agree before the homework assignment that if the patient does not engage in the homework assignment, then part of the next session will be spent reviewing the issue of noncompliance. In fact, a very effective technique is to use part of the next session to actually engage in the homework assigned: thus, if the patient has not completed an Activity Schedule, then the first 10 minutes of the next session can be focused on completing the Activity Schedule.

Evaluating and Changing Other Contingencies

The patient may have others in her life who provide reward for noncompliance with the therapeutic goals agreed on. For example, a single woman who wanted to develop more productive relationships with men spent a good part of her leisure time socializing with an embittered and envious woman friend, who characterized all men as untrustworthy and exploitative. The patient began to realize that whenever she described positive steps that she was taking to improve her own social life with men, her friend would undermine her efforts. Consequently, the contingency was such that positive social behavior was often punished. Similarly, a male patient who had indicated a desire to decrease his drinking found that his drinking buddies were often critical of him for not drinking. In both of these cases, the reinforcement contingencies dramatically impacted on the patient's ambivalence about the treatment goals.

Changing behaviors within an interpersonal system will often disrupt that system, leading other parties to try to bring the patient back to the problematic behaviors. The patient should examine the costs and benefits of decreasing time spent interacting with these enablers and then attempt to commit to an experiment for a set period of time during which the patient spends less time with the enablers and more time either alone or with others. In the cases of both the patients described above, the commitment to spend less time around the enablers led to an even clearer recognition of how others often did not have the patient's best interests at heart, further motivating the patients to continue independently.

AGENDA SETTING

Following the initial evaluation, during the first session of therapy the patient should be socialized into the cognitive therapy model (Beck et al., 1979; J. Beck, 1996; Leahy, 1996a; Leahy & Holland, 2000). The initial socialization can include a clear description of the need for the patient to set agendas, the focus on here-and-now problem solving, the construction of a problem list, the development of baseline measures, the emphasis on continued evaluation of targeted symptoms or problems, and the expectation that self-help homework will be carried out. The patient should be assigned books or handouts to read that emphasize the cognitive model—such as David Burns's *Feeling Good: The New Mood Therapy* (1980) or *The Feeling Good Handbook* (1990). This conveys the message that therapy is collaborative, problem solving, psychoeducational, and involves self-help.

The construction of a list of problems to be addressed in the course of treatment can be established in the first two sessions. The therapist presents a list of possible problems that the patient may want to address: self-criticism, procrastination, panic, relationship conflict, decision making, and the like. The patient can select the problems—or add problems—to his or her list. The message the therapist wants to convey is, "We will be working on specific problems." The patient is then told:

> "Each session we will set an agenda. I want you to think about what you will put on the agenda before you come to the session. We will have certain items on almost every agenda—for example, reviewing your feelings and thoughts about the previous session, reviewing your self-help assignments—and then we will address the current topic that you wish to put on the agenda. We will complete the session by reviewing what we covered and I will ask you for feedback."

My experience is that limiting each session's agenda to one or two problems is more realistic than covering three or more.

• *Patient does not have an agenda.* Agenda setting is a clear statement of a problem-solving set. It also represents the expectation that the patient will be responsible for participating in the problem solving. There are numerous reasons why patients do not set agendas. Some are related to the failure of the therapist to socialize the patient into agenda setting. Some may result from the therapist not following the patient's agenda even when the patient does set an agenda. However, a reason more pertinent to the topic of resistance is that the patient may not set the agenda because of schematic issues related to problem solving.

The patient may not have an agenda because the patient does not think about problems as "problems to be solved." For example, many patients view their problems as problems about which they complain. Thus, the patient looks at therapy as validation or as reassurance seeking rather than as a problem-solving experience.

Other patients may believe they are coming to a "doctor" who will guide them to a solution. For example, the dependent patient who has relied on others to protect her and solve her problems may sit passively at the beginning of the session, waiting for the therapist to initiate the discussion. One woman, a dependent personality whose narcissistic husband left her for another woman, would sit passively at the beginning of the session and would respond to the therapist's question about the agenda with a litany of complaints. Her view of therapy was that the therapist would listen to her complaints and somehow magically make her feel better.

Another reason for not having an agenda is that it implies responsibility for solving problems. For example, one patient, who habitually did not have an agenda, was asked: "What are the advantages of not having an agenda?" He answered: "If I have an agenda, I then have to be responsible for solving a problem. I don't want to solve these problems." Another patient indicated that the reason she did not have an agenda is that she felt her problems were so overwhelming that no agenda would do justice to her plight. It would trivialize her experience.

• *Patient requests that the therapist set the agenda.* Not uncommonly the patient may say something like: "I don't have an agenda. I thought maybe you could set the agenda today." Such an attempt to get the therapist to set the agenda may involve a number of "hidden agendas." First, the patient may believe he is incapable of solving or even identifying his problems and that only the therapist (or someone else) will be able to solve these problems for him. Second, the patient may wish to "test" the therapist to see if the therapist "really understands me." For example, one patient indicated she did not have an agenda. She then insisted that the therapist set the agenda. The therapist indicated that his experience suggested it was better for the patient to set agendas, since he might set an agenda the patient did not wish to follow. The patient then said: "Let's talk about what we talked about last time. Can you summarize what we covered?" The therapist then referred to his (obsessive) notes, summarizing the major points of the previous session. The patient then got angry and shouted: "Why do you have to refer to your notes? Are you too busy to remember who I am and what my problems are?"

This self-defeating "victim" behavior led to a discussion of the patient's self-defeating narcissism:

THERAPIST: It seems that you asked me to summarize our previous session, and then you got angry at me for doing what you asked me to do. Was your goal to test me and then fail me on your test?

PATIENT: Oh, Dr. Jones [her former therapist] was much better. She really cared about me. Do you really know anything about my problem—obsessive–compulsive disorder?

THERAPIST: Is your goal to prove that I am incompetent and therefore can't help you?

PATIENT: Maybe.

THERAPIST: Before you came in today, were you thinking of putting me to the test?

PATIENT: (*smiling*) Yes. I actually wanted you to fail.

THERAPIST: Why would it be important to you to make me fail?

PATIENT: You're so busy. It's hard to get an appointment with you. I don't have millions of dollars like your other patients do.

THERAPIST: What does that make you think?

PATIENT: That you won't think I'm important enough to care about.

THERAPIST: So, if I fail your test, does that mean I'm not important enough to be your therapist?

PATIENT: (*smiling*) Maybe.

Here, the patient's refusal to set the agenda and then her demand that the therapist set the agenda was actually a "hidden agenda": to fail the therapist so that the patient would feel "victorious" over someone she believed considered her not important enough to be a patient.

The hidden agenda for this patient—focusing on the therapist's inadequacies rather than her own feelings of worthlessness—was uncovered by directly examining her investment in "failing the therapist." The patient confessed that she always felt like she did not get enough attention from her parents and that she was always in competition with her brothers. Moreover, her belief was that the only way she could compete was to be perfect—that is, to look perfect, achieve great success, and always please men. This led to her perception that life was "all-or-nothing": either she would deprive herself of food or binge, either she would have the best job or not work, and either she would be the best patient or not be a patient at all.

• *Patient places too many items on the agenda.* As I indicated above, working on one problem for the session should be sufficient. However, some patients may place five or six items on the agenda. When asked to prioritize them, the patient often has difficulty. The underlying assumptions guiding this "overwhelming agenda" approach include the following: "I have many problems. If I don't work on all of them, then we are not going to get anywhere"; "It's essential that I solve my problems now"; "The therapist has to hear all my problems to understand me completely. If he doesn't understand me completely, then he can't help me at all"; or, "The therapist is an expert who can help me with everything. I should tell him everything, he'll have all the answers, and then I will get better."

For example, a woman would begin the session with five items: "I'd like to talk about my father, my work, my friend Susan, this guy I'm dating, and how I'm feeling physically." Although initially she agreed to prioritize the first two as the problems to work on, she eventually shifted to the other topics. Interestingly, she seemed not to listen to the therapist's responses to her questions, but would shift to the next topic. When the therapist pointed this out to her, she indicated that she had too many problems to work on to stop to think and talk about any one problem. In her words, "All of these things are important." This led to a discussion of her hypomanic–narcissistic father who barraged her with questions and judgments, and then rejected all her responses. She indicated that she always felt she could not get a word in edgewise with him. Therapy, for her, was an opportunity to be at center stage and get her needs for validation met.

• *Patient places his or her feelings on the agenda.* The patient may not take a problem-solving approach to therapy, and instead may place her feelings on the agenda: "I'd like to talk about how tired I feel" or "I'd like to talk about my depression." The therapist can follow up on these issues by asking: "Is there something in particular that's making you feel depressed?" or "Can you tell me what's going through your mind when you are depressed?" However, some patients simply wish to talk about how they feel, attempts to take a problem-solving approach with them may result in their feeling invalidated. For example, a bulimic patient indicated that she wanted to talk about how she felt. Knowing that cognitive therapy was problem solving in its orientation, she still refused to focus on how to solve any problems until she could talk about how she felt. The therapist indicated that this was a bit different from the usual agenda:

THERAPIST: As you know, we usually talk about how to solve a problem, but it's interesting that you want to focus on how you feel. How much time should we set aside for that?

PATIENT: Can we talk about my feelings for the first 15 minutes? I don't want to challenge any thoughts or solve any problems—just talk about the way I feel.

THERAPIST: That would be fine. (*Patient then describes her feelings about her mother, the man she was dating, and the pressures of her job, focusing on the issues of not being understood, feeling inadequate, and feeling overwhelmed.*) Why did you think it was important to talk about your feelings rather than to work on solving problems?

PATIENT: I guess it's because I'm never sure what my feelings are. I'm not sure if my feelings make sense.

THERAPIST: Is that something that someone made you think and feel?

PATIENT: Yeah. In my family, you weren't allowed to have feelings. My father was an alcoholic and we weren't allowed to say anything. Mom just made believe that everything was all right.

THERAPIST: But it sounds like it wasn't. How did it make you feel when your mother would make believe that everything is all right?

PATIENT: It made me feel confused and angry.

THERAPIST: Those sound like the kinds of feelings a lot of people will have in that kind of situation. How do you feel when I try to get you to set an agenda and focus on solving problems?

PATIENT: Well, sometimes I think it's a good idea. That's why I'm here. But I also think about whether you're interested in my feelings.

THERAPIST: Does that make you feel anything?

PATIENT: Confused and angry.

• *Patient sets an agenda, but refuses to follow it.* Perhaps most confusing for the therapist is when the patient does set an agenda but then refuses to follow it. There may be several reasons why this occurs. One simple reason is that the patient begins to recognize, in the course of the discussion, that something very important that wasn't on the agenda has come up and needs to be addressed. A second reason is that the patient begins to follow his agenda, but then realizes that the topic is too upsetting. Therefore, he attempts to change the agenda. A third reason is that the patient wishes to "appear" to be cooperating with the process of change, but really does not want to change.

Consider the case in which the patient recognizes that something more important needs to be discussed. So, he changes the agenda. The therapist should recognize that the agenda is being changed and inquire directly why. The patient and the therapist can then agree to discuss the original agenda at the end of the session or to place the item on the next agenda.

In a case in which the agenda is changed because the topic is too upsetting for the patient, the therapist can address this issue directly by noting that the patient is changing the topic and that the patient became upset just before he changed the topic. For example, a woman who believed that her husband did not care about her affection and sexual needs placed these items on the agenda. However, when the therapist began discussing her thoughts and feelings about these issues, she changed the topic to focus on her schedule at work. The therapist noticed that the patient was modifying her original agenda.

THERAPIST: I noticed that we began talking about your needs in your marriage, but then you changed the topic to discuss your schedule at work. What was going through your mind when we were discussing your marriage?

PATIENT: That my needs are not being met, so I changed the subject because it was too upsetting.

THERAPIST: What do you predict will happen if we address these needs in therapy?

PATIENT: I would just get more upset.

THERAPIST: Is this anything like what you do with your husband?

PATIENT: I never think he's going to meet my needs, so I don't like talking about my needs with him.

THERAPIST: It sounds like you are assuming that none of your needs will be met, so you don't bring them up, so they don't get met. Have there been other people in your life that this has been true with?

PATIENT: My mother. She was more interested in her own needs. When I would talk about my feelings, she would tell me I was selfish.

The foregoing clinical exchange illustrates how the cognitive therapist can directly examine transference issues with the patient. Setting the agenda is an assertive act. This act, on the part of the patient, elicits her schemas about validation and emotional deprivation. Just as she believes that discussing her needs in therapy will result in being upset, she also is able to recognize the generality of this problem with her husband and her mother. (It was also operating with her employer and her friends.) Her shift away from her own needs led her and the therapist to set up several experiments in assertion with her husband, her employer, and her mother. In addition, she became more assertive with the therapist, insisting that her needs be placed on the agenda for subsequent sessions.

A third pattern of the patient straying from his own agenda involves "help-rejection" behavior. Here, the patient sets an agenda and then gets annoyed with the therapist for following the agenda. One patient who was continually reluctant to set an agenda finally agreed to an agenda—in this instance, looking for work. When the therapist began discussing this with her, she became more frustrated.

THERAPIST: What are some options for work that you might consider?

PATIENT: I don't know.

THERAPIST: What kind of work have you done in the past?

PATIENT: I worked in an office as an administrator. I also did some telemarketing. I don't know what to do. Do you have any ideas?

THERAPIST: Well, what thoughts do you have about pursuing the work that you used to do?

PATIENT: I don't want to do anything. I don't care. It's not worth it. You know, my parents are always putting pressure on me.

THERAPIST: You said that you don't want to do anything. What is the consequence of that belief?

PATIENT: Look, nothing is going to get better. Even if it did, it's nothing anyway. Why are we talking about this, anyway?

THERAPIST: I thought you put work on the agenda.

PATIENT: It's what *you* want to talk about.

This interaction led to a discussion of the patient's tendency to ask for help—from the therapist, from her parents—and then to criticize the people who helped her. When this was pointed out to her, she then criticized the therapist even more.

THERAPIST: It seems that you are asking for help and then getting angry when someone tries to help you. What about getting help bothers you?

PATIENT: It means that I have to accept whatever I get. It's never going to be as good as I want it to be. You're telling me to *settle*.

This interaction led to a discussion of the patient's perfectionism in almost all areas of her life, and of her belief that she needed to be perfect, which conflicted with her belief that she was incompetent to accomplish anything. Consequently, following any agenda—including her own—resulted in an increase in anxiety and anger, since it activated her feelings of deprivation and invalidation, as well as her recognition that she would not have the "special" existence that she believed she needed (and deserved). Her goal, then, was to defeat all agendas, including her own.

COLLABORATIVE SET

Cognitive therapy is based on the idea that the patient and the therapist are joined together to examine and modify the patient's thoughts, behaviors, and feelings. Beck (Beck et al., 1979; Padesky, 1996) has stressed the importance of the mutual discovery entailed in the Socratic dialogue, where the therapist guides the patient through a series of questions and answers to elicit automatic thoughts and assumptions and examine the logic and evidence that relate to them. The patient is expected to discuss his feelings and thoughts honestly and to work with the therapist to examine their validity.

Some patients wander in their discussion, often bringing up tangential issues. Indeed, there are times when it is difficult to follow what the patient's point is. One of my patients would begin the session with an agenda, but then would go off in different directions on unrelated topics, asides, irrelevant details, and tangential comments about various people in her life with whom I was unfamiliar. I commented on the fact that her discussions were tangential and difficult to follow and wondered what the reason for this might be.

This led to a discussion of the fact that the patient's alcoholic father and narcissistic mother never seemed to listen to the patient's needs when she was a child. Consequently, she never knew what was important to talk about and what was not important, since nothing seemed to matter to her parents consistently. What appeared to allow her to hold the floor in her family was to tell interesting anecdotes. This was something she continued to do in therapy (and in life). Her feelings of not being heard were further reinforced by her husband's coolness toward her and his constant criticism of her. I was able to give her the following feedback in a manner that did not appear critical: "Because your needs and feelings are important to me, I'd like to be able to follow the important points that you are trying to make. Perhaps because you are so much more familiar with the details and the people involved, you may forget that I do not know as much as you do. It will help me to understand you better if you could edit what you say to the major point so that I do not get lost. That way you will be able to feel heard and cared about."

This validation of her feelings and needs was very different from the withdrawal or criticism that she had experienced with her parents and her husband. Subsequently, much of her therapy was focused on identifying her needs and her rights and teaching her how to assert herself without having the need to get the approval of people around her. In fact, her "off-task" behavior was not "resistance" in any oppositional way, but rather reflected her need to learn new skills in articulating her main needs. Ironically, like many people who have difficulty articulating their needs, she was very good at meeting the needs of other people.

Another aspect of the collaborative set is that both patient and therapist should be able to give each other feedback and recommendations for change. The therapist may encourage this kind of interaction during sessions by requesting feedback at the end of the session, both directly or through self-report forms that elicit specific feedback (Beck et al., 1979; Burns, 1989). The therapeutic rationale for eliciting feedback from the patient is that the patient's assertion may help the therapist better tailor the therapy to the patient's specific needs. The therapist should demonstrate an empathic and helpful style in listening to the feedback, but should encourage the patient to suggest some problem-solving strategies that can be utilized. For example, a patient complained that too much of therapy was focused on identifying and changing thoughts and behaviors and not enough time was allowed for the patient to express her emotions. The therapist suggested the following: "What would be a good way of structuring our sessions so that we can do both of those things for you?" The patient recommended that sessions be divided into "thirds," with a third focused on emotions, thoughts, and new behaviors, respectively. Resistance to change may be decreased when direct feedback is elicited and followed with a problem-solving strategy.

HOMEWORK COMPLIANCE

As I indicated in the previous chapter, self-help compliance may be enhanced by breaking down assignments into their simplest units of behavior. The therapist can also model the appropriate self-help during the session, showing the patient how he (the therapist) would fill out appropriate forms or by having the patient fill out these forms in the session under the therapist's supervision. Assigning specific behavior (e.g., write down one thought each day and challenge it) may increase compliance. Furthermore, homework compliance can be increased by arranging reinforcements that maintain the homework.

Some perfectionistic patients may view self-help as a "test" that they will fail, which will then disappoint the therapist. These issues may be addressed by framing homework as practice and learning, rather than as evaluating. Indeed, doing no homework is practice in doing nothing—the patient can find out what happens when he does nothing. (Indeed, with noncompliant patients I have assigned "doing nothing" as part of their homework, so that on certain days during the week we could find out how they felt when they were inactive.)

The cognitive therapist can utilize many of the traditional self-help techniques to evaluate the automatic thoughts that contribute to noncompliance with homework. Thus, the patient who does not do any homework may be asked the following:

THERAPIST: Let's see. You did not do any of the written homework last week. Let's look at this. At the top of the page, write "Did not do homework." Let's do a cost–benefit analysis on this. What are the costs and benefits of doing no homework?

PATIENT: The costs are that I don't get to change my negative thoughts and I probably won't get better. The benefits? I don't spend my time on something that might not work. I get to do other things. (*He determines that the costs outweigh the benefits by 80% to 20%.*)

THERAPIST: OK. Try to finish this sentence, "When I think of writing down my thoughts and challenging them I hesitate because I think. . . . "

PATIENT: It won't work. It's trivial.

THERAPIST: All right. We certainly don't want to spend our time doing things that are useless. But let's look at these thoughts. How much do you believe from 0 to 100% that doing homework won't help?

PATIENT: When I'm not doing homework? 100%!

THERAPIST: OK. So you are predicting that if you write down your thoughts and try to challenge them that you will not have any change in your feeling?

PATIENT: I know it sounds ridiculous. But that's how I feel when I'm at home.

THERAPIST: Let's look at the evidence. In the past, in sessions with me or at home, when you have written down your thoughts and challenged them, have you ever felt better?

PATIENT: Actually, I generally feel somewhat better. (*He then rerates his belief that self-help won't help as 10%.*)

Specific automatic thoughts can be examined as a basis of resistance to homework compliance. These include fortune telling ("It won't work"), all-or-nothing thinking ("I'm not all better"), discounting the positive ("It's not as big a change as I need"), labeling ("Only losers do this kind of thing"), emotional reasoning ("I just don't feel like doing it"), or overgeneralizing ("I didn't feel better when I challenged one of my thoughts, so it won't work for the other thoughts"). The therapist can challenge and test these thoughts by examining the costs and benefits of each belief, looking at the evidence for and against the belief, setting up "experiments" in- and outside of sessions, and asking the patient what advice he would give a friend. Examples of noncompliance with homework and rational responses to these negative thoughts are shown in Table 3.1.

We can also evaluate noncompliance either from the perspective of

TABLE 3.1. Rational Responses to Reasons Not to Do Homework

Automatic thought	Rational response
"It won't help."	"You never know unless you try. Let's set up an experiment. Let's do some of the homework in the session and see if you feel any change in your mood. Why not try it for a week and see if it helps at all?"
"I can do it in my head."	"Many people think they can, but you might find it's more effective to write it down. It's like the difference between taking notes at a lecture and just trying to remember it."
"This is for losers."	"If you get better, then you are not a loser. Is exercise just for losers?"
"I don't have the time."	"How much time do you think it will take? Why not assign a limited amount of time for the homework, but still do some of it. How much time do you take up being depressed/ anxious?"
"This is just rationalization."	" 'Rationalizing' refers to making up stories that aren't true. Homework is trying to collect the facts and practice positive behavior."
"I must be a loser because I need to do this."	"You are more effective if you do homework. 'Losing' would mean losing out on being able to help yourself."
"My problems are real."	"Your problems may be partly real and partly how you're handling real problems. Self-help can help you deal with real problems. If you have 'real' problems, then you need to help yourself even more."
"I shouldn't have to do this."	"You are under no moral obligation to help yourself or not help yourself. Just as there is no obligation to do exercise. It's your choice."
"If I do homework, you may judge me."	"Homework is an opportunity to collect information about how you think and how you behave. The goal is to improve what you do. The therapist is not here to judge you. He or she is here to provide you with guidance and direction. If your accountant asked you to collect information, would you refuse to do so because you felt embarrassed?"

schematic resistance or from the perspective of the patient's personality disorder. For example, consider this homework assignment: "Write down your negative thoughts in the left column and your rational responses in the right column." What could be some reasons for noncompliance?

1. *Special person.* The narcissistic patient believes that he is a unique, superior person, and that homework must "rise to the occasion" of his superior ego. Often, for the narcissist, cognitive and behavioral

interventions—or popular books on cognitive therapy—may elicit thoughts that "this is trivial" and "my problems are more complicated and require a more specialized and sophisticated approach." The therapist can indicate that the patient needs to find his special way of approaching his thoughts by learning how to tailor his rational responses to his special thoughts and problems.

2. *Emotional regulation.* Patients whose schema reflects problems of emotional regulation may view homework as irrelevant to their emotional needs, which are primary to them. Thus, a rational or problem-solving approach may not appear to address the problems of intense emotion. The therapist can indicate that the patient's emotions are so important that they can best be heard once the patient has been able to moderate these emotions and express them in the most effective manner. This will become one of the goals of homework assignments.

3. *Abandonment.* For the patient concerned about abandonment and dependency issues, homework may seem irrelevant since the problem is viewed as the total lack of a person in the patient's life or the danger of losing such a person: "How will writing down my thoughts help me find a partner?" Or the patient may say: "How will challenging my beliefs keep her in the relationship with me?" The therapist may indicate that having better control over moods and behavior will help the patient in developing better relationships and in being better able to function in between relationships.

4. *Demanding standards.* The obsessive–compulsive patient may hesitate to do self-help because he believes it is not worth doing unless it is done perfectly. These patients will sometimes call between sessions to "check up" on how the homework should be done. Further, if the homework does not yield a perfect solution, it may be viewed as worthless. The therapist can indicate that perfection is a goal for the patient, but learning and practice are the process. The patient can be encouraged to learn from his imperfect homework that progress can be made imperfectly, thereby helping him modify his need to be perfect in everything.

CONTINUITY OF APPOINTMENTS

A common factor with resistance in therapy is that the patient does not maintain continuity in treatment. Of course, there are practical factors that may interfere with treatment, such as scheduling and financial cost, but many patients demonstrate their ambivalence about treatment simply by not showing up for appointments or by showing up late. In some cases, the patient may attempt to demonstrate his independence or, in fact, his wish to punish the therapist by aggressively withholding his presence in treatment. This is most clear in the case of patients who have agreed to a cancellation policy whereby they pay for unannounced no-shows, but who refuse to pay for the missed session.

The therapist should establish the expectations for continuity from the beginning of treatment by indicating that the patient is expected to come weekly (in some cases, twice per week). If the patient indicates an unwillingness to contract for continuity, the therapist can inquire as to the reasons, for example, cost, inconvenience, or ambivalence. In some cases, issues of cost may be examined with a problem-solving approach. For example, the patient may be expecting that the commitment to continuity means that he will be promising to come every week for years, whereas the contract may target 10 sessions. Or the patient may overlook resources, such as insurance coverage or savings, that may ease the financial burden of therapy. In many cases, the patient may need a referral to a lower fee therapist. Many people are ashamed to disclose their true financial limitations for fear that the therapist will think less of them. Many people believe that a less expensive therapist is an inferior therapist. These issues can be addressed directly: "Do you have any feelings about talking about financial limitations?" or "Do you have any feelings about seeing a less expensive therapist?"

However, in cases in which the patient's inconsistent attendance is not attributable to these problems, the problem needs to be directly examined: "I've noticed that you've cancelled several appointments. Is there some problem you are having with the idea of coming on a weekly basis?" The patient may indicate practical problems—money, scheduling, or work and family demands—and then both therapist and patient may examine possible solutions to these problems. Absent these practical issues, the therapist may directly ask, "Are you having any mixed feelings about treatment?" A variety of responses may follow from this inquiry: "I'm thinking that this therapy isn't working"; "I think it's self-indulgent for me to talk about my problems"; "I don't like the idea of getting too dependent on you"; "My husband doesn't think I should be seeing you." One patient who feared her growing dependence on the therapist also feared being rejected by him. Her strategy was to show up late (so he "would wait for me") and to miss whole sessions on occasion. She indicated she wanted him to feel like he needed her as much as she needed him.

ABUSIVE OR SEDUCTIVE BEHAVIOR TOWARD THE THERAPIST

Abusive Behavior toward the Therapist

Some patients act out their pathology by abusing the therapist. Abuse includes physical or sexual threats against the therapist, threats of lawsuits, abusive language, intimidating yelling or shouting in sessions, repeated demanding phone calls, and threats not to pay. The therapist should try to address any hostile or demeaning behavior at its first appearance. Therapists who are afraid of offending patients or of losing the patient's business may hesitate in setting limits on patients. Other self-sacrificing, even masochistic, therapists believe their own needs and rights are far inferior to the demands of the patient. At the other extreme are therapists who themselves become retaliatory and punitive when the patient expresses any hostility. These therapists, often with narcissistic issues of their own, will respond with sarcastic, humiliating, even threatening behavior.

Therapists are not whipping posts. We are not to be used for abuse. By allowing our patients to engage in abusive behavior toward us we demean ourselves and we reinforce pathological destructive behavior on the part of the patient.

Linehan (1993) has provided excellent guidelines for setting limits on acting-out behavior with patients—including limits on phone calls, suicide threats, and lack of continuity in attendance. To supplement Linehan's excellent guidelines, I would like to add the following comments. First, therapists are human beings who have the right to work in a nonabusive environment. We have the right to be free from sexual, physical, and psychological harassment. Second, patients have a right to professional treatment, but patients themselves have *obligations*. These obligations include paying for services, not abusing phone privileges, not using abusive language toward the therapist (or the support staff), and not engaging in any behavior with the therapist that would constitute harassment in any workplace. For example, patients who make demeaning and harassing comments about the therapist's ethnicity, the therapist's family, or the therapist's religious beliefs should be told that these comments are not acceptable. The *motivation* for such disparaging comments can be examined, but the harassing *behavior* itself should not be tolerated. Patients who refer to the therapist as a "bitch" or a "whore" should be told that continued use of such language will lead to termination of the session and, if necessary, termination of treatment. Patients who take a physically intimidating posture toward the therapist should be warned: "I find that I cannot work with people who express their anger in this fashion. I will not be able to continue to see you unless you are able to express your anger in a more acceptable and controlled manner."

A patient began to abuse phone privileges by frequently leaving messages on the therapist's answering machine. Initially, the therapist noted that while he understood that the patient's feelings were important, his answering machine should only be used for very serious problems or medical emergencies. The patient continued to test the therapist's limits by showing up an hour early and then staying in the waiting room an hour longer after the session. As this behavior increased in intensity and frequency, and as the patient failed to respond to each point of limit setting, the therapist decided to provide the patient with a written list of rules for being a patient: "No phone calls between sessions unless they are medical emergencies. You must not stay in the waiting room more than 15 minutes after the session. Insulting or abusive language toward the therapist is not tolerated. Failure to follow these guidelines may lead to termination of treatment."

Presenting the patient with such guidelines is a sensitive and difficult issue. The first questions the therapist should ask are: "Am I simply acting out of anger? Am I trying to punish the patient?" In the foregoing example, the therapist admitted to himself that he was angry, but he recognized that these guidelines were necessary in order to provide the patient with a model of appropriate patient behavior. These guidelines would help both the patient and the therapist. The therapist's assertiveness, or limit setting, should be proportional to the behavior of the patient. Many patients will get angry, questioning the therapist's credentials, sensitivity, and approach. However, abusive and destructive behavior on the part of the patient requires appropriate assertion from the therapist. This should include a specification of the out-of-bounds behavior, a description of appropriate behavior, an acknowledgment that the patient is upset and that his feelings are important issues in therapy, and a direct acknowledgment that the therapist believes that he has rights too. I feel comfortable telling patients something like this: "I understand that you have a need and a right to talk about your feelings, but I also want to tell you that I have a right to be treated with respect as a human being." Sometimes, patients may respond, "You're my therapist! I pay you to listen to this!" My response is: "You pay me to provide professional services for you, not to be abused by you. In order for this treatment to work for you, it also has to be something that I am willing to do with you. I will try to provide you with the best treatment I can, but I also believe that you have a responsibility to think about making this treatment something that I want to work on with you." I often ask the patient, "If you were me—the therapist—and you had a patient saying or doing these things, what would you do?" Another question to ask the patient is, "It seems that we have a dilemma. You are coming to me for help—and I want to help you. But how will it help you get what you need if you act this way? How will I want to help you if you are abusing me? Is it in your long-term interests to do this?"

After describing the guidelines for the patient, I suggest we examine the patient's negative and positive feelings about what has been said.

Negative responses include statements like: "You're rigid. You don't care. All you care about is yourself. You're like my father. How can I be honest about my feelings if I have to think about your feelings?" Positive responses include: "I know I was losing control. I'll try to control myself." One patient was relieved to learn that the therapist was willing to talk about the patient's abusive behavior rather than attack the patient and dismiss him. This resulted in a tearful session for the patient where he indicated that he always expected that people close to him would reject him for his bad behavior. The collaborative, but assertive, approach that the therapist utilized assisted the patient in maintaining the therapeutic relationship.

Seductive Behavior toward the Therapist

Therapists are human beings, and the relationship between patient and therapist is a powerful emotional experience. Some patients may develop an erotic transference with the therapist. The attraction that the patient may develop for the therapist may be a natural consequence of the feeling of attraction between two people in a strongly emotional relationship. However, in most cases the attraction is a consequence of the increased dependency of the patient. The patient's schemas may be activated, resulting in the idealization of the therapist. For example, the schema "others will take care of me" may lead the patient to idealize the therapist as someone who will rescue the patient from his or her problem. The patient's selective knowledge and filter about the therapist should not lead the therapist to flatter his or her own ego in thinking that he or she is irresistible. Usually, the attraction says more about the patient than it does about the therapist.

In some cases, the erotic transference may reflect the patient's attempt to seduce the therapist down from a position of power. In these cases, the patient may perceive the therapist as a controlling and powerful figure, whom he or she simultaneously fears and desires. The fantasy may be to possess the therapist as a lover, so that his or her power is taken away and thereby becomes the patient's power. For example, a female patient made sexually seductive poses toward her male therapist in the context of her discussion of how she had been victimized by men. In these discussions, she described how she had enjoyed being an erotic dancer in the past because it made her feel powerful and contemptuous toward men that "needed me but couldn't have me." She then leaned forward toward the therapist, in her sexually provocative clothing, and said, "I wonder why men allow women to do oral sex on them. It makes the man so vulnerable." This provocative and seductive behavior on her part led the therapist to make a transference interpretation: "I wonder why you feel the need to control men and make them want you."

This then led to a discussion of how she had felt when she was an adolescent—that she was unattractive and fat and that no boy wanted her. She indicated that she felt she always had to compensate for these feelings by being seductive. She confessed that she had married a man who, she believed, needed her more than she needed him. She did this, she said, because she was always afraid that men would leave her because she was not lovable. Thus, a potentially seductive interaction in the session was turned into a productive discussion of her sexual schemas.

Some patients push the limits of appropriate behavior, making lewd and suggestive comments and even directly propositioning the therapist. Initially, transference interpretations may be helpful, as they were in the foregoing case. However, in some cases the patient's behavior continues to be provocative and unacceptable. In these instances limits need to be set. A male patient who continued to sexually harass his female therapist by indicating that he had masturbation fantasies about her was told that these comments were not appropriate for therapy. When the patient said that he masturbated in the office bathroom while thinking about the therapist, the therapist indicated that she would not be able to see the patient any more if he continued such behavior and confessed such thoughts and feelings. (Moreover, since the therapist was operating in a group practice, she was able to assure herself that other staff were always present in the office setting when this patient came to sessions.) This assertion was useful in moving the therapy forward toward more productive and less hostile and inappropriate behavior.

Sometimes the patient's erotic transference is not workable. Some patients may feel that the therapist reminds them so strongly of someone they have known—or someone they would want—that the patient cannot control his or her behavior. In these cases, a direct discussion of these issues should be made: "Do you think that these feelings are too strong for you to continue to work with me?" The patient may claim that she can continue to work with the therapist, but the real test will be the degree to which the patient refrains from the inappropriate behavior. The therapist can indicate that the patient's intentions to change may be present, but that it is not working. In such cases, a transfer of the patient to another therapist may be appropriate.

SPLITTING THE TRANSFERENCE

Patients in therapy often have more than one person to whom they turn for help. It is not uncommon for a patient to have one practitioner for therapy and another for medication. In some cases, the other practitioner may be another therapist who is providing a different kind of treatment. For example, the cognitive therapist may be providing treatment to someone who also has a psychodynamic therapist. In other cases, the other therapist is providing couple or family therapy. A patient recently out of the hospital may be in group therapy in a day program. It is good practice to contact the other practitioner and attempt to coordinate treatment. However, even with the best of efforts and best of intentions, the patient may either create or find himself in conflicts between practitioners.

A common source of split in the transference occurs when the patient has one doctor for medication and another for therapy. The patient may believe that he is getting two conflicting views of his "illness": a biological view and a cognitive-behavioral view. I attempt to offset this confusion by indicating to the patient that depression, for example, is usually the result of a number of factors: biological makeup, childhood experience, current relationships, stress, rewards, and the way we think about things. Rather than viewing depression as entirely biological or entirely cognitive, one can think of it as the interaction of both these factors. I find that the example of high blood pressure (hypertension) helps to illustrate such interactions: "If you had hypertension, there would be a number of things that you could do to control it. You could take medication, but you could also use a number of lifestyle changes. For example, you might cut back on drinking and smoking, you might exercise and lose weight, and you might practice relaxation to reduce your stress. Each one of these things could be helpful. Indeed, you might want to use all of them."

However, in some cases the patient feels caught between a physician, who believes that everything is biological, and the work in cognitive-behavioral treatment. The therapist should contact the doctor who is prescribing medication and determine what the doctor is actually saying to the patient. It is possible that the patient may be misrepresenting the doctor's position. In any case, it can be helpful to inform the doctor that the patient is indicating that his doctor is saying that therapy is unnecessary. Some doctors may back down from their unilateral view, others may not. If the doctor's position is that therapy is useless, then the therapist should be assertive. He should indicate that the doctor's opinion is creating problems for the patient and undermining the work of the therapist. (Some nonmedical therapists appear to be intimidated by medical doctors who prescribe. My view is that the patient's welfare is the primary goal and that, if a doctor is alienated by appropriate assertion and a demand for professional conduct, then it is more the doctor's problem than the patient's.)

If the therapist finds that the patient's doctor does not refrain from making undermining statements, then the therapist should discuss the patient's feelings of being caught in the middle. The patient may indicate that he feels guilty about challenging the other doctor, or intimidated. These automatic thoughts and assumptions may be challenged by focusing on the patient's right to treatment choices.

In some cases, the patient may be referred for treatment by a therapist with a different orientation—for example, by a psychodynamic therapist. The cognitive therapist should discuss with the other therapist the advantages and disadvantages of having two therapists. My experience is that it is almost always a disadvantage. If possible, the patient should be given the option of discontinuing the other therapy while in the current cognitive therapy. Dependent, avoidant, passive–aggressive, borderline, and narcissistic patients are especially undermined by dual therapy. The dependent or avoidant patient fears alienating any source of support, and therefore feels unable to choose the orientation to follow. The passive–aggressive patient may use one therapist as a means to resist "pressure" from the other therapist. Borderline patients are notorious for splitting the transference—sometimes by making one therapist into the "good cop" and the other into the "bad cop." The patient may say: "My other therapist says that this is superficial and won't help" or "My other therapist really cares about my feelings." The narcissistic patient may surround himself with "adulating" therapists, who serve as an audience rather than as a source of change. Several years ago, a patient was referred to me for cognitive therapy. She was already seeing a doctor for medication, a psychoanalyst for traditional analytic treatment, and a psychodynamic therapist for "regular therapy," and now she wanted to see me twice a week for cognitive therapy. She announced in the first session that she had no intention of doing any homework assignments and that if she was going to get better it was going to be in the session. Therapy had become her life. Her husband paid little attention to her and two of her therapists appeared to provide her with special privileges: extended sessions, frequent phone calls, and personal anecdotes about themselves. She dropped out of cognitive therapy with me after 2 weeks, apparently realizing that cognitive therapy would not provide her with a surrogate life.

These splits in transference should be discussed between therapists. Unfortunately, many therapists are financially dependent on patients and are reluctant to encourage a patient to pursue help elsewhere. Other therapists believe that their approach is superior. The patient is caught in the middle of the countertransference fears of another therapist. If the conflicts cannot be resolved between the therapists, then the cognitive therapist may examine the patient's beliefs about the conflict. For example, the therapist may ask the following:

"What thoughts and feelings do you have about this?"

"What are your goals in treatment?"

"What would you prefer to happen? What would you like me to do and what would you like Dr. Jones to do?"

"What are the costs and benefits of telling me and Dr. Jones what you prefer?"

"What are the costs and benefits of deciding to drop one treatment for a while?"

Patients may have a range of thoughts and feelings about feeling caught in the middle. Some patients feel guilty and confused—for example, they may feel that they will alienate the other doctor and that the other doctor may not be there if things do not work out with the therapist. Other patients fear retaliation—that the other therapist will criticize and humiliate them. Still others like being in the middle: they feel important, needed by the doctor and therapist, and in control. They may enjoy watching the two doctors "fight" over them. It may also allow them to punish one therapist without directly being accountable: "My other doctor says that this cognitive therapy is a waste of time."

Guilt and confusion about the split transference can be examined by determining what the goal is for the patient: supporting the therapist or getting better. The double-standard technique is a useful intervention, since patients are often far more willing to encourage assertiveness in others than to practice it themselves. Unexpressed, or thinly veiled, anger may be elicited: "A lot of times patients in therapy find themselves angry and disappointed with their therapist. It would be natural for you to have some of these feelings with me or with your other doctor. Can you tell me about these thoughts and feelings? How do you feel about telling doctors that you are angry? What kind of automatic thoughts do you have?" Some patients may believe they cannot directly express their anger with one doctor unless they have arranged to have another doctor in the "wings."

PREMATURE TERMINATION

Many terminations seem premature to the therapist, but not premature to the patient. Other therapists, afraid of acknowledging rejection, may have a narcissistic interpretation of termination: "She terminated treatment because I cured her of her panic attacks in one session!" Of course, the real question is "What constitutes premature termination?"

There are no definitive rules for this. Timeliness of termination may be determined by a number of factors—not all valid. These include the following:

1. The patient has decided he does not need more treatment.
2. The patient's symptoms have abated.
3. The patient is not making any more progress.
4. The patient has adequately identified and challenged his cognitive distortions and assumptions.
5. The patient is able to use cognitive therapy techniques on his own.

Unfortunately, in the real world, termination may have more to do with the patient's managed care policy than with therapeutic goals.

Each of these factors is relevant to termination. Patients can think of treatment in a variety of ways—each of them legitimate.

- Treatment is crisis intervention.
- Treatment is reduction of symptoms.
- Treatment is acquiring insight and self-help skills.
- Treatment is personal growth.

When patients think of terminating, they should be supported for their assertion: "It's good that you feel able to tell me that you want to make a change. Let's examine what you came here to accomplish and how you have been doing." The patient can be referred back to the problem list developed in the first few sessions of treatment, or to problems that have come up during the course of treatment. For example, the therapist can say: "Let's look at the problems that you wanted to work on in treatment. You listed depression, anxiety, self-criticism, procrastination, and your relationships with people at work. Let's examine how much progress you feel that you have made in each of these areas."

In some cases, the patient only wanted crisis intervention. This is a legitimate goal, but the therapist can ask, "Are there any factors that might account for this crisis that might reoccur for you?"

The desire to leave treatment prematurely may be related to a number of schematic issues: fear of becoming dependent, the belief that therapy is self-indulgent and that the patient is not worth it, fear of uncovering disturbing material, fear of being controlled and humiliated, and fear of being abandoned and rejected by the therapist. For example, one patient thought of terminating therapy even though she recognized that there were a number of important issues she could still work on. As she examined the costs and benefits of continuing in treatment, she indicated that she was afraid she would become too dependent on the therapist and that this set her up for disappointment should he lose interest in her or not meet her needs. This then led to a discussion of how her mother seldom attended to her needs, leaving her with the additional belief that her needs were not important and that therapy was self-indulgent. She was able to reframe continuing in treatment as an exercise in assertiveness—that is, pursuing *her* needs.

Another patient, who had come to treatment for panic disorder, indicated that she wanted to terminate treatment, even though she was still very anxious and was unhappy in her sexless marriage. As she examined the costs and benefits of continuing in treatment she indicated that she was afraid that she would become too "emotional" in her relationship with the therapist. As we examined the evidence for and against this belief, she disclosed that she had been sexually involved with a therapist years before and that she feared having any sexual feelings toward any doctors in authority. (This was especially problematic for her since she worked in a hospital.) Discussion of her fears of arousal—and her fear that she would not be able to control herself—led to her ability to challenge her guilty thoughts about past exploitation by her therapist. This then led to her ability to begin couple meetings with the therapist and her husband and to improvement in their marital relationship.

Finally, a narcissistic man began therapy by both challenging and idealizing the therapist. As therapy progressed, he discussed his feelings of anger at and emotional deprivation from his mother, with whom he still lived. On one occasion, he began the session in a defensive and angry manner, leading the therapist to question if there was anything he had done to offend the patient. The patient shouted, "I'll reject you before you reject me!" When the therapist indicated that he had no plans of rejecting the patient and wondered what made him think he would be rejected, the patient answered, "I've become too dependent on you." In the next session, the patient began in silence and, when asked by the therapist what was on his mind, the patient responded: "I'm not taking this shit anymore!" He then walked out. The patient's agenda truly was to reject anyone that he had become dependent on since his assumption was that no one who knew him could stand him. Unfortunately, this patient never returned to treatment, even though the therapist attempted to contact him.

SUMMARY

I have examined several aspects of procedural resistance in cognitive-behavioral therapy. Resistance in therapy can take the form of problems in agenda setting, collaborative set, homework compliance, lack of continuity of appointments, abusive or seductive behavior, splitting the transference with other therapists, and premature termination. I have suggested some interventions that might be helpful in addressing each of these problems in therapy.

In Part II, I shall develop a multidimensional model of different modes of resistance. Certainly, each of the aspects of procedural resistance I have discussed here is relevant to addressing each of the dimensions of resistance described in this volume. However, as I hope will become clear, the clinician needs to recognize that there are many differences in why people resist change. Therefore, it is essential to know which processes of resistance are operating with a specific patient at a given time.

PART II
Dimensions of Resistance

4

Validation Resistance

And he said unto him, Son, thou art ever with me,
and all that I have is thine. It was meet that we should
make merry, and be glad: for this thy brother was dead,
and is alive again; and was lost, and is found.
                                        —LUKE 15:31–32

*T*he Spanish philosopher and novelist Miguel de Unamuno (1921/ 1990) observed that the modern era seems to be marked by the belief that the problems of life can be solved with rationality and technology. Yet much of life eludes problem solving, and many situations are incontrovertibly sad and tragic. Unamuno offers the following story: A young man, walking along the road, finds an old man sitting by the side of the road weeping. He says, "Old man. Why do you weep?" The old man replies, "My son has died. I weep over the death of my son." The young man, in his rationality, responds: "But weeping avails nothing. Your son is dead." And the old man replies, "I weep precisely because weeping avails nothing. We must learn how to weep for the plague, not just cure it."

Unamuno (1921/1990) describes this attitude as the "tragic sense of life." In the tragic sense of life, we recognize that, while we may search for solutions, we are still confronted by losses and dilemmas. In the tragic sense of life, we are witnesses to the suffering of others. We give it "meaning" by sharing the experience of the other's dilemma. The literary critic George Steiner, in *The Death of Tragedy* (1980), describes this moment of the inconsolable. In Bertolt Brecht's play *Mother Courage and Her Children* (1941/1991), which Steiner saw in East Berlin, Courage (the mother) must identify the body of her dead son. She looks down at the body, shaking her head in "mute denial." The body is carried off

57

and Courage looks away, with her mouth wide open, as if screaming—but the audience hears no sound. Steiner remarks: "The sound that came out was raw and terrible beyond any description I could give of it. But, in fact, there was no sound. Nothing. The sound was total silence." The audience sat in silence, lowering its collective head. The totality of the loss was overwhelming—it was so much that there were no words to express it or describe it.

Some cognitive-behavioral therapists claim that nothing is awful, nothing is really terrible—because, after all, one can still go on. But the word *awful* does not mean that one cannot go on. Indeed, *awful* means "awe-inspiring": that you stand alone, confronted by an experience, feeling for the moment smaller, overwhelmed, amazed, moved. The death of loved ones—or one's own impending death—and the loss of meaningful relationships are experiences in life that inspire awe. We must distinguish among the "rational, irrational, and the nonrational" (Otto, 1923/1950). That which we stand in awe of is often beyond the realm of rationality and is thus nonrational. It is not logical—it is *moving*. It creates dread, fear, a sense of being overwhelmed.

It is this aspect of the human condition, the recognition that "we must learn to weep for the plague, not just cure it," that is an essential component of meaningful therapy and meaningful relationships. When we experience what seems awful and horrible in our lives, we often take solace in knowing that another person understands, or, at least, is attempting to understand, our pain.

THE LIMITS OF COGNITIVE THERAPY

The cognitive-behavioral approach to therapy is often criticized as a model that does not adequately address the patient's emotions. Patients, and therapists from psychodynamic, Rogerian, and experiential orientations, argue that the cognitive therapist ignores the need of the patient to ventilate his or her emotions and to have these emotions understood and validated by the therapist. *Validation resistance* is the demand for understanding, empathy, and care from the therapist—often to the exclusion of problem solving or a rational perspective.

The cognitive model is based on the *rational principle*, that is, the assumption that people will be motivated to change their beliefs to be consistent with facts and logic. This rational principle assumption, derived from the optimism of the Enlightenment, implies that the "truth shall set you free." If one reads either professional or popular writings in cognitive therapy, one gets the impression that individuals who are suffering simply look at the costs and benefits of their beliefs, examine the

evidence, and change. Thinking and change seem tidy, simple, and obvious. Similar to many Enlightenment models of human nature, such as
the views advanced by David Hume, John Locke, John Stuart Mill, and
Adam Smith, people are viewed as conducting a hedonic calculus and an
empirical investigation to solve their problems. They are driven by
pleasure–pain principles, and they are convinced by rationality.

Problems are viewed as errors, distortions, and biases that, when
corrected, cease to be problems. To describe someone's thinking as "distorted" is not far from implying that he or she is less intelligent than the
person doing the describing. For individuals who already see themselves
as defective, a therapeutic focus on distortions in thinking may be interpreted by them as invalidation.

Some cognitive-behavioral therapists believe that everything has a
solution: getting better is simply a matter of applying the technology and
techniques of the therapeutic model. The therapist may intercede too
quickly, asking, "How can you solve that problem?," without first ap-
preciating that the problem matters very deeply to the patient. As one
colleague, critical of the cognitive approach, said to me: "Some people
think that if there isn't a solution, then there isn't a problem."

THEORETICAL APPROACHES TO EMPATHY
AND VALIDATION IN THERAPY

Indeed, there is considerable theoretical, clinical, and empirical support
for the importance of the elicitation of emotion and empathy in therapy.
Attachment models, stressing the importance of a secure attachment relationship in the development of emotional regulation, suggest that the
therapist should develop a secure and predictable relationship with the
patient such that the patient perceives that his or her emotions are understood, reflected back, and valued by the therapist (Bowlby, 1969;
Guidano & Liotti, 1983; Safran & Segal, 1990; Safran, 1998). According to attachment systems models, such as Bowlby's, the individual will
persist in expressing a distressful emotion until the therapist responds
with empathy and support. The therapist's failure to respond with empathy will result either in the escalation of the negative emotion or in the
patient leaving the relationship.

According to Rogers (1950, 1965), neurotic problems are the result
of the disparity between an extreme ideal self-image and a deflated real
self-image (self-esteem). The goal of therapy is to reduce this self-image
disparity through a process of nonjudgmental, unconditional positive regard. Although there is considerable evidence that improvement in therapy is related to the patient's perception that the therapist is empathic,

DeRubeis and Feeley (1990) found that improvement by the patient *pre-ceded* the patient's perception that the therapist was empathic. This suggests that patients believe that therapists really care about them only after the patient has gotten better: in looking back, we like people who have helped us and we think they cared about us.

From an object-relations perspective, empathic failures are almost an inevitable occurrence in therapy, resulting in the patient's belief that the therapist cannot help him (Kohut, 1971, 1977). The patient's initial idealization of therapy may result in a dichotomization to the other extreme, such that the patient who stresses validation and empathy may become demoralized when it does not occur. Kohut (1971, 1977) has suggested that certain personality disorders—such as those suffered by borderline and narcissistic individuals—are especially affected by the need for "mirroring"—that is, the desire for an almost perfect empathic ability on the part of the therapist.

Linehan (1993) has proposed a dialectical model of validation and change in which she argues that the patient and the therapist are confronted with the (ironic) apparent conflict that therapy requires change, but that the patient needs to be validated for what she or he is now. According to Linehan, these individuals have been told conflicting things about themselves—for example, that they are incompetent, but that great things are expected of them. In the approach I advocate in this book, I have attempted to utilize the "truth" of a dialectical approach in helping the patient understand the dilemma that the patient and therapist are in. This dilemma implies that there is a need for change, but also a need to validate the patient's perception and feelings. Therapy, from this perspective, entails the ability to balance the internal tensions of change and validation.

Greenberg and Paivio (1997) have advanced an experiential approach that incorporates gestalt therapy techniques, Rogerian therapy, and their own integration of cognitive therapy. They refer to this therapeutic model as "emotionally focused therapy." According to Greenberg and Paivio, some affective and anxiety disorders may result from, or be maintained by, disturbances in the processing of emotional content (see also Foa & Kozak, 1991; Pennebaker, 1995; Kennedy-Moore & Watson, 1999; and Wegner, 1989). These problems in emotional processing include overcontrol (through suppression or inhibition of affect) and undercontrol (through excessive expression or feeling overwhelmed by emotions). Greenberg and Paivio argue that the activation of the emotional content or emotional schemas associated with negative thoughts may be important in modifying the underlying thoughts and emotions. Their approach stresses elicitation of affect, through experiential techniques such as streaming and imagery, and restructuring of both emotional and cognitive schemas. They stress the importance of empathy and validation in the therapeutic encounter because they facilitate the patient's recognition of legitimate emotional needs.

Similarly, Safran (1998) and his colleagues have stressed the importance of the therapeutic alliance, in which empathy, collaboration, and repairing injuries in the therapeutic relationship are viewed as essential. According to Safran's cognitive-interpersonal model, the patient's progress in therapy is not reducible to rational disputation of thoughts. It also requires the therapist and the patient to work at recognizing and repairing important "ruptures" in their therapeutic alliance. Here, validation, empathy, and collaboration with the patient to maintain the working bond are placed at the center of therapy. I recognize the importance of this therapeutic alliance in directing the therapist and the patient toward focusing on how the patient's emotional needs and needs for validation may be addressed. These aspects of the therapeutic alliance are relevant to several aspects of resistance—specifically, validation, emotional dysregulation, victim roles, and schematic resistance—and to countertransference issues that I discuss in Chapters 11 and 12.

However, an overfocus on validation to the exclusion of change may result in a therapeutic impasse. For example, some patients may view the entire function of therapy as ventilation and validation. From this perspective, the therapeutic session should consist of the patient ventilating his complaints and emotions and the therapist reflecting back to the patient how awful life is for the patient. Simply "being understood" becomes the goal of therapy. As I suggest later in this chapter, this ventilation–validation model may result in the persistence of the "victim script" in therapy: the patient repeatedly focuses on how his or her life is really difficult, and the therapist becomes an audience and supporter for this view. The consequence is that the patient feels understood, but also feels helpless to change.

Patients who are overfocused on validation often have a set of underlying assumptions about how disagreement is not only invalidating, but a sign of betrayal and hostility. Consider the following examples:

A patient who had been hospitalized prior to therapy for psychotic depression and who received electroconvulsive therapy entered cognitive therapy and was helped to overcome much of her daily anxiety about memory loss. However, as she continued to work with the therapist on issues relating to her work, she claimed that the therapist could not understand what her experiences were like since he (the therapist) had never experienced a psychotic depression. She became angrier with the therapist and requested a referral to "a therapist who has dealt with his own psychosis in the past." The patient's emphasis on validation was so extreme that she believed that the therapist must be similar to the patient in pathology in order to understand and help the patient.

A borderline patient, who viewed her work situation as hopeless, became angry when the therapist suggested some possible changes in her work life—such as becoming more assertive with her supervisor and acquiring new skills. The therapist elicited the following automatic thoughts from the patient regarding her anger at the suggestion of change: "You don't understand me. I really am trapped. If you don't understand that (and agree with that) then you can't help me. If you can't help me, no one can help me. If you aren't helping me, then I hate you because you're going to hurt me."

PATHOLOGICAL STRATEGIES
TO ELICIT VALIDATION

Patients who demand validation and do not receive it may resort to a variety of strategies to elicit validation from the therapist. These strategies include rumination, escalation of intensity, devaluation of the therapist, emotional distancing, splitting the transference, and noncompliance with homework.

The first strategy is to *ruminate* about how awful things are. By repeating his or her complaints and refusing to consider other topics of discussion, the patient hopes to get the therapist to recognize that things really are terrible. For example, one patient constantly fixated on his "financial problems," even though he was affluent. Whenever the therapist attempted to point out that he was financially well-off, the patient dwelled even more on his fears of poverty.

A second strategy is to *escalate the intensity* of the complaint. This can take the form either of raising the voice (to the point of yelling at the therapist) or of arguing that things are even worse than the patient first stated they were. Thus, the patient becomes "interpersonally invested" in catastrophizing: "If I can prove that things are awful, then you will understand how I feel."

A third strategy is to try to elicit *negative feelings* from the therapist by punishing or devaluing him or her. For example, the patient may belittle the therapist: "You're not helping me," "I'm wasting my money and time with you," "You're incompetent," or "I'm not going to come back." I have observed that the patient who feels incompetent is more likely to complain that the therapist is incompetent, whereas the patient who fears being rejected by the therapist is apt to reject the therapist first.

A fourth strategy involves *emotional distancing*. The patient may become taciturn in sessions or even refuse to talk at all. Unlike the patient who directly ventilates her emotions, the emotionally distancing patient acts as if she is saying, "If you want to know how I feel, you will have to ask me." The patient's total silence or reluctance to speak reflects the belief that the therapist will not be able to appreciate what the patient is feeling, so "why bother?"

A fifth strategy to elicit validation is to *split the transference* between two therapists or between the therapist and someone else in the patient's life. For example, the patient who argues that it is "impossible for me to do anything when I'm depressed" reports that the psychiatrist that provides him with medication agrees with him that he cannot do anything when he is depressed. Or the patient may report that another therapist "really understands me and you don't." Many patients with validation resistance surround themselves with friends who reinforce their beliefs that things are awful and who help the patient to focus on how bad he or she feels. When the patient says, "My friend [therapist, husband, wife] thinks this therapy is useless," the patient may be expressing his own doubts without having to defend them.

Finally, the patient with validation resistance will often reject standard cognitive-behavioral interventions and *not comply with homework*. Attempts to look at the evidence for and against a belief are viewed as trivial, and cost–benefit analyses are rejected as irrelevant because "this is how I feel, it's not what I want." The patient views behavioral assignments as unrealistic, since "you don't understand that I really can't change." Therapeutic suggestions that there are alternative ways of viewing the situation are viewed as naive, invalidating, critical, and hostile.

SELF-INVALIDATION

Just as demands for validation may constitute resistance in cognitive-behavioral therapy, so also can a patient's *refusal to accept his or her own needs*. Self-invalidation is a central impediment to therapy, since therapy is intended to *meet needs*. The individual who has difficulty identifying and accepting the legitimacy of her needs will find therapy meaningless, if not disturbing.

Furthermore, overregulation of emotions, especially deliberate attempts to inhibit negative feelings or images, may contribute to the continued anxiety or depression of the patient (Greenberg & Paivio, 1997; Kennedy-Moore & Watson, 1999; Traue & Pennebaker, 1993). Indeed, Greenberg and Paivio (1997) propose a sequential process of (1) allowing hurt feelings, (2) reowning them, and then (3) recognizing the legitimacy of unmet needs. Thus an individual may inhibit her feelings of being hurt and humiliated and not legitimize her unmet need to be treated respectfully. Greenberg and Paivio's "emotionally focused therapy" provides a context in which the reworking of emotions through elicitation and validation may lead to the emergence of self-affirming beliefs such as "I need to be understood" or "I need to have a trusting relationship."

Many individuals who have been invalidated during childhood, adolescence, and adulthood have learned to anticipate invalidation. Therefore, they try to blunt it or deny the need for validation. This self-sacrificing style is an attempt to avoid disappointment or punishment for having needs. Some patients exhibit their invalidation by describing themselves as "whiny" or as "complaining," while others view therapy as "a luxury that I don't need to indulge myself with." The patient may indicate that he expects the therapist to view him as a "crybaby" or "pathetic" for complaining about his needs. Many of these patients believe they are spending too much money and time on therapy "they don't really need." When one takes a history on some of these patients, one is struck by the fact that they have sought little in the way of psychological or medical consultation despite a long history of depression and relational conflict.

Many of these patients utilize classic psychodynamic defenses of isolation, intellectualization, and denial (A. Freud, 1946). In *isolation*, the patient separates out a feeling or need and attaches little emotional import to it. For example, a patient talks about the lack of affection in her marriage in a monotone, showing no awareness that it might be a deprivation. Using *intellectualization*, the patient finds a facile explanation that minimizes the importance of the need or event that would generally be disturbing to others. For example, the patient "rationalizes" her husband's verbally abusive behavior by saying that she has her work to do and she does not really care what he says when he is upset. She may even view her explanation as a successful utilization of cognitive therapy. In *denial*, the most primitive of these defenses, the patient simply represses any feeling that the need is important, even refusing to acknowledge the need. For example, a woman claims that she does not really need sex in her marriage because she does not have any sexual desire.

Some of the more common expressions of self-invalidation are the following:

- Unwillingness to talk about needs
- Viewing needs as weakness
- Using cognitive-behavioral therapy as a defense against needs

- Apologizing for needs
- Inability to process information about needs
- Dissociation
- Attempts to lower expectations
- Somatization

Let us briefly examine each of these strategies of self-invalidation.

Unwillingness to Talk about Needs

The patient may simply refuse to talk about her needs in the session. She may fall silent, turn to trivial issues, comment on the therapist's office or appearance, or change the subject when her needs are brought up. The therapist should be alert to these avoidant patterns and should address them directly: "It seems that we are not talking about your important needs here. You seem to change the subject when we begin talking about your relationship with your husband. How do you feel about your needs in this relationship? What does it make you think when we talk about your needs?" Some patients indicate that talking about their needs makes them feel sad and anxious because they believe that their needs are not legitimate or will never be met.

Viewing Needs as Weakness

Some people have learned to "cope" with their unmet needs by adapting either a defensive or an offensive strategy. They view personal needs as weakness, vulnerability, or inferiority. A male patient, who had been threatened at gunpoint by his mother when he was a child, viewed being in therapy as a sign of failure. He became expert in karate and viewed himself as physically invulnerable (see Leahy, 1992, 1996a). He viewed having emotional needs as unmanly; his rule was "I should never be vulnerable or weak." Exploration of this schema led to his recognition that having any needs of his own was associated in his thinking with the risk of being killed. He adapted a "counterphobic" strategy of placing himself in positions of physical danger so as to prove to himself that he was invulnerable.

Using Cognitive-Behavioral Therapy as a Defense against Needs

Unfortunately, cognitive therapy can often lend itself to a shallow, glib, and minimizing approach to life. Some patients who wish to escape from the recognition of their vulnerability and need are attracted to the practical-technique approach of cognitive therapy. Some of these people will recite rational responses as if a formulaic approach to life will make life better. The patient may cheerfully say, "Oh, I know that I am labeling when I call myself a 'loser.' The incongruity of the cheerful recognition of the right answer with the self-labeling as a loser reveals that the patient does not wish to confront the more profound and disturbing meaning to him of being a loser. Some patients do cognitive therapy homework as a ritual in which they find the "right" answer—"I am not a loser. I have several good points. I have friends, and people like me"— much like the caricature character Stuart Smalley on *Saturday Night Live*. Their approach to their needs is shallow and glib, they seldom allow themselves the freedom to cry in sessions, and they continue in relationships where their needs go unmet.

The therapist can assist such patients by indicating that cognitive therapy often can seem shallow and superficial and that the patient needs to be aware of the risk of trivializing his needs. When I have asked these patients how their needs were trivialized or ridiculed when they were younger, the patient may respond with surprise (and anxiety): "You're not supposed to talk about childhood in here. That's Freudian!" The patient can be told that cognitive therapy has expanded considerably to recognize the importance of earlier experiences. The real question that needs to be addressed is, "What is it that we will talk about that will make you so upset?"

Apologizing for Needs

Some patients apologize for having needs, viewing their needs as excessive, inappropriate and, most significantly, disgusting or pathetic in the eyes of others. The patient may say: "You probably think I'm a loser for being depressed" or "I know I sound like a complainer." Such comments reflect the reality that others continuously invalidate the patient, telling the patient to "grow up" or "snap out of it." One woman vacillated between demands for reassurance—for example, by making frequent phone calls between sessions—and self-denigration of her needs within session. She would often punctuate her conversation with "Is that OK?," thereby questioning the legitimacy of her needs. She was extraordinarily afraid of talking about her anger toward me, anticipating that I would not want to keep her as a patient. The issue for her, of course, was *trust*, which was consistent with the double binds she faced in her family of origin. Her mother would tell her that her needs were excessive and unreasonable and, at the same time, indicate that mother was the only person she could rely on.

Inability to Process Information about Needs

Some patients have difficulty remembering what was just said when it refers to their needs. For example, a highly intelligent patient could not remember what the therapist had just said about her needs for affection and respect. She required several repetitions for the therapist to get his point across. For some self-denigrating, self-invalidating patients, talking about their needs almost seems like trying to speak in an unknown language. This inability is a rudimentary form of protective dissociation, to which I turn now.

Dissociation

Dissociation takes many forms, ranging from mild unawareness of immediate stimuli to distinct multiple personalities. Although distinct multiple personality is rare in clinical practice, a variety of dissociative experiences are common in and out of therapy. One patient appeared to "space out" during sessions, her attention drifting into empty air, becoming nonresponsive to what was being said by the therapist. When I commented on this, she said she had often been told she spaced out. We decided to observe when this happened in sessions and found that it occurred when we discussed her needs for affection, understanding, and sexuality in her marriage. We examined the costs and benefits of spacing out during these discussions, which led to her observation that her needs were seldom met as a child. She had been told that she was selfish and whiny. Her assumption was "I will be punished for my needs." I asked her to observe in therapy if she was being punished or supported for her needs and to test out how she could assert herself with her husband in a manner that was different from assertion with her mother. As we focused more on the dissociation in session and on assertion and recognition of needs outside of session, her dissociative response diminished.

Lowering Expectations

Some patients attempt to avoid disappointment by lowering their expectations that their needs will be met in therapy. The patient may say: "I know you're too busy," "My problems really are nothing compared to the problems other people have," or "I really don't expect very much from therapy." These patients have lived lives in which other people have consistently failed to validate and satisfy their needs, so they have developed a generalized low expectation of need gratification. When the patient finds that the therapist does validate the patient's needs and attempts to support the patient, even when the patient is angry, it creates dissonance for the patient. She may become anxious, fearing that she will trust the therapist more, become more vulnerable, and therefore suffer greater disappointment later. One patient asked, "Why are you being so nice to me?," and then claimed "I'm not used to this." The patient may feel more familiar with the predictable world in which his needs are not being met and may even try to provoke the therapist into invalidating the patient, thereby allowing the patient to retreat to the familiar ground of invalidation and rejection.

Somatization

It is easier and more socially acceptable in our culture to seek assistance for physical-medical problems than for psychological problems. There are a variety of causal pathways to somatic complaints, but one advantage of focusing extensively on somatic complaints is that they are a "legitimate" means of seeking attention. The self-denying, self-invalidating patient may find it more acceptable to seek medical attention for supposed heart irregularities, concerns about possible infection of sexually transmitted diseases, and worries about cancer—especially when the medical grounds for these worries are close to nonexistent. Guidano and Liotti (1983) view these somatic concerns as protecting the patient from recognizing core schematic issues of vulnerability and preventing the patient from developing the insight into relational conflicts and psychological vulnerabilities.

A component of somatization is the excessive placebo effect for some of these patients. Some somaticizing, self-denying patients report feeling "immediately better" after taking a subclinical dose of an antidepressant medication. The perceived/imagined medical cause of their problems allows them to have a "legitimate" need due to biochemical imbalance, but has little implication for their interpersonal deprivation and invalidation. Similarly, these patients are often quite sensitive to side effects of medications, often reporting the expected side effects on trace doses of psychotropic medication. Again, it is more acceptable for them to complain about a physical side effect than to examine what their needs are and why they are not being met in their personal lives.

CLINICAL INTERVENTIONS
FOR VALIDATION RESISTANCE

Therapists often find validation resistance to be frustrating. They will describe patients who focus on validation as "complainers," "help rejectors," "self-defeating," or just unpleasant to work with. Some therapists simply give up and claim the patient is not ready to change. An alternative view is to observe that the patient *is* ready to be validated. Perhaps change will come later.

The therapist confronted with validation resistance may find herself in a dilemma: "If I constantly agree with the patient's negativity, nothing will change, but if I challenge the negativity, then the patient will view me as invalidating and hostile." The strategy in approaching the validation resistance is not to change it, but to join it.

Accept the Validation Resistance

Wanting the patient to be different is not going to change the situation. The patient will continue to demand validation no matter what you, the therapist, want. Accepting the validation resistance is like doing a *realistic diagnosis*. It is the given of the relationship. Some therapists complain about the validation resistance. They believe that the patient's "complaining and whining" won't help the patient. But complaining and whining about the validation resistance won't get the therapist anywhere, either. The therapist can minimize his or her frustration with such patients by realizing that if the therapist does not accept the patient's validation needs, then the patient will not accept the therapy.

Some therapists resist the patient's validation resistance. They ignore the complaints of the patient, and sometimes even remain silent. Or they criticize the patient for complaining rather than trying to solve problems. This criticism, of course, promotes the patient's belief that the therapist does not understand how bad things are. Consequently, the patient complains even more. Attempts to change the patient, who has yet to feel validated, often result in the patient trying to prove he cannot change.

First, in order to accept the validation resistance, the therapist must learn to respect the need for validation. As change agents, armed with our techniques and treatment plans, we are often in opposition to the patient's need for validation. Some therapists feel smothered by, overwhelmed by, or bored with validation needs. They understand the need for grief and mourning, the need for a ceremony to mark the death of someone we care about, the need for compassionate talk when someone has been diagnosed with cancer, but they fail to appreciate the need for validation.

Second, the therapist must abandon, for the moment, the attempt to change the patient. Change implies letting go. When we ask the patient to change her thoughts and feelings, we are telling her to leave them behind because they are no longer valid. To have these thoughts and feelings accepted, rather than disputed, affirms for the patient that she is valued and respected as a person. How can I feel respected by you if I believe that my feelings seem strange or trivial to you? Imagine how a child would feel if she believed her mother never heard her when she cried. Moving too quickly to change the patient may result in the patient believing that the therapist cannot lead the patient forward because the therapist does not know where or who the patient is now.

Third, the therapist must communicate an authentic curiosity about the need for validation. Simply saying "I accept the need to validate you as my patient" may be interpreted by the patient as "He'll tolerate my neurosis." The patient does not want to be accepted as a necessary, but inconvenient, time-wasting annoyance. However, if the therapist focuses on developing a curiosity about validation, that he can share with the patient, then the patient may believe that both are on the same side. Focusing on curiosity, rather than change or rationality, allows both therapist and patient to explore how the patient can achieve validation, how this need has been frustrated, and how the patient feels about having this need.

Help the Patient Identify the Need to Be Validated

Rather than looking at the patient's need to be validated as another problem the patient has (which is an invalidating approach), I find it useful to join with the patient who wants to be validated. Patients with this need often alternate between demanding validation and criticizing themselves for their need to be validated. Thus they invalidate themselves. If the therapist is critical or withholding, the patient may conclude that the therapist can never meet these needs, that no one cares about the patient, and that no help will be available. The therapist can help the patient normalize his or her need.

It is helpful to tell patients something like this: "It is absolutely important that you feel understood and cared about. This is a basic human need. When you are feeling hurt, upset, or all alone, it's essential that I, as your therapist, try to appreciate what it is like for you." In contrast to challenging the patient's thinking, it may be more helpful to say: "It sounds like it really hurt you when that happened" or "That sounds really upsetting." The therapist who is familiar with the patient's thinking and vulnerabilities might say, "Of course it was upsetting for you when that happened."

One patient believed she was a complainer when she described her frustration. Her husband was invalidating at home, and her supervisor was invalidating at work. She, herself, was very validating to her friends and to her employees. She believed that to assert herself was selfish and that it would only cause inconvenience to others. Her rejection of validation was, ironically, a form of resistance: she was resisting getting her needs met, because she thought it was selfish.

Consequently, therapy needed to focus on validating her need for validation. When she was a child, she was told she was selfish for expressing her needs. She was told she should "just snap out of it." Her mother used her as a sounding board for her own needs and criticized any signs of independent functioning. Therapy for this woman focused on developing a "Bill of Rights," such as the right to be cared for, the right to have sex in her marriage, the right to communicate her frustrations, the right to have pleasure, the right to set limits on the number of hours she worked, and the right to get angry. The treatment of this patient illustrates that in order *to motivate the patient to solve the problem, the patient must first accept that she has a right to have a problem.*

Recognize and Identify Your Own Negative Thoughts and Feelings about the Validation

The therapist may find herself frustrated, angry, anxious, or threatened by the patient's demand for validation. The therapist who is eager to intervene and change the patient's thoughts and feelings may be the most susceptible to a negative response to validation resistance. This therapist may feel frustrated and angry. Later, she may recognize that her own automatic thoughts about the patient are much like the following: "This patient doesn't really want to get better. All she wants to do is whine. She's keeping me from getting my job done. I'm going to look like I'm incompetent because she won't do what she should do. This patient is just irrational. She shouldn't be irrational."

I have found that in supervising therapists and in examining my own irrational thoughts that it is immensely stress reducing and helpful to the patient's therapy when the therapist can identify and challenge these negative countertransference thoughts. Challenges to these thoughts include the following:

"All of us need validation some of the time."
"Never to need validation could be a sign of a schizoid personality."
"It's irrational to think people should be rational all the time."
"The patient isn't here to help me do my job. The patient is here to feel cared about and to feel better."
"Some people get better by feeling that they are understood first."
"Reflecting, caring, showing curiosity and respect, and being a good listener are interventions."

Examine the Patient's Past and Current Invalidating Environment

People who have high needs for validation often describe their parents as invalidating (Linehan, 1993). Typical memories for these individuals include experiences of being told not to have a feeling, being criticized for crying, and being told that they were selfish whenever they expressed their needs. Often, the child was used by a parent as a confidante for the parent's own problems, frequently in families in which one parent formed an alliance with the child to the exclusion of the other parent. In some families, secrets were kept from the child but the child still knew there were secrets. When the child tried to learn what the truth was, he or she was criticized for not respecting other people's privacy.

Some invalidating early (and current) environments are marked by conflicting messages. For example, in several families of origin the child (now an adult) was told alternately "You are superior to other people. We expect great things from you" and "You are incompetent." In some families, the child (now an adult) was told "Your life is a living hell. How can you stand it?" and "Why don't you just snap out of it?" A patient of mine, who had been complaining of how invalidating her parents were, had a mastectomy. When I visited her in the hospital, her parents were also in her room. They then proceeded to tell me about the problems they were having in their condominium in Florida.

Validate That the Model Is Invalidating

People seek out cognitive therapy because of its reported efficacy and its empowerment of the patient. Yet many patients complain that the model seems to trivialize emotions and make it seem that everything can be easily solved. Attempts in therapy to do cost–benefit analyses on thoughts or to look at the evidence for and against a belief often strike patients as naive, "power-of-positive-thinking," facile ploys. The patient often believes something like this: "Here I'm coming in feeling absolutely terrible and this therapist is acting as if all I have to do is *choose* to think, feel, and act differently. How ridiculous! How could he ever help me?" Or, when the patient claims "I'll never have another relationship again," and the therapist directs the patient toward evidence of past relationships and positive personal qualities in the patient that might lead to future relationships, the patient may think "But I feel terrible and he's trying to make me think everything will be OK."

In fact, the cognitive model can be quite validating for these individuals. Nonetheless, there is some truth in the view that when you are feeling terrible, "testing negative thoughts" may seem dismissive. The internal conflict for the therapist and the patient is that getting better may ultimately involve changing beliefs and behavior, but the therapist urging the patient to do this may appear trivializing to the patient. I have found it helpful to openly acknowledge this irony as an intrinsic and unavoidable problem with the model: "Sometimes cognitive therapy can feel invalidating—sometimes it comes across as treating your problems as if they aren't real to you. Your problems are very real to you and real things have happened that may be really bad. The dilemma is that for you to get better it may be helpful for you to find some additional ways of dealing with your problems, but this does not mean that your feelings are unimportant or that your problems don't hurt you."

When the therapist voices the patient's own doubts, the patient feels validated and the therapy gains credibility. It also directs both participants to a recognition that there is a reality to the patient's suffering. The therapist might find it useful to say something like this: "It's hard at times to get around this internal conflict of cognitive therapy. When I ask you to examine the way you're thinking, it may feel like I am implying your thinking is wrong or distorted. It might be better to say there are *different ways* of thinking about this, each with its own truth. There's a little bit of truth in each thought. And there's always truth in how you feel."

Acknowledge Dilemmas

Consistent with recognizing that testing or challenging the patient's thinking may feel invalidating to the patient, the therapist should recognize that there are interpersonal conflicts in which both participants share some of the truth. *Dilemmas* are situations in which an individual is faced with two alternatives, each with significant cost: whatever choice she makes, there is the chance that it will be more costly than beneficial. Take the example of a man terminating his marriage: his dilemma is that he feels unhappy living with his partner, but he recognizes that he will see his children much less if he gets divorced. There is no right or simple alternative. Recognizing dilemmas implies that the truth is not found in one position, in one fact, or in one perspective. Truth is partly a construction in which the person's schemas or needs are manifested. Truth may change as one recognizes new facts or as one's needs are met. The therapist can indicate that she will validate the truth as the patient sees it and experiences it, but she should also indicate that there are additional truths that hang in the balance.

For example, a woman who wavers about leaving her husband holds onto the "truth" that she is in a loveless marriage and that her husband is too different from her to satisfy her needs. But she also has another truth that she is attached to her husband and he is the father of their two children. And she recognizes that she has contributed to the problems in the marriage. She may vacillate between thinking her husband is awful, she is a terrible wife, and she doesn't want to hurt her children. As Kierkegaard (1843/1954b) commented in *Either/Or* about the difficulty of making a decision: "If you do it, you'll regret it. If you don't do it, you'll regret it." When the therapist validates for this woman that her dilemma points to important truths on both sides, then she implies that the decision is difficult and open to question. Consequently, the patient recognizes that the goal is not to dichotomize the decision ("I'm right, he's wrong"), but *to learn to make a decision in the face of a dilemma*. There is no right or wrong, rational or irrational decision. It is a true dilemma—there is truth on all sides. The patient can be directed to view the goal as learning to live with conflicting truths, learning to accept that there are significant costs to either choice.

Acknowledge Your Own Failures in Validating

One of the most powerful interventions I use is to acknowledge to a patient that I have failed him or her because of my own shortcomings. There are times when I become defensive, or stuck on a technique, or simply want to prove that I'm right. The patient defends herself and rejects the techniques, and we find ourselves at an impasse. One patient, who alternated among anger, silence, and transparent vulnerability, repeated that I just did not understand how hard it was for her. Rigidly, I fell back on my cognitive techniques, asking her to examine the evidence that it was too hard for her and suggesting that we set up an experiment. This not only fell on deaf ears, but even seemed to blow up in my face: "Goddamn it! It *is* too hard! When are you going to get it?"

After stewing in my own failure to get the patient to be rational and cooperate, I decided to work with the patient rather than have her follow my rigid rules.

THERAPIST: I think that I have failed you in the last couple of sessions.

PATIENT: (*looking suspiciously*) What do you mean?

THERAPIST: I haven't really been listening and hearing how hard it is for you. I've been pushing my own agenda. I've been trying to get you to change, rather than trying to understand how hard it is for you to just get through the day.

PATIENT: That's right (*still suspicious*).

THERAPIST: You know, we've been talking about your issues a lot. But let me tell you about my issue—with myself. My problem is that I'm always trying to fix things and make things better. Maybe it's part of my grandiose sense of myself. So I get frustrated when you're not getting better. I take it too personally.

PATIENT: Yeah. A lot of the time you don't listen.

THERAPIST: That's right. A lot of the time I'm pushing my thing. What I have to realize is that you have been having these problems before you met me. I shouldn't be pushing you so hard.

PATIENT: You know, I have been doing a lot to help myself lately.

THERAPIST: I know. But when I get onto this thing of getting you to change, I don't appreciate all these things that you have been doing. You've been taking public transportation—and just a month ago you were too afraid to do that.

PATIENT: And I applied for a job.

THERAPIST: And, if I really thought about it—from your point of view— I'd recognize how incredibly hard that must have been for you.

PATIENT: It was hard. But I decided to do it anyway.

THERAPIST: You know, it must be really hard at times having me as your therapist. I guess I can be really pushy.

PATIENT: You are pushy. I really appreciate your talking like this to me.

THERAPIST: I guess I still have a lot to learn. I wonder if you can let me know when I'm connecting with you and when I'm not.

PATIENT: It's a deal.

This patient commented in the next session that this acknowledgment of my failure in empathizing and understanding was one of the most important things that I had done. She felt we were relating as two human beings, not as doctor–patient, and working together rather than against each other. For my part, it was an enormous relief not to be stuck with defending my own rigid behavior.

Examine Empathic Failures and Degrees of Validation

Some patients who have experienced considerable invalidation in their early and current life view validation as an all-or-nothing phenomenon: "Either you agree with me entirely or you don't understand me." "Either you appreciate all of my feelings or you don't care about or understand me." Kohut (1971, 1977) described these experiences as "empathic failures." He viewed them as inevitable in the process of therapy. The utopian nirvana of emotional mirroring that some patients seek is like all utopias: it exists nowhere. Yet, because of the invalidating environments these individuals have emerged from, their deprivation results in a "hunger" or striving for complete validation. Inevitably the therapist will fail the patient.

The therapist can achieve partial inoculation for this failure by telling the patient that it will occur—that is, that the patient will feel the therapist has let her down and failed to understand and appreciate her feelings and needs at some time. This prediction of empathic failure may come as a surprise to the patient—since she has been hoping she would get the validation she needs. But it will also serve to validate what the patient already knows to be true: "People let me down." This shared recognition of the empathic failure is validating to the patient: "The therapist knows she'll let me down. Well, at least she knows what I need and what her shortcomings are."

Ironically, the therapist may imply that the patient can trust her precisely because they both already know how the therapist will disappoint the patient. The expectations have been lowered enough to be consistent with reality: the patient will be disappointed sometimes. The question that both can turn to next is "How can the two of us deal with this disappointment?" By acknowledging that the therapist will never provide the patient with 100% validation, the patient is invited to examine how much validation will feel sufficient. "Since I will fail to always validate you, I wonder if we could examine some less-than-perfect ways that I could validate you." The patient is invited to look at validation along a continuum: "What would be some 50% examples of my validating you in the future? How about some 80% examples? How about 10% examples?" The therapist could ask: "Sometimes in our discussions I'll talk about changing things and this could feel invalidating to you. How would you feel if part of the session were spent on discussing some things that feel invalidating?"

This negotiated partial validation may seem unusual to the patient. Since the patient's prior demands or protests about validation may have resulted in previous therapists or current friends criticizing the patient, this discussion may be unique. When the patient has complained to another therapist, saying something like "You don't understand!," that therapist may have responded: "No one can satisfy you!" This feedback, of course, convinced the patient that there was no validation at all. Unfortunately, the patient's prior demands for validation have resulted in invalidation.

One patient complained that she was "the sickest patient you've ever seen." She indicated she would feel outraged at AA meetings because she could not stand listening to other people talk about how bad their problems are: "My problems are much worse." She would try to get her father's attention by calling him and telling him that she was so upset with him that she was going to put her head in the gas oven. Her father would vacillate between responding sympathetically to these emergencies, criticizing her for her feelings, and telling her to "snap out of it!" After several weeks in which my attempts to use traditional cognitive therapy failed miserably, I decided to surrender my role of trying to change her and attempt to validate her.

THERAPIST: You know when you've been saying that you're the sickest person I've ever seen, I think I haven't been hearing you the way you need to be heard.

PATIENT: What do you mean?

THERAPIST: I've been trying to convince you that you have a lot of good qualities—I've been acting like a cheerleader.

PATIENT: You don't understand how bad I feel.

THERAPIST: That's very true. I've tried to think about how bad you feel. I've tried to think about the worst sadness that you have. And I think that you're right. It's impossible for me to understand how bad it is for you. I've never felt anything like the way you feel. I can only imagine that it is terrible, but I don't know what that feeling is like.

PATIENT: That's right. Life is so easy for you.

THERAPIST: It may seem that way. In comparison to these terrible feelings that you have, I can't imagine how bad that is. I can only hope you can let me in so that I can see some of what it feels like to you. But I know that I'll never understand exactly how you feel.

PATIENT: Now you understand me.

Overcoming empathic failure involves sharing the failure with the patient. When the therapist says "I don't understand how badly you feel," the patient thinks "You at least understand that I feel worse than you can imagine." This may be the point the patient is trying to make: "My feelings are not the same as yours. What do I have to do to get this point across? Do I have to stick my head in the oven?" The patient and the therapist can acknowledge the therapist's inevitable empathic failure and put it in its place as the therapist's limitation rather than as an intentional withholding of needed care.

Validate How the Pain Reflects Meaning

People feel loss and suffer because they have lost something meaningful. We tend not to feel upset when we abandon trivial things. The existential approach suggests that absence points to the importance of what is no longer there (Kierkegaard, 1843/1954a, 1843/1954b; Sartre, 1956/ 1964). It is one thing to lose a relationship, it is even worse to lose the belief that relationships are meaningful. Through the loss the patient experiences, higher, more enduring meanings may be affirmed (Frankl, 1959). Indeed, this is the point Greenberg and Paivio (1997) make about emerging valid or adaptive needs.

A man contemplating separation from his wife finally came to the conclusion that it was time for him to move out. He moved out and was overcome with the sense of loss of his children. Even though he would continue to see his children, he felt he would not see them enough. He then commented, "I know it's ridiculous for me to be upset over this. I'm so irrational." The therapist reflected, "Do you want to be the kind of man who does not miss his children? Doesn't your sadness indicate how important your love for them is? Doesn't it reflect the kind of father you really are—a father who loves his children?"

The suffering of the loss would only last for a while, but the meaning—the value—of loving his children would endure. He may have lost some time with his children, but he did not lose the meaning of being their father. The existential approach—finding meaning where emptiness and loss exist—directs the patient to more central personal goals. With this patient, he could hold onto his respect for his values and for himself. The therapist not only validated that he felt badly, but also validated, and valued, his meaning.

Identify Feeling Validated and Invalidated

Once the therapist and the patient recognize and accept the need to feel validated, the patient can begin to self-monitor experiences of being validated and invalidated. This process can begin in the session: "I'd like you to tell me, when we are talking, when you feel like I'm really connecting with you and understanding you and when you feel I am failing to do so." For example, one patient who believed himself to be especially invalidated by the therapist felt relieved to be able to tell the therapist, "I don't think you're understanding what I'm feeling right now." This "collaborative permission" to identify invalidation allowed both therapist and patient to engage in clarifying communication. On the therapist's part, this involved acknowledging the patient's need and right to be understood, accepting that a lack of validation was frustrating for the patient, and inquiring further about the patient's feelings and intentions.

Self-monitoring of invalidation can continue outside the session. Family members are often invalidating—even when they think they are being helpful. For example, one patient commented that her husband would criticize her about feeling bad. Therapist examination revealed that the husband was disputing her negative thinking, minimizing how bad things were, and offering solutions. This, of course, was invalidating—although the husband indicated, in a joint session, that he was "just trying to get her to feel better." Both spouses were urged to read Deborah Tannen's (1990) *You Just Don't Understand,* which is an excellent description of gender differences in communication styles (although I have observed many role reversals in these styles). They recognized that she had a need to express and share her problems, while his style was to minimize and solve problems. Of course, both styles have legitimacy. After counseling, she could understand that his intention was not to invalidate, and he could understand that he needed first to validate before they could discuss problem solving. The therapist suggested that the person with the problem could announce what his or her need was: either to be heard or to solve a problem. This clarification of communication styles, and the permission and direction to be assertive about what one wanted, was helpful in reducing her feelings of invalidation.

Use Vertical Descent Regarding Validation

Being validated or invalidated may mean different things to different people. Some patients do not wish to spend much time receiving validation. They may view therapy primarily as the place to acquire skills to be used in "real life." Others may believe validation is the primary or even the sole function of relating. With these individuals, the therapist should examine the meaning of invalidation by asking a question like: "What does it mean to you when I do not connect up with your feelings?" or "What are you concerned would happen if I did not see things the way you see them?"

The therapist may then use "vertical descent": "What would happen next? And, if that happened [or if that were true], what would that mean?" One patient indicated the following:

"If you don't understand how I feel, then you can't be trusted."
"Then you will hurt me."
"I'll be destroyed."

Another patient had the following automatic thoughts:

> "If you don't see things the way I do, then you can't help me."
> "If you can't help me, no one can help me."
> "I'm all alone."
> "I'm hopeless."

These feelings of betrayal, hopelessness, and vulnerability led these patients to escalate their emotions in the session. One patient said, "I've got to make you recognize how bad it is for me so that you'll pay attention." The other patient, who expressed considerable anger, said, "I've got to make you feel as bad as I do so that you'll understand how I feel." Ironically, some patients who use this approach of trying to elicit the same negative feelings in others find that they are continually criticized and invalidated—precisely for these attempts to seek validation. As I indicate below, these individuals can be helped to seek validation more adaptively.

There are numerous underlying assumptions that patients hold when they feel invalidated:

> "If you don't validate me each time I feel bad, then you can't be trusted. You're incompetent. You won't help me."
> "If you don't agree that things are awful, then you are my enemy. I must punish you."
> "You don't care about me or my feelings."
> "You're condescending. You're criticizing me. You're telling me I shouldn't feel the way I do."
> "I'm all alone. No one can help me. You're just like everyone else who doesn't understand me."
> "You think that everything is so easy. You're different from me. How could you help me?"

The therapist can assist the patient in examining these assumptions by first validating them. For example, the therapist can say: "I can understand that if you feel I can't be trusted, then I would not be able to help you" or "I can see that if I didn't care about you it would make you angry and you might want me to know how angry you are."

I have found it helpful to examine these assumptions by turning the focus away from the therapist initially to help the patient recognize other empathic failures the patient has experienced. This refocusing assists the patient in recognizing that there are some good reasons for having these beliefs and, at the same time, that the therapist is validating that there is some "truth" in holding beliefs that can be examined and modified. For example, a woman who claimed the therapist could not be trusted with her feelings was able to recognize that she was not able to trust her mother with her feelings, since her mother's narcissism prevented her from understanding the patient's needs when she was a child. When the therapist shifts to this transference interpretation, the patient feels validated. Similar parallels in empathic failure may be observed in other relationships.

Subsequently, the therapist may introduce a "deprivation–hunger" model of validation: "If you have been deprived of validation early in your life, you develop a greater than average hunger for it later. You feel you need it more than most people will need it. When you don't get it, you may feel that you will starve emotionally." Most of us can appreciate how hard it is to keep things in perspective when we are starving.

The patient can examine what consequences follow from needing complete and perfect validation. What are the costs and benefits? What would be the advantage in accepting some validation rather than requiring total validation? How can the patient learn how to validate her own needs and feelings? Are there any signs of support and care in therapy? What is the evidence that the therapist does not care?

Examine the Dialectic of Validation and Change

Change requires the willingness to leave behind a feeling and a perception (Kegan, 1982). It is a "letting go" of something that one has focused on. Many patients protest this letting-go aspect of change and view it as invalidation: "You're telling me to just forget it and move on. I can't just forget it!" The therapist then faces a dilemma with the patient: if he encourages change, he is invalidating, but if he does not encourage change, he may join in the patient's helplessness. The therapist and the patient can transcend this dilemma by first recognizing it, and then finding the lesson in it.

As I have indicated several times in this chapter, it is legitimate to identify the limitations of cognitive therapy directly with the patient: "The cognitive model often feels invalidating. That is one of the limitations of the model." Accepting the limits of the model obviates the patient's need to protest it. I have found that many patients feel relieved with this. A young college student, whose father was overly rational, initially resisted the cognitive model because he thought it did not recognize feelings. It was helpful to him when I indicated that this is a legitimate criticism of the approach and that I hoped we could both be creative enough not to be limited by rationality. I indicated that my goal with him would be to find his "unique, personal emotional truth." Since

I had joined his protest, he felt little need to continue to resist the treatment on these grounds.

The second aspect of this dialectic is to learn to *recognize the loss, but learn the lesson.* In fact, to say "Forget about it, move on" would be in contradiction to "learning from all experiences." Thus the patient who experiences regret and sadness from the end of a relationship is not told to "move on and put it behind you." Rather, the relationship is identified as something that will always be important, since the patient had strong feelings about this person. The patient is urged to discuss the meaning of the relationship and the loss and what it reflects about his needs.

PATIENT: It really hurts when I think about the fact that it is over.

THERAPIST: Yes, of course it hurts. It hurts because you loved him and it did not work out. It shows, I think, your capacity to love and to care. But it also hurts to have that ability.

PATIENT: I don't think I'll ever feel that way again.

THERAPIST: Right now it may be important for you to protect yourself with that feeling. Perhaps we can look at what you have learned about yourself and your needs and the kind of man who would be right for you.

PATIENT: What do you mean?

THERAPIST: I mean that you have a great ability to love. But what can you learn about what you need in a man that [Tom] lacked?

PATIENT: I guess I learned not to get involved with a married man.

THERAPIST: What do you think led you to think you'd be able to handle being involved with a married man?

PATIENT: Well, after my marriage ended, I guess I didn't want to get too attached. So I thought that being involved with someone who is married would keep me from being hurt.

THERAPIST: Perhaps you've learned that you have such a strong ability to love that you can't compartmentalize your feelings that way.

This dialogue illustrates how the patient's loss can be validated and included in her adaptation to future relationships. She may have suffered a loss in a relationship, but she has gained more understanding about her real needs.

Learn How to Ask for Support

As Linehan (1993) has indicated, many patients need assistance in asking for help. I have found it useful to help patients develop the responsible assertive skills necessary to seek validation from others. Some patients who demand validation from others utilize behaviors that ultimately lead to criticism from and withdrawal by others. These validation-seeking behaviors include yelling, cursing, repetitive calls, complaining, telling people "You don't understand" or "You don't care," catastrophizing ("I can't stand it!"), threatening self-mutilation or suicide, withdrawing, not returning phone calls, or excessive crying. As Coyne and Pepper (1998) have indicated, these behaviors lead to the withdrawal of support and criticism of the patient, further adding to the patient's depression.

Some patients, when told their help-seeking behaviors may need to be changed, respond with all-or-nothing thinking: "OK. I just won't bother you or anyone else again." The patient should be told that asking and receiving support are essential components of being a human being. The therapist can indicate that the important thing is to be *effective* in seeking support. Here are some useful guidelines for seeking support:

1. "Indicate clearly that 'I need to spend a few minutes talking about my feelings so I can get your support. Is this OK with you?' "
2. "Focus on your feelings and the actual facts. Try not to catastrophize or make it seem worse than it really is."
3. "If you believe that the other person has not understood you, ask him or her to rephrase what you just said."
4. "Limit the amount of time that you talk about your problems. Focus on positive things about the other person or positive things that you can do."
5. "Describe, if possible, some positive steps that you can take to solve a problem."
6. "Don't punish or criticize people you are seeking support from."
7. "When people are helpful to you, tell them what they did that you appreciate: 'It was really helpful to get your feedback on my problems at work.' "
8. "Before you call someone, think about how you can use some self-help skills to make progress on your problems. Are there behaviors to change, problems to solve, ways in which you can examine your thoughts?"

OVERVIEW OF VALIDATION CONCERNS

Given the possible priority of validation concerns in therapy, and the risk that the cognitive-behavioral approach may seem especially invali-

TABLE 4.1. Validation Assumptions

Assumptions

"If you don't feel what I feel, you don't care about me."

"I need you to care about me—in order to be helped by you, in order to trust you, in order to feel safe."

"If you ask me to change, then you are invalidating my feelings."

"No one can understand me."

Interventions

Identify validation needs in therapeutic relationship.

Normalize the need to be validated.

Use active listening skills: rephrase, empathize, validate, inquire, ask for feedback.

Indicate the potential for conflict between validation and change.

Engage patient in problem solving how both therapist and patient can be sure that validation occurs but that change is also the goal.

Examine transference origins of validation needs: feeling invalidated in family of origin, significant others, friends, etc.

Examine meaning of invalidation in past: "My feelings don't make sense," "I'm different from everyone," or "No one cares."

Ask patient to give feedback in sessions of when he or she feels validated/ invalidated. Examine "validation" along a continuum.

dating, the therapist may wish to refer to Table 4.1 to assess validation issues with patients.

In addition to the foregoing validation concerns, emotional dysregulation—that is, the undercontrol or overcontrol of emotions—may interfere with obtaining help, interacting with others, utilizing insight, and developing more adaptive emotional and personal schemas. Examples of emotional dysregulation include volatile affect, difficulty modulating anxiety, anger, mania or depressed mood, dissociation, distraction from emotion, avoidance, and escape. Again, the clinician may use the brief guidelines in Table 4.2 to determine the nature of emotional dysregulation, assumptions, and relevant interventions.

SUMMARY

Patients in therapy are attempting to get help. If patients utilize maladaptive behaviors outside of therapy, they will continue such behaviors

TABLE 4.2. Emotional Dysregulation Assumptions

Assumptions

"I can't control my feelings."

"If I lose control, terrible things will happen ('I'll go crazy,' 'Make a fool of myself,' 'Hurt someone,' 'Hurt myself')."

"I've got to get rid of any negative feelings."

"It's urgent/essential that I change this feeling [or get what I want]."

"These negative feelings will never stop."

"I've got to express any negative feelings."

"I should act on my feelings."

Interventions

Identify difficulty in and out of session in regulating emotions.

Identify "escape" or "avoidance" processes in therapy: dissociating, changing the subject, blunted affect, inability to cry, trivializing the content of therapy, "forgetting" to do homework, and not coming to sessions.

Examine costs and benefits of acting on emotions (e.g., drinking, bingeing, acting out anger, avoidance, and escape).

Examine evidence for and against the assumptions (above) about emotions: "What will happen if you don't get rid of an emotion immediately?"

Self-monitor emotions and situations (functional analysis): Which situations elicit which emotions at what intensity? Do emotions rise and fall?

Why do certain situations elicit high levels of affect? What thoughts are activated in these situations? How can you prepare for these "stressors" by identifying and challenging your negative thoughts?

Are high levels of emotion associated with skill deficits? For example, can the patient learn to be more assertive, engage in problem solving, or use "time-out"?

Practice tolerating or experiencing various degrees of emotion *without acting out. Write out and challenge thoughts about urgency, necessity, or danger of having an emotion.*

Examine transference origins of emotional dysregulation: "How did your parents [others] respond to your emotions?" "What did this make you think?"

Practice relaxation and breathing exercises to moderate emotions.

Use "flash-cards" to self-instruct during intense emotions—for example, "I am feeling aroused or emotional right now. These feelings will rise and fall on their own. They are unpleasant but not terrible. What thoughts am I having right now? Am I thinking that I have no control, that I have to act out, that this is terrible? But I do have control, I don't always act out, and nothing terrible will happen to me if I have a strong feeling." Use self-reward for self-instruction.

in therapy. Simply setting limits will not help the patient understand why he or she has these needs for validation, nor will it help him or her learn how to elicit support outside of therapy. Validation means different things to different people. Individuals who value autonomy may place a low value on validation: they want a set of tools with which they can solve their problems and, in fact, they may view validation as condescending or too intrusive. However, many patients may believe empathy and validation are essential components of getting help; indeed, some may believe validation by itself is sufficient.

Cognitive-behavioral therapists may find that the very interventions they employ to help the patient appear invalidating to that patient. My experience has been that, when all else seems to be failing, I should return to validating and empathizing, rather than continue with trying to change the patient. The therapy can focus on the patient's experience of not feeling supported. That focus may open the window to the patient's schemas, past experiences, current interpersonal world, and ability to collaborate directly with the therapist. In fact, I have found validation is so important that I find myself returning to it even when it does not seem necessary. Even when the traditional interventions of cognitive therapy appear to be working, I attempt to find some truth in the patient's position. As with many experiences in communication, to find the other's truth allows her to accept my truth.

5

Self-Consistency

*T*herapy is about change—or, at least, we hope it is. Yet considerable evidence from cognitive-social psychology indicates that individuals are often motivated to maintain consistency. One may be driven to achieving balance or consistency in one's beliefs, maintaining stability in one's roles, avoiding surprise, maintaining control, or committing to sunk-costs.

Consider the following: A woman has been involved with a married man for 2 years. He has continually suggested that he will leave his wife, but he has made no attempts to leave her. During this period, the woman has foregone opportunities with other men and has grown accustomed to seeing her paramour only when it is convenient for him. As time has passed, however, she has become more frustrated with this arrangement and their arguments have increased. He tells her that he is talking with his wife about separation, but that now is not the right time. The woman has threatened to break off with him, complaining that he is never going to leave his wife, so "why should she bother to stay?"

Her own marriage had ended in divorce. Her husband had been unfaithful with many partners over several years. She was devastated and promised herself that she would never let this happen to her again. She indicates now that, with the married man, at least there are no surprises. Getting into the relationship, she already knew that he was involved with someone else. She believed she could compartmentalize her life with him, see him when she wanted to, but not be betrayed as she had been with her ex-husband. Now, however, she is frustrated and angry at her lover, and she claims she knows it has to end.

But she nonetheless finds herself trying to convince him that he will not leave his wife. She confesses to her therapist that she hopes in these arguments that her lover will convince her that he actually will leave his wife, but of course he never does. She claims, "If he did leave her, it would prove I was right for having been with him these last 2 years. It would not have been wasted time."

Why would an intelligent, attractive, personable woman stay in a no-win situation for so long? Her experience demonstrates the power of the consistency of one's beliefs, maintaining stability in one's roles, avoiding surprise, maintaining control, and commitment to sunk-costs. She is consistent in her belief that it is worthwhile. She is able to maintain a fixed role with which she is familiar and, at times, comfortable. There are no surprises, since she discounted the downside of the relationship from the start. She had felt that she was in control, since she knew "exactly" what she was doing. But she had invested a lot of time, energy and, among friends, her reputation in this affair, so now she was overcommitted to sunk-costs. She was trapped by her past behavior.

COGNITIVE CONSISTENCY

Familiarity does not always breed contempt. In many cases, familiarity results in comfort, decrease in anxiety, and liking of others. This same attraction to familiarity is found among chronically depressed patients who find their negative thinking familiar, consistent, and predictable. Swann (1983; Swann, Stein-Seroussi, & Giesler, 1992) has proposed a *self-verification* model that suggests that individuals seek out information that verifies their self-concept—regardless of the positivity or negativity of the self-concept. Individuals are motivated to pursue the familiar and the consistent.

Most of us want our belief systems to have internal consistency—what Fritz Heider (1958) would have called *cognitive balance*. In fact, we often become anxious and embarrassed when someone points out the inconsistency of our beliefs. (Cognitive therapy draws upon this desire for cognitive consistency, as Socrates did with his students; therapists, like Socrates, promote the desire to change beliefs by pointing our their inconsistency.) Similarly, the depressed patient's negative cognitive biases may become even stronger and more resistant when the patient is confronted with information contradicting their negativity. Rather than change the negative belief, the patient may reject the positive evidence—and perhaps fire the therapist.

The patient's investment in the consistency of his negative beliefs is illustrated by the fact that many chronically depressed patients, when presented with evidence inconsistent with their negative beliefs, will aggressively search out any evidence to support their negative schema, thereby becoming even *more* depressed. One might even view their problem as the *need for negative consistency.*

Why is inconsistency so troubling? First, there may be innate needs for perceptual and cognitive consistency as evidenced by gestalt principles of perception (e.g., closure, fitness, etc.; see Koffka, 1935/1963; Kohler, 1929). Second, structure (such as the negative categories of the depressive schemas) reduces uncertainty and complexity. Evidence from infant perception studies suggests that there may be innate predispositions toward categorical perception of speech sounds, color, and form (Bornstein & Arterberry, 1999; Bornstein, Kessen, & Weiskopf, 1976). The predisposition to *impose categories* on perception and cognition may, for the chronically depressed, result in rigid, categorical, *but consistent,* schemas. Third, stereotypic (or categorical) thinking reduces "information-processing" demands. If most information can be assimilated to a single schema—for example, "failure"—then there is less need to make exceptions, resolve contradictions, or develop differentiated schemas. Consistency makes processing quicker and more efficient, but not necessarily more accurate. Fourth, cognitive consistency may result in the belief that events are predictable and controllable, factors that may be viewed by the perceiver as reducing helplessness (see Peterson, Maier, & Seligman, 1993).

PREDICTABILITY AND MAINTAINING CONTROL

Many people enjoy surprises. They seem to add novelty and excitement to their lives. Others, however, view surprise and change as disturbing, difficult to assimilate, and requiring unwanted adjustments. The idea of surprise or the unexpected has been of interest to behavioral theorists like Berlyne (1978), social-psychodynamic writers like Fromm (1941), and cognitive social psychologists like Langer (1990) and Taylor (1990). The unexpected may increase anxiety, defensive posturing, and withdrawal. One could argue that there may be an innate human resistance to surprise and the unexpected, since the unexpected may confer danger or loss. One can imagine the mixed emotions accompanying hearing someone say "Something unexpected happened." Of course, the unexpected may be a positive windfall, but it can also be a disaster. Patients who are chronically depressed will view the unexpected as a probable negative.

The desire for control is illustrated by the fact that people will tolerate much higher levels of shock if they can administer the shock themselves (Geer, Davison, & Gatchel, 1970; Geer & Maisel, 1972). People will tolerate more pain if they believe it is predictable and that they can control the pain themselves. Depressed individuals believe they are not in control of positive reinforcements, but that they are in control of negatives. Depressed people often blame themselves for negatives, but do not take credit for positives (Abramson, Seligman, & Teasdale, 1978; Alloy, Abramson, Metalsky, & Hartledge, 1988; Abramson, Metalsky, & Alloy, 1989). The depressed individual may attempt to gain some predictability and control in his life by holding to the belief that he is to blame for the negative events that occur—that is, *he controls and produces negatives*. This may be interpreted as a hidden agenda for these patients: they know how to be depressed, they know how to fail, they know how to avoid. The fact that they feel they have some control (even if it is for negatives) may be an added inducement to their investment in resistance and negativity.

One reason change is resisted is that the patient may not believe he will have control over the new situation or the new self that arises from the change. The patient knows how to reject help, complain, and think negatively. He may protest about the consequent depression, but he may also fight the therapist's attempt to control his negativity. Clinicians who have worked with resistant patients sometimes sense that the patient gains some satisfaction and a sense of victory by assuring that his negativity is not adequately modified.

SELF-JUSTIFICATION

Cognitive dissonance theory proposes that individuals are motivated to reconcile their "psychologically" inconsistent beliefs (Festinger, 1957). For example, the individual who has been asked to perform a boring task for very little reward might resolve this "dissonance" by changing his evaluation of the task: "It was interesting. You should try it yourself." Interpretations of dissonance theory (e.g., Aronson, 1995) have emphasized that people are motivated to view themselves as rational, fair, and justly compensated. Consequently, people would be expected to reduce dissonance by viewing their actions as sufficiently justified even when their actions are not sufficiently justified. The dissonance effect, however, does not always hold up for people with low self-esteem: if they are not sufficiently justified, then this is not inconsistent with their view of themselves (see Aronson, 1995, for a discussion of these data). I propose that this may be due to the fact that dissonance studies are designed to create conflict with a "positive self-image," a conflict that the depressed person with low self-esteem will not experience.

How does dissonance theory relate to depression? Consider the depressed person who lacks motivation and interest in activities. He is confronted with the opportunity to go to a party. He decides not to go. How can he justify this decision? Many chronically depressed people will justify such a decision by claiming that the party was not worth going to, that things would have gotten worse, and that they are *better off* to conserve their energy by avoiding parties. Further self-justification might be that the person believes that he lacks the skills or looks to enjoy parties no matter what the occasion.

When the depressed individual is confronted with a choice to do something positive, he can "justify" his decision by devaluing the alternative not chosen (the party), increasing the value of the chosen alternative (staying home to conserve energy), and/or attempting to convince others that he is right (i.e., trying to convince the therapist that the party was a bad idea). For example, an intelligent, successful, attractive male continued to pursue a woman for over a year after she rejected him. He had generally viewed himself as someone who could get whatever he wanted—except her. With each rejection by her he tried to convince the therapist that the woman had "special qualities"—for example, physical and sexual qualities. Or he tried to convince the therapist that he was somehow alienating the ex-girlfriend and that if he could only figure out how, he would be able to win her back. Because the facts were inconsistent with his image that he was an effective person, he tried to reduce the dissonance by idealizing her qualities (so she was worth all the pain) or by blaming himself (he was doing something wrong) so that he could mobilize himself to get her back. This kept him in a continual rejection–reconciliation script for many months.

INTERACTIVE REALITIES

Maintaining control and predictability is not simply an *intrapsychic phenomenon*—that is, something going on inside the patient's head. Most chronically depressed patients have constructed an interpersonal reality that supports their negative thinking. We refer to this as an *interactive reality* (Leahy, 1991). Specifically, the patient selects an interpersonal world that will either allow him to confirm his negative beliefs or to obtain compensation for these beliefs. I view these as *life scripts* (Leahy, 1991, 1995).

Most chronically resistant patients are invested in the consistency of their negativity. Consequently, exposure to information inconsistent with these beliefs is disturbing to them. An examination of the interpersonal networks of resistant patients often indicates that many of their friendships are focused on shared complaining, negativity, and blaming. For example, as noted earlier, a single woman spent hours each week with another woman sharing negative impressions of the "men in New York." When her therapist asked her if she spent any time talking with friends who had a positive view of men, she replied that she did not know people like that. (Similarly, a woman-hating male either isolated himself from friends or spent time with other men who hated women.)

Another manner in which consistency is maintained is through provoking others to conform to the negative belief. For example, a single male who had negative beliefs about women would provoke women he dated by personalizing almost anything that they did. Alternatively, he was able to support his negative view of women by visiting prostitutes, thereby confirming his view that women were inferior.

The interpersonal selectivity of these patients, who reinforce their negative life scripts, is reflected in the fact that they often find it very disturbing to be around people who do not share their views. For example, a woman who had negative views of relationships often felt enraged when she saw "happy lovers." They not only exemplified what she did not have (a positive relationship with a man), but also challenged her "safe" belief that good relationships are a fraud. The cognitive dissonance created by viewing happy couples led her to avoid situations where she would see happy couples or to create stories that would demean their happiness ("They're just shallow yuppies").

Interactive realities may also serve as *compensations* for negative schemas. For example, the dependent person, who views herself as helpless, may seek out powerful, narcissistic men whom she believes will protect her and take care of her. The initial infatuation, however, gives way to being exploited and rejected by the narcissist, further reinforcing her view that she is helpless and alone. Other compensations may involve the reversal of the feared role. For example, a 32-year-old man, who had been abandoned and threatened by his mother when he was a child, became a compulsive caretaker and an expert in martial arts (see Leahy, 1995). His caretaker role and martial arts skills served as compensations for his underlying sense of abandonment, distrust, helplessness, and vulnerability. He would select people who would become financially dependent on him so that he would not need to confront his own dependence and so that he could "guarantee" that they would never abandon him.

Because interactive realities and life scripts of negativity are so powerful, the chronically depressed patient may have considerable evidence that people really do reject him or treat him unfairly. In other words, many of their automatic thoughts are true: "I've been rejected," "All my relationships failed," "People take advantage of me." Rather than giving the patient a pollyannish interpretation that he is viewing events too negatively, the therapist should accept the truth that his view is valid.

The questions that arise then are: "What is this person doing to confirm his underlying negative views?" and "What is the negative point that he is trying to prove?"

SUNK-COSTS

Ideally, in making a decision, we consider the future benefits that may result from a course of action. However, substantial evidence indicates that individuals may place greater emphasis on their prior costs and use these costs to determine whether they will continue to pursue action that already has proven to be unrewarding (Staw, 1976, 1981; Staw & Ross, 1987; Thaler, 1980, 1992). Moreover, the greater the investment (sunk-cost), the greater the tendency to reinvest in the initial commitment.

For example, the patient described at the beginning of this chapter had already committed substantial behavior, at high cost, to a relationship with a married man that seemed to be going nowhere. Classical learning theories, guided by a reinforcement or extinction model, suggest that she would abandon the relationship, even if no other rewarding relationship was available. From reinforcement theory, the reinforcements would be seen as diminishing as the costs increased. Longer learning history in the relationship would predict even greater impetus to abandon the relationship. However, she resisted abandoning the high-cost, long-history relationship.

Individuals are not always guided by reinforcement history, nor are they easily convinced by cost–benefit analysis. Her current decision point—whether to continue or to quit—is determined by her prior investment in the relationship. Research and theory on the *sunk-cost effect* indicates that individuals are more likely to continue in a course of behavior the *greater* the prior cost has been (Arkes & Blumer, 1985; Garland, 1990). Furthermore, if she views a change as having a high cost relative to her existing "assets," she will continue longer in the behavior (Garland & Newport, 1991; Kahneman & Tversky, 1979). The longer she is in a costly relationship, the *fewer* her remaining assets may be, since the relationship undermines her self-esteem and decreases her opportunities to pursue alternatives.

Commitment to Sunk-Costs

According to normative models of decision making, that is, how a rational person would make a decision, individuals should evaluate future utility in making current decisions. Thus, an individual deciding to sell her house should ignore the money she spent on improving her house and should consider the current market for selling the house. If Susan bought the house for $200,000 and put $50,000 into improving the house, she should not demand that she get *at least* $250,000 in the sale of the house. Rather, she should try to get what the market will pay— say, $225,000. However, individuals often act as if their past investments—sunk-costs—demand recovery, thereby leading many people to stick with a losing proposition.

Consider this example from one of several studies by Arkes and Blumer (1985). Subjects are told the following:

> "As the president of a company you have invested 10 million dollars of the company's money into a research project [a plane that cannot be detected by radar]. . . . When the project is 90% completed, another firm begins marketing a plane that cannot be detected by radar. Also, it is apparent that their plane is much faster and far more economical than the plane your company is building. The question is: should you invest the last 10% of the research funds to finish your radar-blind plane?"

The authors found that 85% of the subjects in the study recommended finishing the airplane. However, another group, who was not told about the prior investment, overwhelmingly decided not to invest the money. For most people, making a prior investment that was a mistake became an overwhelming justification for adding to the bad investment.

There have been a number of attempts to explain the sunk-cost effect. Honoring sunk-costs has been explained by commitment theory (Kiesler, 1969), cognitive-dissonance, self-perception theory, and cognitive bias (see Arkes, 1991, 1996; Arkes & Blumer, 1985; Arkes & Ayton, 1999; Baron, 1994). Furthermore, some have argued that individuals do not want to appear "wasteful" (Arkes & Blumer, 1985), and therefore may continue in a losing course of action in order to demonstrate that they still have an option to make it work out. Increasing the individual's sense of personal responsibility for the original action increases the sunk-cost effect (Staw, 1976; Whyte, 1993). Conversely, if the individual is able to attribute part of the responsibility to someone else, then he is less likely to honor the sunk-cost. Staw and Ross (1987) found that bifurcating (or separating) the initial and subsequent decision making for a project decreased sunk-cost effects, presumably because the individual considered the utility functions of each decision independently of the other.

Over the short term, taking action to change the status quo is more likely to result in regret than remaining inactive (Gilovich, Medvec, & Chen, 1995). Thus the individual who is already prone to regret may be more likely to avoid a change in order to avoid further regret. Some individuals clearly articulate their commitment to sunk-costs: "I can't walk away. I've invested too much"; "If it's so easy to change, then why didn't I change before? This would make me look like an idiot"; "Giving up now would mean that I had wasted all that time"; or "I have a responsibility to make it work out."

There may be some validity in many of these concerns. If the individual can "easily" change now, then it does raise questions about why the change did not occur earlier. Many people have difficulty integrating the idea that intelligent people can make foolish decisions. The therapist can help the patient by pointing out that making a decision that does not work out does not mean that one is a fool, nor does it mean that all one's decision making is impaired. Furthermore, since the original decision may not have been based on all the information the patient knows now, it may have been a reasonable decision given what he knew at the time. Moreover, conditions change over time, thereby leading one to continually reevaluate further costs and benefits.

It is an unusual course of action that does not have some benefits, no matter what the costs. The woman involved with the married man, did derive substantial benefits from the relationship, but was now faced with diminishing returns given the higher costs. Finally, it is also true that absorbing sunk-costs and moving on may lead to a decrease in reputation among others, since the public admission of a mistake may result in criticism. This is especially true for politicians, who are loath to admit that prior decisions to invest tax money may have been misguided. Perhaps this is why there is no federally sponsored dam that was left incomplete, regardless of the costs and the utility of the project.

Backward-Looking Decisions

The sunk-cost is the hidden agenda from which the individual cannot escape. In fact, the sunk-cost creates even greater future sunk-costs in a sequential, debt-building model or escalation of commitment (see Leahy 2000b). Current decisions become ever more backward-looking. The Vietnam War is a tragic example of a sunk-cost that resulted in heightened resistance to change. In contrast to a reward–punishment model that would suggest a greater inclination to pull out with a greater cost, there was overwhelming popular support for a president (Nixon) who maintained the war past his first administration. American justifications for the war changed each year, always "honoring" the sunk-costs of previous commitments.

Individuals may attempt to redeem themselves from sunk-costs by trying to make the unworkable finally work. Thus the woman whose relationship with a married man continued to be a source of depression for her described how she argued frequently with him about how he would never leave his wife. He would argue that he would leave the wife and the woman would insist that he would not. When I asked her what motivated these arguments—that is, how did she want them to turn out—she indicated that she wanted to lose the argument and be convinced that he would leave his wife. If she could lose the argument, she reasoned, then she had not wasted all her time in a no-win relationship.

Reversing Sunk-Cost Traps

As blinding as sunk-costs may be to the decision maker, many individuals are able to recognize the power of their commitment to prior decisions.

  • *Explain the concept of sunk-costs.* Most people understand the concept of "throwing good money after bad money." They understand the experience of having a car whose increasing need for expensive repairs eventually exceeds the cost of buying a new car. They understand how difficult it is to walk away from something they have invested in— that is, an *investment trap.* And they understand the simple question, "If you had to do it over again, what would you do?"

  • *Contrast sunk-costs with future costs and benefits (future utility).* The investment trap of sunk-costs implies that the individual is *retrospective* in deciding about costs, rather than *prospective* about costs and benefits. Expected utility theory proposes that individuals (should) consider the costs and benefits for the future for a current decision. The patient can examine the costs and benefits of basing current decisions on past sunk-costs versus the costs and benefits of basing these decisions on future utility ratios. Furthermore, the therapist can ask the patient, "Would you feel comfortable if the current situation continued for 1 year? Where would you like to be a year from now?" By extricating the individual from the experience of a recent sunk-cost, the therapist can help the patient make a decision that is more prospective than retrospective. Future backward looking is more effective than current backward ties.

  • *Contrast past and future utility ratios.* A woman who was attached to a man who was an alcoholic and with whom she shared a 6-year relationship had difficulty ending the relationship:

THERAPIST: What would it mean to accept that the relationship is not worth continuing?

PATIENT: It would mean that I've wasted all that time, all those years.

Here, as is true with many people committed to a sunk-cost, the patient's perception is about dichotomized gains and losses: "If I accept it's not working, then it was a total waste." Regret often entails all-or-nothing thinking about a past behavior—as if there were no rewards in the relationship.

THERAPIST: So, if you decided now that the relationship was not worth pursuing, then it means that it was entirely a waste of time. That sounds like all-or-nothing thinking. I wonder if you can think of a shifting balance of positives eventually outweighed by negatives? (*Draws the graph shown in Figure 5.1 for the patient.*) If we look at the graph, it seems that the positives outweighed the negatives for much of the relationship. How is that consistent with the idea that it was a waste of time?

PATIENT: I guess that's true. There were many positives. But I feel sad when I think of that, because I no longer have those positives.

THERAPIST: Well, you still have some of them, but it seems that the negatives have outweighed the positives for some time now.

PATIENT: That's true.

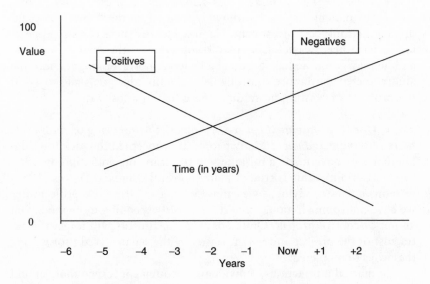

FIGURE 5.1. Graphing utility ratios.

THERAPIST: And, if we extend the graph into the future, then that difference between positives and negatives might even get greater.

PATIENT: Yeah. Things seem to be getting worse.

THERAPIST: So, if we look at the graph, it seems that the past had many positives—especially in the beginning—but that these positives have declined and the negatives have gotten greater.

PATIENT: I wish I could have the things that we used to have.

THERAPIST: But if you had more positives than negatives for part of the relationship, then that doesn't seem consistent with the idea of "total waste."

PATIENT: Right.

THERAPIST: So, the question would be, "What will the difference be between future costs and benefits in the relationship?"

PATIENT: I'd be better off without it. That's pretty clear. I can't go on like this.

THERAPIST: Sometimes we make decisions based on the past, sometimes we make decisions based on what will be good for us in the future. What would be good for you in the future?

PATIENT: To move out and get my own place.

• *What are the advantages and disadvantages of abandoning sunk-costs?* The patient may be inordinately focused on the "costs" of abandoning the sunk-cost investment. He may identify these costs as appearing to have been wasteful, he may recognize that the goal is hopeless, and he may admit he has failed. The benefits, however, might entail the ability to change to more controllable and achievable goals and to avoid the problem of wasting more time and effort in a lost cause.

• *Does the individual believe he "owes" the honoring of sunk-costs to an observing audience?* Many people are concerned that acknowledging that they have made a mistake will result in condemnation by other people. Certainly, this is true in many political contexts. Dawes (1987) recounts a senator saying, "We cannot walk away from this project after we have put so much money into it," to justify spending more money on an out-of-control project. Quite possibly constituents will forget the extra cost of the project and will at least give the senator credit for getting the project completed.

In marital interactions, individuals are often concerned that, should they admit to their partner that their own past behavior was wrong, their partner will use this information to punish them. In some cases this concern is not altogether ungrounded. The therapist can examine with the "observing partner" the costs and benefits of allowing the partner to acknowledge a past mistake without having to continue being punished for it.

Sometimes the individual finds himself engaging in maladaptive behavior that he knows is maladaptive. He has made a commitment to something he knows will not work. Now, finding himself out on a limb with a maladaptive response, he thinks, "Either I acknowledge that I'm acting like an idiot or I must prove that I was really right."

- *Challenge self-justifying sunk-costs as a "need to win."* Consider the following "self-justifying sunk-cost" script. John is arguing with his wife, Katherine. In the middle of the argument, he realizes that he is wrong. However, he believes that he must "win" and that he should never "acknowledge defeat." The dilemma is that if he continues to hold tight to his absurd position, his wife will win. He resolves this dilemma by bringing up past "mistakes" that Katherine made that are unrelated to the current issue. By doing this, he is able to provoke Katherine into a defensive position, distracting both of them from his current absurd position, and "rescue" himself. As a consequence, he is able to justify his anger toward Katherine by provoking new defensive behavior in her and by bringing up past "wrongs."

Many of us are highly invested in "being right," which to many of us means that our partner must be "wrong." Couples who are locked in prosecutor–defendant scripts generally find it difficult to acknowledge their role in the problem, thereby making it difficult to produce change. Being committed to defending a lost cause results in replaying old accusations and, often, escalating the conflict in order to provoke the partner so that the previous resentment and anger can be justified.

The therapist can use a *"stop-frame"* intervention to demonstrate the patient's investment in "proving a point" rather than making a change. For example, Ron and Ellen were constantly in conflicts. As I observed their typical prosecutor–defendant–judge script, I saw that both of them felt self-righteously "right" about their positions, even though their relationship was collapsing. I asked each of them to describe to me a typical recent argument. As Rob described "I said–she said," I stopped him at one point where he recalled saying, "You're just a crazy bitch."

THERAPIST: What would you predict would happen when you label Ellen as a "crazy bitch"?

RON: She'll get angry at me and maybe hit me.

THERAPIST: So, it might be fair to say you know by telling her that she's a "crazy bitch" that she will act like she's out of control?

RON: And I was right—she did.

THERAPIST: So, why is it more important for you to be "right" than to avoid having Ellen act out of control?

RON: (*long pause*) Because I know that I've failed her in a lot of ways. I know that I've been acting like a jerk.

THERAPIST: Sometimes we get ourselves involved in defending a past mistake by getting our partner to make a bigger mistake.

RON: I do that all the time.

ELLEN: He's always doing that. Provoking me.

THERAPIST: Let's take a short pause right now. I'd like each of you to write down the mistakes you have made and are making even now. Don't focus on your partner's mistakes, just list your own mistakes.

After Ron and Ellen wrote down their respective mistakes I asked each of them to read their statements to the other. This "confessional" intervention was helpful in getting them past the "no-win" script of provoking the partner to justify a past mistake.

   • *Does the individual believe that accepting a sunk-cost implies he cannot make any decisions?* Some people believe that finalizing the sunk-cost and moving on is a statement that "I cannot make any good decisions." For example, one individual, ruminating about a past relationship that did not work out, said: "The fact that the relationship did not work means I can't trust my judgment. Therefore, how could I have any other relationships in the future? How could I trust my judgment?" The rational response that worked for this person was: "Even people who are good at many things—including making decisions—make mistakes." The patient can be told that good decision makers are good at recognizing their mistakes and extricating themselves from the mistake.

   • *If you went back in a time machine to the initial decision to make the investment or decision to enter into the sunk-cost, would you make the decision to get involved?* Current decisions to change are often predicated on the justification of a sequence of prior decisions that form a trap, a kind of "magnet to the past." The therapist can ask the patient to imagine going back in time, with the value of hindsight knowledge, and ask, "Would you make the decision to get involved, knowing what you know now?" For example, a man who was involved with a married woman, and who complained that he felt caught in a trap, described his lover as selfish, unpredictable, dishonest, and demeaning. The therapist suggested that the patient enter a time machine that went back in time. He was now reading a personal ad that said "Married woman who will not leave her husband is dishonest, unpredictable, selfish, and demeaning. Seeks kind and sensitive man for a no-win relationship." The patient laughed, recognizing that he would never get involved.

• *If you allowed three other people to make the decision for you, what would be their likely decision?* The advantage of arbitrating the decision by bringing in new "deciders" is that other people are not committed to honoring the sunk-costs. The patient may object: "But they haven't gone through what I have. They don't have the commitment that I've built up. They aren't as attached as I am. They don't have my *history!*" These objections highlight precisely why arbitrating the decision is useful. Since the other person has not gone through what the patient has gone through, he or she can look toward future utility rather than backward to sunk-costs. Further, the purpose in making a decision is to determine whether commitments are worth keeping. If the reason for a commitment to a sunk-cost is simply that a commitment has been made, then no change would be possible. The real question should be, "Is it worth maintaining these commitments in the future?"

• *Is the sunk-cost related to a core schema?* Many people get trapped by sunk-costs in one area of their lives, but not others, because the sunk-cost activates a core schema. For example, the woman "trapped" by the sunk-cost intimate relationship with a married man recognized she was not similarly trapped by sunk-costs at work. She was able to cut her losses on business projects and even move from job to job. However, her sunk-cost risk in relationships was the result of her core schema that she was undesirable as a woman—especially, her view that she was not attractive, interesting, or enticing to a man. Ironically, staying in relationships in which she was a second choice for the man reinforced and maintained her core schema. Thus, it is often helpful to have the patient examine how sunk-cost traps are schematically related, since it assures the patient that not all sunk-costs are traps.

• *Examining opportunity costs from sunk-costs.* Backward-looking decisions, in which the individual attempts to redeem and recover a loss, often overlook the prospect of future opportunity costs. Again, the irony is that staying in a bad relationship, as an example of a sunk-cost, can not only cut off realistic opportunities for other more rewarding relationships, but it can also undermine the ability to perceive that an opportunity could be achieved elsewhere. A woman who stays in an abusive relationship experiences a drop in self-esteem and general feelings of efficacy, thereby further discouraging her from the belief that other men would want her—or from the belief that she would be better off without a man. The question of opportunity cost can be addressed by asking the patient the following questions: (1) "If you were not pursuing this sunk-cost, what opportunities for reward would be available?"; (2) "How does staying in this sunk-cost perpetuate the belief that you are not able to produce other positives in your life? How does it reduce your perception of yourself as an effective person?" The therapist can suggest that the patient has been banging her head against the wall for a long period of time. It is now time to walk around the wall and pursue other goals.

• *Does the patient believe the acceptance of loss in giving up on a sunk-cost will result in overwhelming affect?* Some people believe they will never recover from the sense of sadness they feel when they abandon the sunk-cost. The patient may believe he will be overcome with depression and hopelessness, and these feelings will last forever and destroy him. The therapist can remind the patient of how he was able to give up on other lost causes and that his experience of loss was temporary and not overwhelming. Furthermore, by pointing out other decisions to abandon sunk-costs, the therapist may ask, "What would your life have been like if you had continued in [the other] sunk-cost?" The therapist can compare the sudden and quick pain of pulling a splinter out versus the long steady pain of leaving it in. The therapist can ask, "How would you feel 1 week, 1 month, 6 months from now, if you gave up on this?"

• *Expand social support for positive change.* The patient can examine alternative sources of support for positive change. For example, encourage the substance abuser to enter a 12-step program, rather than spend time with friends in bars. The patient can examine her support network to determine which friends or family members facilitate change and which seem to deter it. The patient can assign more time to spend with facilitators of positive change.

• *Identify specific steps toward change.* Similar to the model advocated in motivational interviewing (Miller & Rollnick, 1991), the therapist should help the patient to problem solve specific behaviors and discover resources necessary to produce change. For example, the patient who has been relying on alcohol to reduce his anxiety should be trained in anxiety-management techniques (Barlow & Craske, 1988) and should be encouraged to reduce sources of unnecessary stress. By adapting a problem-solving strategy to modify past negative consistency, the therapist can focus the patient on achievable goals. This strategy may assist the patient in overcoming feelings of helplessness and low self-esteem. For example, a woman who was focused on how terrible it would be to leave her husband (a major sunk-cost!) was able to refocus on taking specific steps toward change such as arranging her finances independently of him, getting a new place to live, and renewing her contact with friends. This approach diverted her thinking away from the uncontrollable qualities of her husband and toward behaviors and outcomes she could control.

SUMMARY

Social-cognitive processes focusing on self-consistency, predictability, control, and interactive realities also result in resistance in that the depressed patient may be highly invested in maintaining the stability, internal consistency, and control that his negative thinking allows him. The attempt to maintain consistency in behavior may be related to backward-looking decision making focused on sunk-cost effects.

In this chapter, I examined the tendency of individuals to honor sunk-costs, thereby continuing them in a condition of hopelessness. The sunk-cost process appears to allow the individual to maintain some hope that failures, which are not final, can be redeemed as a success sometime in the future. Thus, the individual may appear to discount future opportunities for change and for reward, focusing more on the disutility of his prior mistakes.

I have examined a number of interventions that allow the patient to examine the meaning of a sunk-cost and his resistance to giving up on behaviors that no longer are effective. In the next chapter I will discuss how individuals become trapped in resistance due to their personal and interpersonal schemas.

6

Schematic Resistance

I'll see it when I believe it.
—ANONYMOUS

SCHEMATIC PROCESSING

Not only will a schema direct attention, but it will also affect the *reconstructive* aspect of memory (see Hastie, 1981; Loftus & Ketcham, 1994). Psychoanalysts tend to think of the memory process as one that involves removing layers of repression designed to cover suppressed memories—as if the memory traces are permanently, veridically impressed in the brain cells. In contrast, the *reconstructive model* proposes that memory is an active process, indeed, an *interactive process*, in which current schemas (or concepts) may determine what is *falsely recalled*. For example, research on schematic memory indicates that people invent memories that are consistent with a current schema—that is, they *falsely recall*. (This is the basis of the criticisms raised by Loftus & Ketcham, 1994, regarding so-called repressed memory.) The point of reconstructive memory is that the current schema (or mood) will determine selective recall of schema-consistent information and even the invention of information consistent with the current schema. Thus, autobiographical memory may be determined by the individual's current mood or experience and may often be a "narrative" about the past that makes sense of the present (see Belli & Loftus, 1997; Bower, 1981; Conway & Rubin, 1993).

Schematic Processing and Psychopathology

George Kelly (1955) proposed that we construct our world through personal constructs, or concepts, that reflect our idiosyncratic way of viewing experience. These constructs, which we now call schemas, are "bipolar"—that is, they are marked by contrasts. However, the polarity of a construct is individually determined—for example, the male patient may believe that the opposite of "strong" is "feminine." Personal constructs differ in terms of their range of application, their "permeability or openness" to new information, their differentiation, the degree to which they are superordinate or subordinate, and their relationship to a system of other personal constructs. Kelly's therapeutic model stressed the collaboration of therapist and patient in uncovering the pieces of the personal construct system and in directly modifying these constructs through direct disputation and behavioral assignments.

Beck (1976; Beck et al., 1979) draws on the tradition of research and theory on schematic processing and on the work of Kelly and others in advancing his schema model. In his earlier work, Beck indicated that depression is often the result of or is maintained by selective attention and selective memory concerning information consistent with the schema. Beck's (Beck et al., 1979, 1990) model of psychopathology proposes that each diagnostic entity—depression, anxiety, anger, personality disorders, mania—reflects underlying structural differences in information processing.

In his earlier formulations on depression and anxiety, Beck (Beck et al., 1979, 1985) proposed that affective and anxiety disorders are characterized by biases in thinking, focused on loss and threat, respectively. According to Beck's model, individuals prone to depression have established early maladaptive schemas that orient the individual toward information consistent with a view of loss, deprivation, or failure. These schemas are viewed as relatively enduring organizing structures, which may lie dormant until activated by stressful life events (see Alford & Beck, 1997; Clark, Beck, & Alford, 1999; Ingram et al., 1998). Thus, the individual with a prepotent schema of "incompetence" may appear to think of himself as relatively competent when events are going well, but if a stressful life event activates his incompetence schema, it will precipitate a major depressive episode focused on the patient's belief that he is a total failure.

Beck and his colleagues (Beck et al., 1990; Clark et al., 1999) indicate that individuals have a variety of schemas—emotional, decisional, physical, relational—each of which includes a set of rules that direct the individual in specific situations. Impairment in functioning may be manifested in any one of these schematic processes. Beck (Beck, 1997; Clark et al., 1999) has suggested that a *superordinate*, or organizing, structure stands over and above these schemas. This superordinate structure is referred to as a "mode," and includes anger, depressive, and anxiety modes.

Guidano and Liotti (1983; Guidano, 1987) have extended the schema model into a developmentally integrative model. Their model stresses the early developmental origins of "core beliefs" and schemas, focusing on the attachment processes elucidated by Bowlby (1969). Central issues of vulnerability, such as abandonment or control, mark the content of the early maladaptive schemas, with considerable stress placed on the effects of parenting and early communication. Guidano and Liotti proposed that these schematic vulnerabilities are "defended" by a "protective belt" of cognitions, behaviors, and emotional patterns. Thus, attempts to "remove" the defensive maneuvers, or protective belt, may result in resistance to change, insofar as the patient attempts to defend against direct vulnerability of the schema. For example, attempts to modify dependent behavior—by clinging and reassurance seeking—will result in an increase in other dependent behaviors, in that the patient attempts to avoid confronting schemas of abandonment and helplessness. Guidano and Liotti stress the importance of a developmental reconstructive therapy in which therapist and patient explore the manner in which early maladaptive schemas were established and how the protective belt of defensive maneuvers has maintained the schema.

Beck et al. (1990) expanded the cognitive model to focus specifically on a variety of personality disorders that are characterized by various schematic issues and adaptations. According to this model, each personality disorder may be characterized by the specific content of the dominant schema—for the compulsive personality, for example, the dominant schemas are control and rationality. These "overdeveloped" areas are contrasted with the "underdeveloped" areas of emotional expression and flexibility. Beck et al. (1990) propose that individuals either attempt to avoid situations that may threaten their schema or they may attempt to compensate for their fears of the undeveloped polarity. For example, the compulsive individual, fearing loss of control, may attempt to exercise extreme control over his environment through hoarding and organizing minutiae. These extreme attempts at compensation give rise to depression or anxiety when they fail to adequately control the feared polarity.

Since personality disorders are enduring, Beck et al. propose that the individual has consistently employed these avoidant and compensatory "adaptations," presumably warding off the threat of full exposure to his or her schema. Thus the compulsive personality has warded off confrontation with the experience that he is "really completely out of control" or "really completely irrational and crazy" by avoiding situations that he cannot control or by using magical attempts to control his environment. These ideas of avoidance and compensation are not completely dissimilar to Freud's (1912/1958, 1917/1963, 1923/1961) view that "defenses" are the "economical" solution to the underlying anxiety—that is, they have developed as a method to prevent the breakthrough of anxiety, but they also carry with them their own costs in terms of pathology. Although the cognitive model may share this similarity with the psychodynamic defense model, the course of therapy is different.

The Beck–Freeman schema model attempts to modify the risk of depression and anxiety in the personality disorders by first conducting a cognitive assessment with the patient (see also J. Beck, 1996, for a discussion of cognitive assessment). The patient's automatic thoughts are linked to underlying assumptions and conditional beliefs. For example, the automatic thought "I am losing control" is linked to a conditional belief: "If I do not have complete control, then I have no control." This is then linked to an underlying assumption: "I must be in total control at all times." The underlying core schema is identified as "out of control."

Young (1990) has also proposed a schema model in which he places emphasis on individual schemas, independent of personality disorders. Young has suggested that there are several dimensions of schematic content. He has derived a "schema questionnaire" to assess these dimensions. Further, he has attempted to integrate a range of theoretical perspectives, such as object relations theory and gestalt theory, with a cognitive model. According to this model, individuals engage in three adaptations to their "early maladaptive schemas": avoidance, compensation, or schema maintenance. The latter adaptation simply refers to the fact that individuals may pursue experiences that reinforce their schema. For example, the narcissistic individual may pursue relationships that reinforce her belief that she is special and unique. Young's model differs from the Beck–Freeman model in three ways: (1) his schemas are not entirely related to personality disorders; (2) he introduces the idea of schema maintenance (similar to Safran & Segal, 1990); and (3) he integrates other theoretical models and other therapeutic techniques, such as gestalt therapy, into this therapeutic model. In the model I propose, I borrow from both the Beck–Freeman and the Young models and attempt to relate these approaches to the issue of resistance.

Schematic Themes of Resistance

Individuals differ as to which issues or themes are of concern to them. Almost all of us experience stressful life events, but most of us do not develop chronic, severe, or resistant depressions. The *meaning* attached to events is the key to why the individual became depressed in the first place. For example, the therapist may question the patient who says, "The reason I am depressed is that I am alone a lot of the time." The naive therapist might conclude, as does the patient, that being alone is a sufficient cause of depression. However, the real therapeutic question should be, "What does being alone mean to you?" This question addresses the idiosyncratic meaning for the patient of the state of being alone. "Being alone" may mean a number of things to different people. It may have negative connotations, signifying failure, unlovability, hopelessness, and the inability to take care of oneself. For others, it may have such positive connotations as independence, freedom from pressure, and the opportunity to relax.

The idea that people have different need systems is not new to cognitive therapy. Over 50 years ago Henry Murray (1938) and David McClelland (1951) identified a variety of motivational or need systems. For example, Murray categorized individual need systems, such as need for affiliation, for achievement, and for dominance. These need systems were viewed as part of a *drive theory*: similar to hunger drive, individuals could be deprived or satiated in these needs.

The cognitive model of schemas is similar to the Murray or McClelland model of different need systems, but, unlike the need model, the cognitive model does not assume drive theory. The cognitive model of schemas emphasizes that schemas direct information search and storage—that is, the individual will selectively attend to and recall information consistent with a schema. The emphasis is on information processing and attempts to cope with the schema—for example, by avoiding information that activates the schema or compensating for inadequacies exemplified by the schema (see Beck et al., 1990; Bowlby, 1980; Leahy, 1985, 1991, 1995, 1996a; Young, 1990). Although cognitive therapists do not refer to drive theory (e.g., Bowlby explicitly rejects the drive theory of attachment), the idea that individuals differ in the content of their schemas and that this affects their perception of situations is not dissimilar to classic studies in social perception by Bruner (1992) known as *the new look in perception*. According to the "new look" theory, individuals distort information so that their perception will match their need system. The cognitive therapy model of schematic processing is similar to the new look theory, but differs from the classical theory in that cognitive theorists make no assumptions about drive reduction or deprivation affecting perception.

Developmental Fixation of Schemas

Beck (1976; Beck et al., 1979) proposed that early maladaptive schemas—such as loss, failure, and unlovability—are established during childhood, although the mechanisms by which this occurs are left unclear. Bowlby (1980), in his discussion of the etiology of depression, places considerable emphasis on schemas of loss and abandonment, although other schemas, such as control and perfection, may also be established during early childhood (Guidano & Liotti, 1983). Developmental psychologists may speculate as to the means of transmission of schematic content—for example, imitation of the parental schemas or child-rearing practices involving warmth, control, punishment, rationality, threats of abandonment, conflicting standards, entitlement, or lack of mirroring (Bowlby, 1980; Guidano & Liotti, 1983; Kernberg, 1975; Leahy, 1983; Masterson, 1981).

One source of schematic resistance is due to the structural limitations, or regressivity, of schemas. The therapist who utilizes rational disputation or Socratic dialogues may become frustrated when the patient does not modify his beliefs. In this section, I review the developmental foundations of schema development, arguing that the therapist must keep in mind that schemas are often formed at early stages of cognitive development and that these schemas retain the structural primitivism of these stages.

Themes of Early Schemas

Schemas, or categories, established during very early childhood would be expected to focus on issues relevant to biological integrity, such as the ability to survive, the reliability of caretakers, abandonment, and direct physical danger to the self. It is Bowlby's (1969; 1980) contention that these categories underlie attachment issues during infancy since the infant's helplessness can only be overcome by secure attachments to love objects. Disturbances during this early phase would be expected to affect future information processing, in that the infant, and later the child or adult, would be vulnerable to threats of abandonment and threats to biological survival (Bowlby, 1969). The infant may attempt to maintain the attachment by clinging behavior or protests (such as crying) or, in some cases, by physically attacking the love object when she returns. The attack on the love object is presumed to function as a punishment of the parent so that the parent will be less likely to abandon (or leave) the child in the future. This "system" of attachment behaviors on the part of infant and parent will be activated if disruptions occur. The child establishes an object concept (or schema) which serves as a prototype or model for later interpersonal relationships (Bowlby, 1969). Thus, the infant who has an insecure attachment will come to view other attachments in later life as insecure, resulting in his greater vulnerability.

Structural Primitivism and Centration

Beck et al. (1979) proposed that when the patient becomes depressed, early maladaptive schemas are activated that direct information processing. For example, the depression may activate early beliefs that the self is incompetent, helpless, or physically vulnerable. These early maladaptive schemas are *structurally primitive* in that they are formed during early childhood and function during the depressive episode on a preoperational level of intelligence (Leahy, 1985, 1995). Similar to Piaget's (1970a, 1970b) description of preoperational thinking, early maladaptive schemas are *dichotomous* (all-or-nothing thinking). They are based on *moral realism* (one's intention does not count), *imminent justice* ("Bad things happen to bad people; therefore, if you are depressed, you must be bad"), and *egocentric causality* ("I must be the cause of what is happening, especially if it is negative") (Leahy, 2000a).

Piaget (1970a, 1970b) described the structural process of this thinking as *centration* (or centering). In centering, the individual focuses on one dimension—usually something that is immediate and salient—and is unable to coordinate other perspectives or dimensions. Furthermore, the person overly focuses on what is immediately observable, rather than considering possible covert or internal factors (such as the subjective state of other people). In social cognition, centering is reflected in an emphasis on *proximal*, or immediate, causes, rather than on possible *distal*, or remote, causes (Leahy, 2000c). For example, in explaining personality differences, younger children have difficulty considering how earlier life experiences can determine current behavior: they focus entirely on the immediate situation (see Leahy & Shirk, 1984). Consider the following examples.

MIND READING

Mind reading involves centering or egocentrism in that the individual does not distinguish his perspective from that of others. The depressive assumes that because he has a negative view of himself, everyone shares this view. Furthermore, he does not recognize that others do not have the same (subjective) information that the self has. For example, the social phobic, who directly experiences his own anxiety, has difficulty recognizing that others do not have access to his subjective feelings.

NEGATIVE FILTER, OVERGENERALIZING, LABELING,
AND ALL-OR-NOTHING THINKING

Negative filter, overgeneralizing, labeling, and all-or-nothing thinking are other examples of centration. In these cases, the individual does not consider the variation of his (or others') behaviors. Similar to the preoperational child, he focuses on one dimension (or behavior) and forms a global conclusion from that information. Since his schema is negative, his conclusions are negative. In negative labeling of the self, he does not consider the variation of his behavior across time and situations, nor does he consider his behavior along a continuum. (Continua involve *seriation*—that is, the ability to order things in a series of increasing or relative units. This ability for seriation appears at the stage of concrete operations.)

ABSOLUTISTIC IMPERATIVES

Centration is involved in the lack of an ability to consider mitigating factors (such as duress, lack of foresight, situational constraints, provocation, or history of positive behavior). Thus, depressive moralistic thinking is absolute, rigid, and without consideration of situational factors: "If you did something that had a negative consequence, then you are bad." Furthermore, since centered thinking is so focused on the external or visible, rather than the "covert" or internal processes of persons (such as motives, ambivalence, or history that are not immediately available), the individual has little ability to recognize that negative consequences can often be the result of positive intentions. The preoperational thinker concludes that if a bad event occurred, then it was intended. Furthermore, even given information that the action was *not intended*, the preoperational thinker discounts intention and only considers consequences. Piaget (1934) labels this as *moral realism* (and contrasts this with moral relativism) since the young child focuses on absolute rules and absolute consequences rather than the idea that rules can be modified and that individuals differ in their intentions. "Negative events are performed by bad people" is the moral assumption of the moral realist.

PERSONALIZING

Finally, centering is reflected in personalization: the individual focuses on the self as the sole cause of an event, rather than considering alternative causes (such as other people). The depressed person who takes the entire blame for a divorce fails to decenter from his role in the problem to consider his wife's contribution. Further, he focuses only on his negative behavior and fails to refocus on other examples of his positive behavior.

I view this kind of thinking as *structural fixation*—that is, the early schemas are formed and fixated at an early developmental level characterized by rigid, absolutistic, moral realism (Leahy, 1991, 1995, 2000c). Because early negative schemas are structurally limited by centering, the resistant depressed patient may, at times, be unable to stand back from his thinking to gain the perspective of the *observing ego*.

Young children and chronically depressed patients both lack the ability to make their own cognitions a focus of their own analysis.

Whereas psychoanalytic models of resistance stress fixation due to frustration at an early age, the current model proposes both frustration and structural fixation. Thus, the adult who is able to function well in certain areas of his life may demonstrate structural primitivism or structural fixation regarding the content of his earlier frustration. The child who is blamed for having needs (resulting in frustration) will continue to process this blame at a primitive level of cognitive functioning. The *introject* (or internal self-image) of being viewed as "selfish" will be processed at an early level of functioning. This primitivism will be reflected in the fusion of thought and feeling, dichotomous thinking, and the inability to self-reflect on the lack of validity of the belief. Indeed, schematic content established at very early levels of functioning or through traumatic events at a young age may be experienced as images, emotions, or somatic complaints, rather than as fully developed thoughts.

Chronicity of Negativity

SCHEMAS AND ASSIMILATION

Piaget (1970a, 1970b) argued that cognitive systems or structures are "conservative" in that they attempt to maintain themselves. Piaget refers to this process as *assimilation* and argues that cognitive structures attempt to "fit" external stimuli into the structure and resist accommodation or self-modification. The earliest example of this is found in *circular reactions* during infancy in which the infant attempts to assimilate a variety of objects into a scheme—for example, the infant attempts to assimilate thumb, blanket, and bottle into the action scheme of sucking. According to Piaget's "biological" model, early cognitive structures gain strength through these circular reactions. By attempting to generalize to other stimuli, the infant increases the range of his experience.

The cognitive model of schemas is similar to this Piagetian structural model. Specifically, schemas attempt to assimilate diverse and schematically conflicting stimuli. Furthermore, there is generalization of the schema beyond the initial application of the schema: schemas are generally not limited to a single small class of stimuli. Finally, schemas resist change and tend to be self-fulfilling.

CHANNELIZED DEVELOPMENT

Ethological developmentalists, interested in the effect of early experience on later development, refer to *genetic landscapes* (Waddington, 1957;

Wilson, 1975). Consider a ball that begins rolling through a wide plain. There is considerable variation during the early moments of its movement: It could move to the left or right. However, as it begins moving forward, the sides of the plain close in, forming a valley with increasingly higher walls along the valley. The ball's movement is more constrained by these walls. Similarly, one might view early development as open to considerable variation, but with increasing movement forward in time (and age), there is greater channelization of expression. In fact, differences between individuals become more pronounced and more stable. The early movements of the ball (or the individual) determine future movements, with increasing limits on variability. This analogy may be applied to the development of early schemas.

Since these early schemas are formed during the preoperational stage of intelligence, the patient may have had many years of approaching experience guided by these schemas. For example, the formation of a rejection-sensitivity schema during childhood may have resulted in years of focus on any signs of rejection. Consequently, the developing individual has selectively processed information consistent with rejection and either not noticed or is unable to recall information inconsistent with the rejection schema. Therefore, the schema will have developed stronger associative networks supporting its negativity.

If we view negative schemas as directing information processing throughout the chronically depressed person's life, we can understand how the persistent selective negative bias has provided the individual with sufficient negative information to support his or her negative schemas. For example, if you spent 20 years of your life focusing almost entirely on collecting evidence that people with blue eyes are unpleasant—and you ignored almost all disconfirming evidence—you could probably build a good case against blue-eyed people. The chronically depressed patient has persistently collected negative evidence against himself, thereby strengthening his negative schema.

It appears that the *threshold for activation* of negative schemas (or moods) becomes lower with recurring episodes. We know that chronic or recurrent depressives become even more negative over time: their subsequent episodes of depression are usually more severe and resistant to treatment than their earlier episodes. Similarly, anxiety, phobia, or trauma may be more easily activated after earlier episodes of anxiety, phobia, or trauma.

Attempts to claim that there is a finite set of schemas or a specific set of issues that capture human nature will likely end with the frustration that Henry Murray (1938) experienced: each day there is a new discovery of new needs. I have identified a number of schematic issues that I believe are relevant, but the reader will certainly recognize that I could have included many other schematic themes (see Beck et al., 1990, or Young, 1990, for descriptions of their schematic models.) In Table 6.1, I have identified 11 schemas that are relevant to procrastination (or to other issues confronting the individual, such as marital conflict or achievement). I have included both schemas (the general issues or themes that the individual focuses on) and the maladaptive assumptions (or rules) that are operative with these schemas.

TABLE 6.1. Procrastination Schemas and Assumptions

Schema	Issue	Example
Entitlement	Special, superior person	"I'm too good to have to do this. I shouldn't have to do this. These rules shouldn't apply to me."
Rejection sensitivity	Undesirable	"If I do this, I'll get rejected. It's terrible if I get rejected. If I get rejected, it means I'm undesirable, worthless."
Dependency	Incompetent, helpless	"Someone else will solve my problems. I should wait for someone to rescue me."
Control	Dominated, spontaneous	"I don't like being told what to do. I shouldn't do anything unless it's on my terms when I want to do it."
Perfectionism	Perfect, rational, above reproach	"I shouldn't do anything unless I can do a perfect job of it. I should only start it if I can get the whole thing done."
Passive-aggressiveness	Need to test others	"Why should I do this if it will please someone else? I can deprive them by not doing it. If they really valued me, they'd accept the fact that I don't do this."
Emotionalizing	Aroused, emotional, spontaneous	"I need to feel inspired—excited—to do this. If I feel it's going to be terrible, then it will be."
Low frustration tolerance	Depleted, exhausted, overwhelmed	"I can't stand doing things that are unpleasant. If I do this, I'll be depleted and exhausted."
Personal inadequacy	Flawed, helpless	"I am helpless and unlovable. Therefore, I can't do this. If I fail, then I should criticize myself."
Past determination	Fatalistic, regretful	"Since I haven't succeeded in the past, nothing will work. I may as well give up. I should criticize myself for my mistakes."
Self-defeat	Undeserving, morally reprehensible	"I really don't deserve to succeed, so why bother?"

Consider how individuals with different schemas and assumptions might respond to the following situation: the individual's supervisor requests that the individual has to submit a report by the end of the week. Individuals with different schemas might respond differently to this requirement, but in each case by procrastinating:

- *Entitlement*: "I shouldn't have to do this. This is beneath me."
- *Control*: "Who is she to tell me what to do? I'm not going to be controlled by her."
- *Perfectionism*: "I've got to do a perfect job. It's going to take me weeks to get all the information for this, but it's due on Friday."
- *Low frustration tolerance*: "I can't stand doing these reports. It makes me anxious. I'd rather watch television."

The cognitive model proposes that individuals differ in the manner in which they process information. For example, personality disorders can be viewed as variations in schematic processing: dependent people focus on abandonment, avoidant people on negative evaluation, paranoids on betrayal, compulsives on control, and narcissists on special status. As I indicated earlier, one might multiply the number of schemas for individuals far beyond this taxonomy.

In analyzing the transference response of the patient, the use of schematic analysis is essential. For example, the therapist proposes that the patient write down his negative thoughts and rational responses over the next week. When patients attempt to comply with this assignment, different schemas will be activated (see Table 6.2).

Self-help assignments may be a useful probe into the patient's schemas. The therapist should ask the patient if he or she had any thoughts about doing the assignments and ask him or her to share them with the therapist. Patients may adapt specific roles in the transference such that these roles will indicate their underlying schemas.

Compensation and Avoidance of Schemas

The idea that people may overly compensate for their feelings of inadequacy is not new. Adler's (1926/1964) theory of social power was precisely based on the view that people who feel inferior and weak may attempt to compensate for these feelings by overachieving or by dominating others. Bowlby's (1980) view is that some individuals who have experienced threats of loss or actual loss may compensate for this by excessive clinging, reassurance seeking, or even compulsive caretaking. The depressed patient who believes that he is basically unlovable may compensate by attempting to be excessively pleasing, deferential, dependent,

TABLE 6.2. Schemas and Responses to Self-Help

Schema	Response
Demanding standards	"I have to do a perfect job or it's not worth doing."
Approval orientation	"My therapist wants me to do this, so I should be sure to do a good job or she'll think less of me."
Helplessness	"I don't know how to do this. I can't help myself. What's the use?"
Control	"Who does she think she is to tell me what to do? I don't take orders."
Special person	"This is trivial and beneath me. Maybe the other patients she has do homework, but not me. I'm too busy."
Betrayal	"What if she uses this against me? I've got to watch what I say or she'll take my thoughts and turn them against me."
Demand for certainty	"I shouldn't do anything unless I know beforehand that it will work. I have to wait until I am sure."

or unassertive. Some will even be self-effacing: in an attempt to avoid others' criticisms, he or she will "beat them to the punch."

Compensations may be attempts to adapt to the negative schema about self and other, but in fact the compensation may not effectively change the schema. For example, a patient who was a senior executive at a major corporation believed he was basically incompetent, even stupid. When the therapist had him examine the evidence of his many years of achievement, he discounted the evidence by claiming that these achievements were not significant—especially in light of the fact that others he knew had achieved more. The therapist engaged him in "developmental cognitive therapy"—that is, going back to his early childhood to examine how he learned he was not competent (Leahy, 1985, 1990, 1995; Young, 1990). It emerged that his mother used to compare him unfavorably to his older, highly achieving brother. The therapist asked him to engage in a role play: he was to imagine that he had returned in a time machine to his childhood, with all his knowledge of his future achievements intact, and now he had to challenge his mother's criticisms with the facts of his actual achievements. Oddly, it had never occurred to him that his mother was wrong. He was still processing this information as a 6-year-old.

In the example above, the executive had gone through his life attending to his inadequacy, not to his success. He also had a *compensatory strategy*: "If I can be perfect, I'll avoid my inadequacy." Since he was not perfect, he would default to his inadequacy schema.

The compensatory strategies seldom are effective in modifying the core beliefs about the self that are activated by negative life events. These compensatory assumptions—"I must be perfect" or "I must always have the love of a man [or woman]"—are rigid, unrealistic, and almost always impossible to achieve. For example, a highly successful businessman, confronted with a serious business mistake, activates his early schema that he is incompetent and stupid when a failure occurs. Or he worries that failure might occur, thereby "proving he really is stupid." He acts (thinks) as if none of his prior success matters, since he has not achieved perfection. Regardless of the individual's prior achievements, his or her negative schemas remain dormant until events catalyze the schemas, resulting in a depressive episode.

The reliance on maladaptive assumptions (conditional rules or schemas)—such as perfectionism, need for approval, and anxiety intolerance—reinforce the patient's belief that he or she must compensate or avoid the underlying negative self-schema (of helplessness or unworthiness). Similar to compulsive behaviors that keep the obsessive from exposure to the feared stimulus, the chronically depressed patient, relying on maladaptive assumptions, may seldom challenge his or her underlying schema. For example, the successful business executive, continually striving for perfection and approval, may think his problem is that he is not "successful enough"—thereby further seeking perfection in his work. Similarly, the patient who believes he is basically unlovable may have a compensatory strategy of trying to get everyone's approval. When he succeeds in gaining approval he reports no problems, but when he fails to get approval he becomes depressed. Since his underlying schema of unlovability is not challenged, he concludes that he must strive even harder to get approval in the future.

For many, if not most, patients, challenging automatic thoughts (e.g., "I'll fail") or challenging assumptions (e.g., "I must be perfect") is sufficient for change. However, for other patients whose resistance is stronger, the underlying schema is protected by their assumptions and automatic thoughts. It is as if the patient is saying, "I can't give up my perfectionism because then my true helplessness will be manifested."

SCHEMAS AND RESISTANCE
TO MODIFYING ASSUMPTIONS

The individual's maladaptive schema has had a long history of self-verification. Because the patient has been selectively focused on information consistent with the schema, and has selectively filtered from memory information inconsistent with the schema, the patient may find it difficult to weigh in the "new evidence" that the therapist provides that challenges the schema. Moreover, the patient may believe the schema is not only veridical, but also protects him from further loss. For example, the patient whose schema about others is that they are exploitative may have a self-schema that reflects weakness. In order to avoid being exploited by others, the patient may avoid any close relationships (e.g., especially in therapy) or may approach relationships with an exaggerated toughness. To give up his belief in the exploitative nature of others would result in a greater threat to his supposed weakness, which can always be obscured by appearing "tough."

Core maladaptive schemas are usually experienced in dichotomous terms rather than in terms of complexity or differentiation. For example, the narcissistic patient, whose surface schema is "I am a special, superior person," has a mirror schema of being empty and worthless. The compulsive personality, whose surface schema is "I am in control" or "I am rational," often reflects an underlying fear of being "out of control" or "crazy." When events threaten the surface schema (e.g., "I am a special person"), the patient may mobilize his cognitive, behavioral, emotional, and interpersonal resources to protect the surface (positive) schema. For example, the narcissistic individual, mobilizing his defenses in the face of possible "failure," may discount the importance of other people, devalue the therapist, act out through drinking or sexual exploitation, or seek reassurance that he really is special. A narcissistic executive, on the brink of losing his job, may mobilize his narcissistic defenses to protect his schema that he, indeed, is superior, even though he is about to be fired. He defends his schema by pointing out to the therapist how inferior his coworkers (especially his boss) are, how ineffective the therapist has been in helping him, and, at the same time, seeks reassurance from the therapist that he, indeed, is a superior individual. The patient then begins a tirade in the session, pointing out all the supposed inferiorities of the therapist.

Patients utilizing these defensive maneuvers to protect the surface schema have difficulty gaining insight in therapy, since any challenge to their view that they are special or in control implies the polar opposite—that is, that they are worthless or completely out of control. Because the patient has either avoided situations that might threaten his schema or has overcompensated so that his schema is not exposed, the patient may fear that abandoning his strategies of avoidance or compensation will lead to core threats. Schemas are seldom put to the test by the patient, since avoidance and compensation maneuvers interfere with direct examination of the validity of the schema. The patient whose core schema may be "I am unlovable" utilizes a conditional rule or assumption: "If I am perfectly pleasing, people may like me." These compensations are similar to the "safety behaviors" of anxious individuals who believe that their magical behaviors protect them from impending disaster (see Wells, 1997). The schema, then, is never directly tested.

Another interference with testing a schema is that the patient has *discounting rules*: "Yes, I let him know more about me and he liked me, but (1) he's different from other people and (2) there are still some things about me he doesn't know." These discounting rules prevent disconfirmation of the schema since the schema is based on overinclusion rules: "If there is a single aspect of me that someone doesn't like, then it means I am unlovable."

Patients often seem remarkably lacking in insight regarding their schemas and the biased cognitive processing that they entail. They may be able to directly access the schema—"Yes, I'm unlovable"—but they seldom spontaneously recognize how their maneuvers have prevented a test of their schema. Like the anxious patient who focuses on threats and safety precautions, the schema-ridden patient focuses on defending himself. His emphasis is on the threat to his schema, not on the validity of the schema. Indeed, some patients may believe that to stop and examine whether their beliefs are unrealistic might actually handicap them in the never-ending task of defending themselves.

MODIFYING SCHEMAS

Therapy cannot rid the patient of his schemas. This would be equivalent to completely eliminating a personality disorder. The approach that I take is more modest, but perhaps more realistic. The goal in therapy is to assist the patient in recognizing how his schema controls his emotional and interpersonal life and to *reduce the effect of the schema* on the patient's daily functioning. Thus, the patient who has the schema that he must be a special person may still hold on to some beliefs about being special, but may set his goal as accepting the truth that he does not have to be better than everyone. The compulsive person may still strive for control, rationality, and fairness, but aim for the ability to have some flexibility in these domains.

Identifying Schematic Content

The patient's schemas can be identified through a variety of assessments. Young's "schema questionnaire" allows the clinician to identify the patient's specific schematic vulnerabilities. Beck et al. (1990) provide an extensive evaluation of schemas. In addition, assessments of personality disorder such as Millon, Davis, Millon, Escovar, and Meagher's (2000) scale, may reveal specific schemas in that the personality disorders are theoretically related to schemas. In addition, schemas are central in affective and anxiety disorders, with the depressive schemas relating to failure, loss, helplessness, and emptiness, and the anxiety schemas related to threat, danger, and imminence (see Beck, 1976; Beck et al., 1979, 1990). These schemas may be identified through the use of vertical descent (the downward-arrow technique): "You said you felt bad about the breakup with Bill. I wonder if you could tell me what it means to you?" The patient responded:

"He didn't want me."
↓
"I'm flawed."
↓
"No one will love me."
↓
"I'll always be alone."
↓
"I'm a loser."

Examining Patterns of Schematic Content

Individuals with personality disorders often recognize that something is pervasively wrong in their lives, but they seldom have true insight into their repetitive schema defenses. The therapist can help the patient gain awareness of these defensive maneuvers by indicating that the patient tries to protect himself through various patterns of thought and behavior. For example, the therapist can explain to the narcissistic individual that his depression and anxiety often follow experiences where he is "threatened" with the belief that he is not "superior to everyone."

THERAPIST: Do you see a pattern to the times that you have been upset? It's when something might go wrong in your business and you think "I'll be exposed as a failure." Or you find yourself comparing yourself to someone who has done extraordinarily well and you think "I'm inferior." Even though you recognize that you have done very well, you discount this, because you believe you must be superior to everyone in order to be worthwhile.

PATIENT: Yes, there's a pattern.

THERAPIST: Let's also see if there's a pattern to what you do when you have these feelings and thoughts.

The therapist was able to illustrate a pattern of anger toward others, depression, and worry. These feelings were accompanied by envy, devaluation of associates, increased drinking, spacing out (dissociating), and reliance on prostitutes. In addition, this patient would sometimes work compulsively in order to compensate for his supposed inferiority. Each of these behaviors or experiences helped "defend" him against the perception that he was inferior. For example, his envy of others led him to devalue the achievements of others and, indeed, to devalue the people he thought might be evaluating him. His drinking and dissociating allowed him to momentarily escape from his negative self-reflection, while his solicitation of prostitutes made him feel superior and nonthreatened. Each of these defensive maneuvers interfered with his ability to gain insight, and thereby modify his core beliefs.

THERAPIST: As long as you rely on these defensive maneuvers, you will have a hard time changing yourself. I would compare this to someone who has four drinks every time he feels anxious. He immediately gets rid of his anxiety, but he never has the ability to stop to think about what is really bothering him. He can never change his mind, because he doesn't take the time to examine his mind.

After identifying schematic patterns, the therapist can ask the patient the "typical" cognitive therapy questions:

"What are the costs and benefits of this schema?"
"How would your life have been different without this schema?"
"What is the evidence for and against the schema?"
"If someone else said they believed what you believe, what advice would you give them?"

Compartmentalizing the Schema

It is essential for the patient to recognize that his identity is not reducible to his schema. A schema may be labeled as a "specific vulnerability": "You have a tendency to focus a lot on the issue of whether you have a right to have needs. But in most other areas of your life you see things fairly clearly. This bias, though, is a specific problem, a specific vulnerability, that may have an impact on how you feel about yourself and other people." The patient should be encouraged to talk about his "schema," referring to it as "my schema" or "it." This establishes an internal dialogue for the patient. Other techniques that are helpful include having the patient write his schema on an index card (e.g., "Schema: Undeserving"), write out examples of thoughts that are derived from the schema

("I'm being selfish talking about my problems"), talking back to the schema ("You are wrong. I do deserve to help myself"), using the empty-chair technique to address the schema, and writing the schema down on a piece of paper and tearing it up.

In addition to compartmentalizing the schema, the therapist may also inquire as to experiences in which the schema does not seem to be powerful. We often assume that schemas are so pervasive and profound that, if the patient thinks she is undeserving (as an example of the schema), we assume that this is true in all situations. However, there may be important exceptions for the patient. Have there been relationships, experiences, or times when the patient did feel deserving? What was different about these experiences? This variability in a schema may highlight the possibility of change and may suggest what the patient needs to make this change possible. For example, the patient with the "undeserving schema" might be capable of feeling deserving if she were with a nurturing, nonjudgmental person or if she "deserved" support in taking care of someone else.

Developing a Case Conceptualization

The importance of the schema in the patient's life is best illustrated by the use of a case conceptualization (Beck et al., 1990; J. Beck, 1996; Leahy, 1996a; Needleman, 1999; Persons, 1989; Young, 1990). There are a variety of models of case conceptualization, but each model stresses the importance of cognitive assessment and life history. A case conceptualization that elucidates the function of schemas would include a thorough cognitive assessment that would identify typical automatic thoughts, how these thoughts are related to the patient's maladaptive assumptions (*should rules*), conditional beliefs ("If I am totally deferential, people will like me"), and core schemas about self and other ("I am helpless" and "Others are supportive"). The therapist can also determine the strategies that the patient has utilized to protect himself or to adapt. These strategies include avoidance and compensation. Moreover, the patient's selection of partners, friends, work goals, and other goals may also reflect underlying schemas. Indeed, many of these choices may have maintained the schema. For example, a dependent woman may be attracted to apparently "confident" men, through whom she expects to obtain security and support. However, their narcissistic qualities may frustrate her, further leading to her negative schema about obtaining support from others and being able to support herself.

The case conceptualization should also identify important childhood experiences that give rise to the current schemas. For example, a well-educated, unemployed woman was able to identify conflicting messages during childhood: "We expect great things from you" and "You are totally incompetent" (see also Linehan, 1993, on "invalidating environments" for borderline personality). As a consequence of these conflicting messages, the woman avoided independent work and instead relied on others to take care of her and protect her from her loneliness. She further attempted to compensate for her double bind through "beauty perfectionism," that is her belief that "If I am beautiful, I will be able to get a man to take care of me."

DISCONFIRMATION EXPERIMENTS

We can view schema maintenance as an attempt to confirm a hypothesis that maintains apparently dysfunctional behavior or thinking. For example, a husband passively withholds any interaction from his wife. His hypothesis is "My wife is a controlling nag. If I interact, she will criticize me." The wife, observing that he is silent, responds: "What's wrong? Why aren't you talking to me?" The husband, anticipating her control, remains silent, reading the paper. The wife then tries to elicit a response from him by saying: "Are you upset?" The husband has now confirmed his belief that she is controlling and he feels further assured that he should withdraw in the future.

The therapist can point out that the husband is seeking confirmation for a negative belief. But this will only maintain his withdrawal and his wife's intrusiveness. The therapist would do better to recommend an experiment like this one: "Bill, every time you find yourself passively withdrawing, I'd like you to immediately change for a few minutes and ask Susan about her activities during the day and her feelings: focus entirely on Susan's thoughts and feelings." This experiment allows the patient to disconfirm his belief that his wife is always controlling him. It is likely that focusing on the wife's report of her experiences will decrease her "intrusion" on Bill, since her "intrusive behavior" has been a response to her husband's withdrawal. *By removing Bill's problem-maintaining solution, we have allowed him to examine the validity of his schema.*

CHALLENGING READINESS DEMANDS

Some patients believe that they should only do things that are spontaneous. These individuals are often high in autonomy and reactance needs, viewing requests for change as interfering with desired personal freedom (see Dowd, 1999; Brehm & Brehm, 1970). Overemphasis on "spontaneity" may result in impasses that maintain chronic dysfunction.

The therapist can explore the patient's beliefs about spontaneity. A typical series of beliefs includes: "I'll lose my freedom. Someone else is in control. If they are in control, then they might mislead me. This makes me a robot. I'll be less of a man [woman]. It won't do any good if I'm not spontaneous."

The therapist can validate the importance of spontaneity: "It's important to be yourself. But sometimes to become better at being yourself, you might end up doing things you don't want to do." The therapist can pose the following question: "What is your highest priority: to always do things spontaneously or to have a more productive life?"

Rational responses to the foregoing thoughts associated with reactance are:

"I can have greater freedom to accomplish healthier goals if I develop self-discipline" (Examples can include the greater freedom and goal attainment made possible by reducing drinking and overeating and by increasing exercise.)

"If I do things that are good for me, I—not someone else—will have greater control." (Examples include following the instruction of a skilled coach or working collaboratively with a client in the patient's business.)

"Following advice is really an experiment. If it doesn't work out, I always have the freedom to change." (Examples include accepting a recommendation to a restaurant. You do not have to return if the meal is mediocre.)

"I am not a robot or less of a human being for doing things nonspontaneously. In fact, I'm more of a human being—more in control of myself—if I do things that require self-direction and self-discipline." (Again, examples from drinking, smoking, overeating, and exercise are important.)

"Positive things occur every day when I'm doing things that are nonspontaneous, but healthful. Positive behavior—even if it is not spontaneous—creates new positive realities." (Examples include health issues, disciplining oneself on the job, time management, and practicing positive behavior toward others—even if you do not "feel" like it. The new *positive realities* that result include better health, increased energy, improved appearance, increased productivity, and positive behaviors from other people.)

Homework assignments can include practicing several "positive behaviors" daily that the patient feels do not "come spontaneously." These might include refraining from overeating or overdrinking, giving compliments, and carrying out other behaviors that the patient does not want to do. The therapist can ask the patient to monitor his responses to the following:

"What are the costs and benefits of doing this?"
"How difficult to predict will this be, rating from 0 to 10?"
"How do you think you'll feel 5 minutes after you do this?"
"Precisely, what do you predict the outcome will be?"

Some patients will predict that they will feel defeated, controlled, childish, "not like themselves," or taken advantage of. They sometimes predict that their partners will make more demands on them and see them as weak. These predictions can be tested along with the therapist's inquiry: "Let's see if you feel more in control, more mature, or more effective. Let's see if your partner nags you *less* and even appreciates the positive things you do."

Issues of autonomy or reactance can also be addressed through the collaborative nature of cognitive therapy. The therapist can identify the "healthy" aspects of autonomy (see Newman, 1994, 1997). Cognitive therapy may be presented to these individuals as a self-help program whereby the therapist and the patient work together. The therapist can emphasize the autonomous aspects of treatment by recommending self-help bibliotherapy, Internet searches for information, homework that the patient self-assigns, emphasis on the patient providing the agenda, and asking the patient for corrective feedback in each session. After the patient has become familiar with the techniques and conceptualizations of cognitive therapy, the therapist can "make the patient the therapist":

THERAPIST: What would you like to work on today?

PATIENT: My procrastination on a project at work.

THERAPIST: I'll tell you what. Let's try something new. I think that you're pretty familiar with what I would do. Let's make believe I'm the patient—with your problem—and you're the therapist. This way you can get practice in your self-help therapy. OK. So I'll start off by being you: "I can't seem to get this project done. Can you help me with this?"

PATIENT: (*as therapist*) What are the next steps in doing the project?

By having the patient adopt the role of giving help, the therapist reduces the patient's reluctance to accept help.

Another approach to reactance is to examine the origins of the schema. For example, the therapist can indicate that the patient places a lot of emphasis on being in control—especially being independent from the control of others, including the therapist's control. The therapist can ask, "When you were a kid, how did your parents relate to you? How about your siblings?" Other relationships in which control was an issue can be explored. How did the patient feel about being controlled: punished, ridiculed, diminished, angry, childish? The patient can be encouraged to access images of specific incidents or memories of being controlled and to indicate his visual or bodily perspective ("I felt like I was small and weak"), automatic thoughts ("She was always nagging me"), and feelings ("I felt humiliated and angry").

The therapist can modify these recollections through imagery re-scripting (Smucker & Dancu, 1999): "Try to replay that memory. But this time you're much bigger and she is much smaller. You're in charge. She has a squeaky voice, barely faint. She's giving you an order, but you're telling *her* 'I'm in charge.' "

These interventions may assist the patient in repairing a sense of autonomy in the original memory. The therapist can then shift to memories of feeling that his autonomy has been threatened in therapy:

THERAPIST: Can you recall feeling like I was controlling you in our work?

PATIENT: Yes. When you challenge my thoughts, it feels like you're humiliating me.

THERAPIST: Sometimes cognitive therapy has that effect on people. That must have been hard for you. It might be helpful to hear the kinds of thoughts and feelings you had. I wonder if you could complete a sentence: "I felt humiliated by you because I thought. . . . "

PATIENT: You just want to have things your way. You want to be in charge.

THERAPIST: And this bothered me because it made me think. . . .

PATIENT: I must be a loser to need other people to tell me what to do.

THERAPIST: Did you have similar feelings and thoughts when you were a kid?

PATIENT: I felt angry and afraid and trapped. I felt like my mother was treating me like I was an idiot.

THERAPIST: So you feel this way now—that I could be treating you like an idiot when I challenge your negative thoughts?

PATIENT: I guess so.

THERAPIST: And what's it like for you when you share these feelings with me, but think "He thinks I'm an idiot?"

PATIENT: It's very hard. It's humiliating.

LINKING THE SCHEMA TO THE TRANSFERENCE

The patient's schema may well interfere with the therapeutic relationship. The therapist may anticipate this problem if the patient describes a series of other therapeutic relationships that have been unsatisfactory. For example, the patient who describes other therapists as exploiting him may be likely to think that the current therapist will also exploit him. After the "honeymoon" period of the patient's initial cooperation and idealization of the therapist, underlying schematic issues may emerge.

After the therapist and patient have identified specific schemas, the therapist should indicate to the patient that he or she should be aware that some of these same issues may manifest themselves in the therapeutic relationship: "This may be an opportunity for us to examine your thoughts and feelings in here so that we can work together to make things better." Emphasis on these "hot cognitions" and "ruptures in the therapeutic alliance" (Safran & Muran, 2000) may enable the therapist and the patient not only to observe the schema in action, but to repair the therapeutic relationship (see Safran, 1998).

The therapist should be sensitive to how the patient "presents" the initial complaint or problem. Does the patient seem hesitant to discuss issues? Does he excessively question the qualifications of the therapist? Does he require reassurance that things will get better? Is he skeptical about therapy? How does he respond to the idea of self-help? The patient's shame about having a problem may reflect schemas of rejection, abandonment, undeservingness, or the need to be special and superior. The therapist should inquire as to the underlying beliefs that give rise to the shame: "You said you felt embarrassed having these problems. I wonder what thoughts you are having about this. Could you complete the following sentence? 'I feel uncomfortable talking about this because I think. . . . ' " Responses to this question vary considerably, depending on the schema: "You will reject me," "I will feel inferior to you," "You will try to tell me what to do and then control me." The therapist may note these thoughts with the patient and indicate that through their "working relationship" they can find out how things will develop.

Schematic issues are also reflected in the patient's perception of the therapist as a person. Abandonment schemas are reflected in the belief that the therapist may be someone the patient can attach to or be abandoned by; schemas of uniqueness and superiority may be reflected by the belief that the therapist is an inferior person (or, alternatively, may be expressed through envy of the perceived superior position of the therapist). In Table 6.3, I have indicated how specific "overdeveloped" schemas, associated with various personality disorders (Beck et al., 1990), are manifested in the transference.

TABLE 6.3. Schemas in the Transference Relationship

Schema	Example
Incompetent (avoidant)	Avoids difficult topics and emotions. Appears vague. Looks for signs that the therapist will reject her. Believes that therapist will criticize her for not doing homework correctly. Reluctant to do behavioral exposure homework assignments.
Helpless (dependent)	Seeks reassurance. Does not have an agenda of problems to solve. Frequently complains about "feelings." Calls frequently between sessions. Wants to prolong sessions. Does not think he can do the homework or believes that homework will not work. Upset when therapist takes vacations.
Vulnerable to control (passive–aggressive)	Comes late to or misses sessions. Views cognitive "challenges" as controlling. Reluctant to express dissatisfaction directly. Vague about goals, feelings, and thoughts—especially as related to therapist and therapy. "Forgets" to do homework or pay bills.
Responsible (obsessive–compulsive)	Feels emotions are "messy" and "irrational." Criticizes himself for being irrational and disorganized. Wants to see immediate results and expresses skepticism about therapy. Views homework as a test to be done perfectly or not at all.
Superior (narcissistic)	Comes late or misses sessions. "Forgets" to pay for sessions. Devalues therapy and the therapist. Expects special arrangements. Feels humiliated to have to talk about problems. Believes that therapy will not work since the problem resides in other people.
Glamorous (histrionic)	Focuses on expressing emotions alternating rapidly from crying, to laughing, to anger. Tries to impress therapist with appearance, feelings, or problems. Rejects the rational approach and demands validation.

RELATING THE THERAPEUTIC TRANSFERENCE
TO OTHER RELATIONSHIPS

It is important that the patient not perceive the therapy relationship as a unique or idiosyncratic experience. Psychoanalytic models stress the essential nature of the transference in therapy (Freud, 1937/1964; Masterson, 1981). The patient's schemas about himself and others will very likely be manifested during therapy. These "in therapy" experiences are often representative of the patient's experiences in many other relationships in the past and the present. For example, a woman became very angry with the therapist, arguing that he "did not listen." If the therapist had responded defensively—"I am listening!"—this would have confirmed the patient's negative schema. However, the therapist chose instead to focus on the patient's current emotions: anger and anxiety (see Greenberg & Paivio, 1997). The core emotions, however, were "behind" these initial emotions.

THERAPIST: How did you feel when you thought I wasn't listening?

PATIENT: I felt really pissed off. Like I wanted to hit you.

THERAPIST: Those are really strong feelings. And it does bother you—as it would anyone—when you are not heard. But I wonder if there's more going on for you in this. Did this remind you of anyone in your past?

PATIENT: Yeah. When I was a kid my mother would always complain about her problems with Dad, and if I had anything to talk about she just told me to be quiet and not complain as much.

THERAPIST: That must have been hard for you. How did you feel?

PATIENT: Like I do now. I felt really angry. Like I wanted to scream.

THERAPIST: But did you feel anything else?

PATIENT: Yes. I felt hurt and humiliated.

The therapist and the patient then examined other relationships in which the patient did not feel heard or understood—such as her relationships with her husband and her best friend. Moreover, her recurrent anger at her mother, from childhood, was quickly activated with other people, leading her to escalate conflicts when she was not heard. This then led other people to either argue with her or withdraw, further supporting her negative schema.

MODIFYING THE SCHEMA BY MODIFYING THE DEFENSES

A central component of schema therapy is to decrease the impact of defensive maneuvers. For example, a woman complained that she was overworked and that her marriage was unfulfilling. She presented with a severe major depressive disorder, with her current episode lasting 2 years. Her previous therapist appeared to have an exploitative approach, asking the patient to do favors for her. During the course of therapy, the patient often dissociated, failing to recognize what we were talking about, often forgetting the train of thought in the sessions. Whenever we discussed her needs in her marriage or at work, she asked for reassurance: "Is that OK for me to want this?" Her core schema in her marriage and at work was that she was "undeserving" and "unlovable." Whenever she thought of asserting herself, she also thought: "I must be selfish. All I think of is myself." Her developmental history indicated that her mother, who received little or no affection from the patient's father, had used the patient as a surrogate for attention and nurturance. Thus, the patient, as a child, would nurture and reassure the mother. Whenever the child/patient expressed any needs, the mother would label her as "selfish."

Since her defensive maneuvers were interfering with her progress, we decided to make the defenses the focus of the treatment for a while. *Defenses* were defined as any experiences or behaviors that interfered with identifying and challenging her belief that she was unlovable and undeserving. The defenses that the therapist and patient identified included the following: spacing out in sessions (dissociating), changing the topic when her needs were being discussed, emotional blunting, talking about someone else's problems, missing sessions, procrastinating on any assertion outside of sessions, allowing work to interfere with her needs, and not getting enough sleep.

Focusing on Cognitive Biases That Maintain the Schema

After the patient recognizes that she engages in behaviors that maintain the schema, the therapist should direct her attention to how her cognitive biases reinforce her negative schema. In the case of this patient, her distortions included minimizing her positives ("I really didn't accomplish much at work"), overgeneralizing a negative experience ("Everything I say is stupid"), fortune telling ("If I assert myself, he'll get enraged"), and labeling ("I'm just selfish"). The therapist can use many standard techniques to challenge these cognitive distortions, attempting to examine how the schema is maintained. These include examining the evidence for and against the thought ("Let's list some things that you have accomplished and some things that are still left to do"), using the double-standard technique ("Would you think that your friend Susan is selfish if she asserted herself? Why not?"), and challenging the logic ("Is it reasonable to think that if someone makes one mistake, then she is 'stupid'?"). The therapist should continue to emphasize the idea that "Because you have these biases and distortions in the way you think, you keep reinforcing this negative belief about yourself that you are undeserving."

EXAMINING HOW THE DEFENSES HAVE WORKED

The patient has now categorized and recognized some of her defensive maneuvers and is aware of the typical automatic thoughts, compensations, avoidance, conditional rules, and schemas. The therapist can next introduce the following idea: "How have your distortions and biases in thinking led you to maintain your negative beliefs about yourself [and others]?" For example, the patient who believes he is a loser can recognize that this belief is maintained by mind reading ("He thinks I'm a loser"), discounting the positives ("Doing well on the exam doesn't count. It was easy"), or all-or-nothing thinking ("I don't do well on anything"). Compensations, such as trying to do a perfect job in order to prove you are not a "loser," can also illustrate the maintenance of the negative schema since the patient may not have attempted to do "just OK" to find out that less-than-perfect is acceptable. The therapist should discuss avoidant strategies, such as procrastinating on tasks or selecting very easy tasks, to illustrate for the patient how he may have avoided any evidence that he can pursue challenging tasks without being perfect—that is, he could have been more successful by pursuing more tasks at less-than-perfect levels of performance. By avoiding tasks (or relationships) he has reinforced his belief that he is a loser. The therapist should indicate, "You are not a loser. You have simply avoided playing the game."

SETTING UP PREDICTIONS TO DISCONFIRM THE SCHEMA

As with confronting any belief or fear, the real "test" for the patient involves participating in behavioral experiments that challenge the schema. Unfortunately, many schemas have not been open to disconfirmation. Because the patient utilizes a "protective belt" of avoidance and compensation, he seldom confronts a challenge to his schema. Moreover, disconfirming the schema is difficult, since contrary evidence is discounted as an aberration. Consequently, the therapist must confront the patient with the fact that he seldom allows his schema to be "tested." The patient and therapist can collaborate to develop "experiments" that will test the validity of the negative schemas—tests that can be stipulated in behavioral terms.

One useful experiment is to conduct a "poll" of friends and colleagues. For example, the patient who believes that she is "undeserving" can conduct a poll of her friends by asking questions such as: "What would you think of me if I told my husband that he wasn't meeting my needs for affection?" or "What would you think of me if I didn't work as hard as I do?" One patient, who believed that he had to be very successful financially to please his girlfriend, was able to test out this belief by asking her, "What would you think of me if I made half as much money?" Another patient, who believed that he always had to appear sexually virile (in order to compensate for his core schema of being "unmanly and weak"), was able to test out his belief by saying to a woman, at an intimate moment, "I sometimes find it takes me a while to feel comfortable sexually. I guess I'm sensitive in that way."

In each of these foregoing cases, the patient was asked to make specific predictions based on the most extreme manifestation of his or her schema: "My friends would think I am selfish and lazy," "My girlfriend will think I'm a failure," or "My partner will think that I'm weak and unmanly—she won't want to be with me again." The patient and the therapist can begin a long process of "schema predictions" and how these predictions stand up to verification.

MODIFYING THE INTERACTIVE REALITY

In each case mentioned above the outcome was quite favorable. But what would happen if the patient predicted a negative outcome and the negative outcome actually occurred? Does this confirm the negative schema? For example, what if the man asked his girlfriend if she would still want him if he made less money, and she said "No"? The therapist should anticipate this possible outcome. The therapist can ask a question: "Are your friends loving and accepting, or do they have some of the same biases in thinking that you have?" A compulsive and narcissistic man, obsessed with material success, anticipated that some of his friends would think less of him if he had less money. This led to a discussion about how his choice of friends reinforced his negative view of himself and others—that is, being worthwhile was equated with financial success. (His situation was compared to that of an alcoholic whose friends are alcoholics who help him to maintain his problem.)

The patient's attempts to experiment and challenge his schema may lead him to examine the "interactive reality" that he lives in. Is he surrounding himself with people who are "schema-consistent"—that is, who maintain his pathology by reflecting his core negative assumptions? The therapist may ask, "What kinds of beliefs about yourself would you have if you had different friends?" One patient, obsessed with material success, indicated that he actually chose friends whom he knew wanted his "friendship" only for business purposes. He indicated that he preferred it this way because he knew how to play the game of being a successful investor—and he knew that he could never trust his "friends" with anything intimate about himself. Thus, his interactive reality was one of narcissistic materialism—but this was a conscious choice to prevent him from being vulnerable to trusting others. As he progressed in therapy, modifying his schema and his depression, his interactive world changed. He began to focus more on old friends who cared about him and he distanced himself from those "friends" who had a parasitic relationship with him.

ANTICIPATING SCHEMATIC RESISTANCE

Once the patient and the therapist have identified specific schemas, they can begin to anticipate how these schemas might interfere with therapy: "Just as your schemas about yourself and others have interfered with your healthy goals in your life, we can expect these schemas to interfere with therapy. How do you think your schema of [being undeserving] will interfere with your getting help from me?" The therapist and the patient can identify how the schema will affect how the patient feels about being heard in therapy ("He'll think my needs are trivial"), setting the agenda ("My problems are not important enough"), doing homework ("I'm focusing too much on my problems"), and continuing in therapy ("This is self-indulgent"). The patient's schemas about others can be identified as potential problems in therapy. For example, the patient who believes that people are judgmental and rejecting will be inclined to think that the therapist will reject him. So the therapist can ask, "What can we anticipate will happen if you think I will be judgmental and rejecting?" The patient might anticipate that he will conceal shameful material from the therapist, try to please the therapist, and not give the therapist negative feedback.

These schemas and automatic thoughts can then be given as homework. The patient can conduct a cost–benefit analysis of approaching therapy with the negative schemas, examine evidence for and against the schemas in therapy, identify how he could disconfirm his schemas through experiments or behavior within therapy, and identify problems to be solved within sessions. *By acting on the schema we can prevent the schema from acting out and acting on us.*

USING DEVELOPMENTAL ANALYSIS

As I indicated earlier, many maladaptive schemas were formed during early childhood. The therapist can explore the meaning of these schemas by asking the patient to identify his or her first memories of feeling bad (as related to the schema). The patient's attention may be drawn toward how these bad feelings are experienced physically, through bodily sensations and feelings (Greenberg & Paivio, 1997). The therapist can ask the patient to recall visual images from childhood that are associated with these bad feelings. Many times the patient recalls feeling small, isolated, alone, or even in the dark. The patient's symbolic language can also be informative: "I felt like I was frozen in my footsteps. That I couldn't move." The therapist can utilize experiential and imagery techniques, such as intensifying the experience and sensations of the bad feelings associated with the schema, asking the patient to provide details of the early images, having the patient repeat the image while being verbally soothed by the therapist, modifying the image through restructuring it so that the patient is victorious, and using the empty-chair technique in which the patient challenges the source of the schema (see Leahy, 1996a; Leahy & Holland, 2000).

As the patient restructures the experience of the early origins of the schema, he may write out a "Bill of Rights" and a letter to the source of the schema, expressing his anger toward the injury or humiliation and identifying the healthy aspects of the self. The patient can then identify the healthy, adaptive needs that he has—for example, the need to be respected, to be cared for, and to be treated fairly. These adaptive needs can then be linked to adaptive functions of therapy—for example, "I can get the respect and understanding that I want in therapy." The patient can also indicate other sources of support in the present: "I can get these needs met with my partner and with my friends and through myself."

Establishing Collaborative Rules

While the patient is making progress on these schematic issues, the therapist and the patient can identify how these needs can be met in therapy. For example, the patient whose schema is one of being undeserving may identify how the adaptive needs of being taken care of can be realized in sessions. The patient can be encouraged to request the therapist to ask about his or her feelings, unfinished business, frustrations, or ways in which he or she has been misunderstood. The therapist may also offer suggestions that will interfere with the negative schema: "Your schema is that you are undeserving. What if I were to ask you periodically, 'Is there anything that you are avoiding bringing up or requesting of me because you doubt your right to do so?' "

Collaborative rules may also include the understanding that both patient and therapist may disappoint the other: "What would you think if I let you down at some point?" The therapist and the patient can collaborate regarding potential disappointments, recognizing that these can be part of the process of working together and that one should not jump to conclusions and label self or other. Furthermore, disappointments can be used as opportunities for assertion, validation, and mutual problem solving, all of which may act in opposition to the schemas.

SUMMARY

The importance of schemas in therapy has been stressed in recent years (Beck et al., 1990; J. Beck, 1996; Leahy, 1996a, 1997d, 1997e, 1997f;

Leahy & Holland, 2000; Needleman, 1999; Tompkins, 1999; Young, 1990). It is beyond the scope of this book to adequately cover the many vicissitudes of schemas in therapy. However, individuals (and couples) may benefit from an understanding of their habitual biases in thinking and how these biases have given rise to avoidant and compensatory mechanisms. Schemas are like closed systems that maintain themselves and exclude from awareness intrusive information that promotes change.

In confronting the patient's schemas, the therapist will be confronting the patient's resistance. Attempts to encourage the dependent patient to become more independent will result in increased clinging. Similarly, attempts to encourage a narcissistic patient to develop realistic expectations may result in increased demands and devaluation of therapy. The therapist will not be successful if she only identifies negative thoughts and distortions. Rather, she must identify the specific content areas of schemas and how these schemas have been established and have become self-fulfilling prophecies.

I have identified numerous interventions and strategies for modifying schemas in this chapter. But, one may look at each chapter in this book as an approach to modifying schemas. For example, validation and emotional dysregulation are related to schema change, just as addressing the victim role may affect the schema. Perhaps the schema is "core," but the approaches to modifying it are varied.

7

Moral Resistance

COMPULSIVE RESPONSIBILITY

MORAL REASONING

Therapists often pride themselves on their moral neutrality, claiming that it is not their business to make moral judgments about what is right or what is wrong. Some clinicians argue that moral rules or imperatives are unscientific or even meaningless because they are neither universal nor open to empirical disconfirmation (Ellis, 1985). Indeed, the therapist may find herself attempting to modify the imperatives the patient uses to judge himself and others. Even though patients hold some imperatives that are difficult or impossible to comply with, they will often adhere to these beliefs, even when these beliefs cause them considerable distress.

The cognitive-behavioral therapist attempts to modify the patient's thinking by guiding the patient to understand the hedonic value or cost involved. The assumption is that the patient can be led to recognize that the costs of a particular belief or action outweigh its benefits. This recognition will motivate the patient to change. Similarly, cognitive therapists attempt to illustrate internal contradictions or the lack of factual evidence to support the patient's beliefs, hoping this appeal to rationality will persuade the patient to modify his thinking and behavior toward more adaptive modes.

Urging individuals to modify their beliefs by appeals to utility and logic is the result of the influence of the Enlightenment on psychotherapy (Mahoney, 1991). Appeals to the "rational principle"—that is, one is drawn toward the logic and facts upholding a belief—are based on an assumption that individuals will prefer rationality over irrationality. Similarly, appeals to utilitarianism—that is, weighing the benefits and costs of beliefs and behaviors—assume that individuals are motivated by the hedonic value of their actions. These pragmatic and rationalistic approaches to psychology may work for some individuals, but many individuals will resist change if they believe there are moral or ethical issues involved. It is irrelevant that the therapist does not perceive that the issues in question are moral or ethical: it is sufficient that the patient labels them so. Certainly, the history of the 20th century, with an estimated 120 million deaths due to state-sponsored violence, is hardly a history of hedonic calculus and rationality. People will suffer enormous hardship in the pursuit of what they believe is a moral or ethical cause.

In this chapter and the next I examine two very different kinds of moral resistance. In the present chapter, I examine the resistance of individual moral responsibility among compulsive individuals—that is, an exaggerated emphasis on the self as cause and responsible agent—and the processes whereby anxious patients view themselves as negligent. Individuals resisting in this way assume too great a responsibility for events. Therapist attempts to modify this moral resistance often result in the patient's belief that the goal of therapy is to make him into a careless and immoral person.

In the next chapter, I examine cases in which the individual blames others for his problem. The victim views moral irresponsibility as residing in other people and feels entitled to special status. These *victim scripts* involve claims that one's problems are enormous, unsolvable by the self, and caused by others, who are now responsible for compensating the patient. Attempts to modify these scripts often provoke claims that the therapist does not care about the patient or understand the degree of pain unfairly suffered by the patient. Further attempts to challenge these victim scripts often result in the patient feeling victimized by the therapist.

Throughout these two chapters, I propose that the clinician will be more effective if he or she enters into the mode of thinking characterized by moral judgment. Many individuals, confronted simply with a cost–benefit analysis of their moral imperatives, will reject the hedonic solution. Indeed, morality judgments are judgments that are not necessarily practical or self-serving—they may often call for sacrifice and responsibility, where one's immediate gratification is deterred. Instead of using a simple pragmatic approach to moral judgments—which will not be convincing to many patients—I will attempt to develop the view that the patient can shift his thinking from "inappropriate" or "self-contradictory" moral rules to "appropriate" and "consistent" moral rules. By adapting the language of the moral mode of thinking, therapists may be better able to influence the resistant patient's use of imperatives. Thus, we do not abandon imperatives, but rather replace them with better imperatives.

INDIVIDUAL MORAL
RESPONSIBILITY AS RESISTANCE

Throughout my discussion in this section I will be referring to "shoulds" that the therapist recognizes as harmful to the patient. These shoulds create guilt, depression, rage, or anxiety in the patient, cause him to set unrealistic goals, and appear to be arbitrarily applied. The goal of cognitive therapy is not to address the entire moral code of the patient. Only when these moral imperatives contribute significantly to the patient's distress—and, here, to the patient's resistance—do we examine these should statements.

Few of us would want to live in a world in which we believed that no one would act responsibly and that no one could be trusted for anything. The legal philosopher Lon Fuller (1931/1967) proposes that a number of "legal fictions" bind us together as a society, allowing us some sense of predictability, continuity, and justification. Legal and moral rules, especially rules of conventional conduct (or etiquette), are not derived from observations of physical reality, nor do they have the same scientific status as laws of physics. Some cognitive-behavioral therapists, such as Ellis (1985; Ellis & Grieger, 1977), have viewed should statements as arbitrary and irrational, and have suggested that these should statements actually constitute preferences. The goal of therapy, according to this model, is to free the individual from the "tyranny of the shoulds."

There are many arbitrary imperatives that contribute to the anxiety, depression, and anger of individuals, but therapists who boldly state to their patients that should statements do not have the same scientific status as propositions in physics may promote even greater resistance on the part of their patients. It can be an excellent therapeutic strategy to point out the arbitrary and self-defeating nature of some shoulds—such as "I should be perfect"—but this strategy can backfire on the therapist if his goal is to get his patient to abandon any sense of responsibility.

Very few people in our society—or any society—do not believe in shoulds (Wilson, 1993). In almost all societies, and among almost all people, there are should statements pertaining to self-control, honesty, innocence, and deservingness (Wilson, 1993). This does not imply that people live up to their ideals, but some have argued convincingly that social relations would be close to impossible without a binding moral code. Many rational therapists who believe that should statements are irrational would quickly express their own should rules if someone lied to them, cheated them, or hurt them. They would respond with outrage, not because they are irrational, but because they are human.

If we attack the very foundation of *any* moral code for our patients, we run the risk of alienating those patients from therapy. Patients who complain that their impression of cognitive therapy is that they have to give up all their moral shoulds will soon make a decision to give up therapy rather than a belief that people (including themselves) should act morally or responsibly. The reflective patient, confronted with the idea that all should statements are irrational, often concludes that the therapist is living in a world that is different from his own world. That patient may fear that his sense of integrity—his belief that he is, at the least, trying to be a "good, decent, moral person"—is threatened by the therapist's complete "moral relativism"—indeed, by the therapist's apparent moral nihilism. Indeed, the should statements may constitute the patient's "ideal self"; abandoning this ideal self may imply to the patient that he or she is an empty, meaningless, amoral individual.

Good Shoulds and Bad Shoulds

Consequently, the strategy that I advocate is to help the patient develop "good shoulds" and to get rid of "bad shoulds." I indicate to the patient that we need moral and ethical rules to guide us—even if we end up falling short of these rules. The goal in therapy is to be able to distinguish between good rules and bad rules. By working together, therapist and patient can develop a set of "tests" of whether a rule is a bad or a good rule. Cognitive therapists often examine rules by looking at the costs and benefits and the evidence for and against a "proposition." Consider lying. The cognitive therapist might help the patient examine the costs and benefits of lying, leading the patient to the conclusion that lying is in his interests. He might then examine the evidence for and against the idea that people should lie by examining the universality of lying. (This, of course, does not imply that lying is right simply because a lot of people lie.) The patient might conclude that he is free to lie whenever he chooses.

Some patients, however, view this kind of reasoning as facile and empty. These individuals respond by saying something like: "You are trying to get me to do things simply because they feel good to me. This is not a moral rule—this is selfishness." Of course, the patient is correct. Simply examining its hedonistic value for the self does not constitute a test of a moral rule. For example, imagine a white male slave owner in the South in 1830. He might conclude that the benefits outweigh the costs of owning a slave. He might point out that many people do own slaves and that the U.S. government condones slave ownership. He might conclude that he is acting morally—and, of course, he would be wrong.

A Preview of Appropriate Shoulds

Throughout this chapter, I will analyze the nature of causal reasoning and judgments of responsibility in an attempt to develop a model of appropriate standards for moral rules. Let me preface this by saying that I am not developing a new "Ten Commandments"; rather, I will outline some general confusions in moral reasoning that may account for the errors in moral logic among individuals who are inappropriately judgmental. The reader may anticipate what the nature of these guidelines are by considering the line of inquiry provided below.

The patient's resistance to changing shoulds is often reduced when the therapist pursues the following line of reasoning:

- It is important to have a moral or ethical guideline for yourself and others. Cognitive therapy does not try to eliminate morality or ethics. There are some things that people should do and other things they should not do.
- One goal in therapy is to be able to determine what should statements you use and how these shoulds are affecting the way you feel and how you react to other people.
- It is important to determine what "good moral or ethical rules" are. In order to do this, I would suggest the following guidelines:

1. Concisely state your should statement. For example, *"I should be more successful than everyone."*
2. What are the consequences for you of having this rule? *"I feel pressured, inferior, competitive, and self-critical, but maybe I'll try harder."*
3. What would the consequences be if everyone thought they should be more successful than everyone else? *"This would be unrealistic. Only one person could do better than everyone, so almost everyone would feel like a failure."*
4. If we made this a universal rule that we applied to everyone, would this enhance human dignity or detract from it? *"It would detract from human dignity because almost everyone would feel miserable."*
5. Would you want to live in a world in which this was a universal rule that had to be applied to everyone at all times? *"No, because I would be miserable and so would everyone else."*
6. What would be a better guideline to apply to everyone? *"People can try to do as well as they can, without putting too much pressure on themselves."*
7. If we apply it to everyone, then we must apply it to you. *"Then I*

would have to conclude that I can try hard, but I don't have to put too much pressure on myself. I don't have to be perfect."

The general guiding principle for testing a moral rule is to ask what the world would be like if we applied this rule to everyone. For example, if we were to think that "lying is OK," then we can ask whether we would want to live in a world in which it was OK for everyone to lie at all times. Similarly, if we thought that "I should be perfect" was a good rule, we can ask, "Would you want to live in a world where everyone had to be perfect?"

Some people believe "acting responsibly" is the same thing as putting enormous pressure on themselves. The obsessive–compulsive patient may believe that checking every possible source of a mistake is the same thing as being responsible. However, if we use the universal-rule guide, we could ask, "Would it be a good rule to demand that everyone in the world should check every possible source of error, even if it makes them miserable?" If this is not a good rule for everyone, then it is irresponsible to apply this rule to yourself. It is not responsible to apply unreasonable rules to people—and the patient him- or herself is a person.

In the pages to follow, I draw upon legal and moral theory to develop distinctions about moral responsibility and negligence. Specific attention is given to how various components of moral reasoning are confused in the minds of judgmental patients. The goal of therapy will be to assist the patient in recognizing these important distinctions and to develop more appropriate and consistent standards of conduct.

NEGLIGENCE RESPONSIBILITY

Possible Cause and Obligation

The patient believes that once he has recognized that he could be a possible cause of a negative outcome, then he is obligated to do whatever he can to prevent that outcome. This belief is reflected in the resistance to change among obsessive–compulsives, hypochondriacs, and generalized anxiety patients. The obsessive–compulsive individual believes that if he thinks he might have made a mistake, then he should check everything. The hypochondriac believes that if it is possible that he could have an illness, then he must do everything to determine with absolute certainty that he does not have the illness. The generalized anxiety patient believes that he should worry about the possibility of highly improbable events that could be prevented (Salkovskis, 1989, 1996; Salkovskis & Kirk, 1997; Wells, 1997).

The foregoing individuals make little distinction among the following factors that affect judgments of responsibility: prior event, prior cause, reasonable cause, and ethical or moral responsibility. (See Table 7.1 for examples of errors in reasoning about responsibility.)

- A *prior event* is an occurrence that happens before another event, but which may not be causal—in the sense that it is not necessary, sufficient, or contributory. For example, I might wear a red tie, walk to my office, and witness a car accident. This does not mean that my tie caused the accident.
- A *prior cause* does not always imply moral responsibility or guilt. For example, if someone owes me money, and I place him in collection, I may be (part of) a prior cause of his distress. However, I am not "responsible" in the moral sense, since he did not fulfill his part of the contract. His nonpayment of a debt is another prior cause that takes precedence over my action to take collection that accounts for the distress of the debtor.
- I make a distinction between a prior cause and a reasonable cause that accounts for our ascription of moral responsibility. The reasonable cause of the distress for the debtor is his or her irresponsibility in not paying the debt.

The obsessive patient does not consider mitigating factors that affect moral responsibility, such as lack of foresight, lack of malicious intention, absence of a contractual obligation, shared responsibility, or other factors. The moral perfectionism of these individuals leads them to take a view of absolute morality—they assume, "No matter what the conditions are, anything I do that could contribute to a negative outcome makes me absolutely responsible." Thus mitigating factors, such as provocation or lack of foresight or lack of malicious intentions, are not considered. In a way similar to Piaget's (1934) description of moral realism, I refer to this exaggerated focus on the self as causal responsible as "egocentric morality." The obsessive is unable to decenter (or refocus) from one possible cause (the self) to other possible, more probable causes that are more relevant to responsibility (see Leahy, 2000d).

Proximate Cause

Obsessive beliefs in responsibility ignore *transitivity of cause* such that one cause, earlier in a sequence, pervades all other causes later in the sequence. Thus, the obsessive believes that his behavior on Monday may have an effect on events on Friday, irrespective of all other events beyond his control that may transpire between Monday and Friday. The importance of transitivity of cause is reflected in concepts of legal responsibil-

TABLE 7.1. Errors in Reasoning about Responsibility (Prior Event, Prior Cause, Reasonable Cause, and Ethical or Moral Responsibility)

Because . . .	Therefore . . .	Error
An event A occurred earlier than event B.	A is a cause of B.	Prior occurrence is not always causal. For example, I had breakfast this morning and a plane crashed this afternoon. The breakfast did not cause the plane crash.
My behavior preceded the event.	I am responsible for the outcome.	1. There may be many other intervening causes of the outcome. [transitivity] 2. The other person may have contributed to the outcome. [contributory negligence]
If I had not done X (prior cause), then Y (outcome) would not have occurred.	1. I am the cause of the outcome. 2. I am morally responsible for the outcome.	1. Not necessarily. There may be many other causes of the outcome that contributed to this. [multiple causality] 2. It is possible for me to be a cause of an outcome that someone else deserves. [deservingness]
I knew it was possible that I could check something.	I am responsible for checking.	Just because something is "possible," it does not follow that I am responsible. The question is, "Would a reasonable person have checked?" Possibility of cause does not mean responsibility for outcome. We cannot be perfect. [reasonable person criteria]
I was ill and I couldn't get out of bed.	I should have gone to work. I am irresponsible.	Illness is a mitigating factor: we excuse people from certain obligations when they have reduced capacity [mitigation]
I did something that someone else did not want me to do.	I am responsible for his feelings.	I had no agreement that I would comply with his wishes. I am free to do what I choose to do. I was not intentionally malicious. [intention; lack of contractual obligation]
It was a terrible outcome.	I am responsible.	Severity of outcome does not determine responsibility—only foresight, intention, and reasonable cause determine my responsibility. [distinction between outcome and responsibility]
It is a terrible thing that this happened and no matter what I did, it made no difference.	I am responsible.	I am only responsible for what I can do, not for the outcome. [responsibility implies capability]

ity. The law identifies the important cause as the *proximate cause,* which is the cause that is viewed as the event, behavior, or omission of behavior that produced the outcome (Hart & Honore, 1985). It is not a simple procedure to determine the proximate cause. There are many possible events, behaviors, or omissions prior to an event. However, in determining the proximate cause, we tend to consider the likelihood of the outcome if the behavior (or omission of behavior) was present versus not present. For example, in the case of the obsessive, (1) not checking the lock for the tenth time, (2) then finding that the house was broken into later, (3) would lead him to conclude that he did not check the locks enough. But few people would consider the omission of checking the locks yet more times as the proximate cause of the break-in. This is because we know that break-ins of houses are not contingent on checking the tenth time: we do not believe that one needs to check a tenth time to assure the safety of the house—once would be sufficient. There are other causes more relevant to the break-in to which we ascribe responsibility—for example, the fact that the house was being surveilled by burglars or that all the neighbors knew you would be out of town for 10 days and the house is isolated from the road.

Another way of questioning whether a behavior or omission is a proximate cause is to examine the *intervening causes.* In the case of the lock checking described above, the intervening causes after the "omission" of checking included the burglars driving through the area, casing houses, planning a break-in, cutting the alarm wires, breaking in, stealing the material, and escaping. These intervening causes are more probable and plausible causes of the burglary. You may check your locks every day, but burglars are not trying to break in every day. Even if you were somewhat obsessive and said, "I did not check my locks enough," you would attribute most of the causality and responsibility to the burglars. Your insurance company would not fault your behavior because you did not check the locks the tenth time.

Contributory Negligence

Related to the idea of proximate cause and intervening causes or events is the idea of *contributory negligence.* In this case, we consider to what extent others who suffered harm may have contributed to their own negative outcome. To take an extreme example, let us say that there is a deep hole on my property. To warn others, I place a fence around the hole and put up a sign to warn people of the potential danger. A guest who has had too much to drink ignores the warning sign, climbs over the fence, and falls into the hole. He has contributed to his own harm and therefore shares some, if not all, of the "fault" for the harm he suffered.

Obsessives ignore the transitivity of causes, intervening causes, reasonable cause, proximate cause, and contributory negligence. To the obsessive, if one's behavior is a prior event, it is therefore a prior cause, which is the proximate cause, regardless of other intervening causes or the contributory negligence of others. I refer to this as *responsibility imperialism* because it reflects the belief in pervasive, overriding responsibility attributed to the self (see also Rachman, 1993).

Take the case of a journalist who was concerned that if he writes an article for the newspaper, it might cause undue emotional harm to an individual who would be mentioned in the article. The article addressed possible housing violations committed by a landlord mentioned in the article. The patient hypothesized that the landlord would then become upset and that this might affect the landlord's marriage.

Here the obsessive–compulsive patient links an event (writing an article) with a supposed outcome (the individual gets upset). Of course, the prior event may have nothing to do with another subsequent event (the individual gets upset). In fact, it is possible that the individual might not get very upset, or that he might get upset because he has a problematic marriage, or that he might get upset because he has to face the consequences of his own misbehavior.

The next link in the chain is to believe that it is not reasonable to write the article if it is *possible* someone might be upset. The question for the nonobsessive patient is, "What is the reasonable thing to do?" Would reasonable journalists avoid writing *any* article that had *any* possibility of affecting *any* person?

Finally, the obsessive patient concludes that he has an ethical or moral responsibility either to avoid writing the article or to be absolutely sure that no one could be affected negatively. The obsessive patient believes that moral responsibility is established by the fact that a prior event *could be* a prior cause, which *could be* a reasonable cause, *which establishes* moral responsibility. He ignores the issues of proximate cause, contributory negligence, and intervening causes. He is the sole cause and the sole responsibility.

RATIONAL RESPONSIBILITY

In contrast to this view that a prior event that could lead to a negative outcome establishes moral responsibility, we should consider how nonobsessive individuals evaluate moral responsibility. Several factors are involved in considering moral responsibility or degree of responsibility (Hare, 1981; Hart, 1968). First, we consider *whether a behavior actually resulted in a negative outcome*. There must be some logical, factual, and causative link between a behavior and an outcome. For example, if I drive my car into the back of someone else's car, then my driving was a logical, factual, and causative event of the damage to the other car. In the journalist case described above, it is not logical to conclude that an article about housing code violations will lead to someone's divorce, it has not been established as a fact, and there are too many hypothesized intervening events to view it as a causative link. In other words, it is hardly a proximate cause of the hypothesized divorce.

Second, we consider *what the reasonable person would know or do* in the same situation. For example, if I am driving along the road and your car runs a stop sign and I hit it, it is unlikely that I will be found culpable: it would not be reasonable for me to *foresee* that you would ignore a stop sign and drive directly in front of my car. This is known as the *reasonable man doctrine* in the law. In the journalist case described above, the reasonable person would not know that an article about housing violations would end in divorce.

A third way of establishing responsibility would be to examine my *contractual obligations* with another person. Contractual obligations are established by a direct or implied statement that each party to the contract derives some stated benefit in the exchange. Both parties need to be aware of the agreement and a benefit (payment) must be paid. For example, if I ask someone to cut my grass and he agrees to come on Monday, but fails to show up, the contract is voided and I do not pay him. Contracts involve a *promise to perform*, where both parties understand what the promise is. If I do not pay the grass cutter, his failure to perform the service as promised voids the contract. If I had paid him beforehand, then the contract is still applicable and I can claim damages (the fee paid).

The obsessive journalist has no contractual obligation with the landlord. He does not even know the landlord, nor have they entered into any agreements. There has been no promise to perform anything for the landlord nor has the landlord paid a fee for good public relations from the journalist. The journalist promised no benefits from his article. Therefore, there is no obligation to be derived from a contract. Furthermore, one could argue that the journalist has an obligation to the publisher and, indirectly, to the readers of his newspaper to write the truth about housing violations.

A fourth factor in establishing responsibility is to examine *conventional expectations*. What would most people in the position of the journalist expect? *Conventions* are socially prescribed agreements as to what is acceptable behavior. Presumably, when one is following conventional agreements, there is some protection against charges of immorality, although this is not a total protection. The obsessive journalist ignores the conventional expectation that journalists write the truth and do not censor their writing because someone might not like what they write. Consequently, there is no moral obligation if there is no conventional expectation that is violated by writing the article.

Fifth, we consider *malicious intention* in evaluating responsibility. (In the law, this is referred to as *mens rea*—which may be loosely translated as *state of mind* or *guilty mind* [Hart & Honore, 1985].) Did the individual fully intend the negative outcome? For example, suppose that I see that you are not slowing down as you approach a stop sign in front of me. I have enough time to stop and avoid hitting your car even if you run the stop sign. But suppose that I am in a particularly bad mood this morning, I have had far too much caffeine, and I am envious of the fact that your car is much more attractive than mine. I say to myself "Who the hell does he think he is?" I accelerate as I go after your car, hit you on the passenger side, and say to myself "That'll teach him!" You might correctly conclude that I had a malicious intention and proceed to have me arrested on assault charges—in fact, assault with a deadly weapon.

But, of course, that is not what happened. I never saw you coming. And lack of foresight—that is, lack of the ability to see what is coming— is a good defense against guilty intentions. Consequently, my inability to see your car as it approached the stop sign and my inability to stop my car in time—as well as your irresponsibility in running the stop sign—results in the legal and moral responsibility falling on your shoulders, not mine. Characteristically, obsessives do not consider the "guilty mind" theory or malicious intention in evaluating their culpability. In the case of the journalist, his intentions were not malicious: it was not his plan to cause harm.

Sixth, we examine *shared responsibility* in determining the assignment of blame. When we think of assigning responsibility for an outcome—for example, divorce—we may wish to consider the relative contributions of each participant. One can say that each was a "cause" of the relationship ending, since each was a participant whose choices, responses, and behaviors were contributory to the relationship.

Finally, when we think of a cause (and consequent) responsibility, we consider whether *the cause is something that is ordinarily* not *present*, but that was present for this particular sequence of events. For example, we would say, in the example of the car accident described above, that *ordinarily* I get into my car, drive along the street, and obey the traffic regulations. However, we would say that *ordinarily it is not true* that you drive your car right through stop signs. This evaluation of cause and effect refers to our sharing knowledge about what is *generally* true—that is, one is usually safe in driving down the street obeying traffic laws and one is often unsafe driving through stop signs without looking. The obsessive ignores the information arising from generalizations about what ordinarily occurs and claims that one can be a cause or have responsibility for particular negative events simply because one's actions are part of a sequence of events prior to the outcome. Thus the obsessive would think that he is responsible for the accident simply by virtue of the fact that he is driving along and, if he had been totally hypervigilant, could have been able to see the car driving through the stop sign.

OBSESSIVE CONCEPTS OF NEGLIGENCE

Obsessive–compulsives and chronic worriers may resist change because they believe they are responsible for preventing negative events once they have thought of a way that they could be avoided (Salkovskis, 1989, 1996; Salkovskis & Kirk, 1997). For example, a hypochondriacal patient indicated that, once she thought a skin discoloration could possibly be cancerous, she had a responsibility to do whatever she could to check it out. Even though she realized that it was highly improbable that it could be cancerous, she claimed that she would be negligent in not checking it out since the knowledge of the possibility implied a responsibility to act. Negligence was defined as the responsibility that follows from an awareness of a possible cause that could possibly be prevented.

Similarly, a hypochondriacal man feared that he had been infected with bat urine while walking through a cave. Even though he believed that the chance of this occurring was close to zero, the knowledge of the *possibility* resulted in his belief that he was now responsible to check it out and consider getting antirabies shots. He indicated that knowing that *he could have done otherwise* meant that *he should do otherwise*.

Again, similar to our discussion of cause and responsibility, we can see that the patient following this line of thinking views moral responsibility in *absolute* terms: he has an absolute responsibility to prevent any possible negative event once he has knowledge of the possibility. In contrast to this view of absolute negligence, nonobsessives view negligence in terms of what the reasonable person would be expected to do and what the probabilities are. According to this more relativistic or reasonable view, people are not negligent if they have followed reasonable precautions as evidenced by considering what most people would do in the situation. Similarly, there is an acceptance of constraints on knowledge and control—that is, the individual recognizes that she cannot know everything and that not everything can be controlled.

The obsessive does not try to reduce risk; rather, she tries to *eliminate controllable* risk. The obsessive views herself as negligent if a

possible risk, which could have been avoided, has not been totally elimi-
nated (Salkovskis, 1989, 1996; Salkovskis & Kirk, 1997). For the obsessive, all risk is seen as controllable, and therefore as requiring elimina-
tion. The obsessive is willing to accept risks that cannot be controlled.
For example, a hypochondriac who constantly checked and sought reassurance for a variety of false-alarm symptoms indicated that he did not
fear getting into a car accident. His reasoning was that he had no control
over the actions of others and that he did not bother with worrying
about events over which he had no control. Since he did have control
over seeing doctors for examinations, he believed he would be negligent
if he did not follow through on these checkups.

The nonobsessive views negligence in terms of the balance between
what is reasonable, given the odds of a negative outcome, and the costs
or discomfort of constantly checking. For example, the nonobsessive cal-
culates that the odds of a discoloration being cancerous are close to zero
and that the costs in terms of money, time, and the like, of going to the
doctor weekly is unacceptable. Of course it is possible that this particular discoloration is cancerous, but the probability is viewed as infini-
testimal. The risk theory of the nonobsessive leads her to conclude that
the risk is worth accepting. Negligence is defined, by this theory, as the
willingness to accept higher risks, which could easily be avoided. Reasonable, or nonnegligent, decisions are defined as the willingness to
accept very low risks where the cost of avoiding them would be higher
than the benefit.

Related to the obsessive's view of negligence is the ideal self-image
of many of these resistant patients. The ideal self-image—what they
strive for—is often dictated by the view that a sign of their being a good
person is that they worry—or "take things seriously." For example, a
woman whose son was a professional claimed that worrying about him
was a sign of a "good mother." Consequently, she resisted challenging
her worries about her son because she believed that to modify her worries would imply that she was willing to accept being less than the "good
mother who worries." We examined alternative definitions of a good
mother, such as one who allows her son independence and responsibility,
one who does not nag her grown son, and one who has provided the son
with an upbringing that has helped him achieve many of the things that
he wished to achieve. By these alternative criteria she was able to recognize that she was a good mother and that worrying was not the same
thing as a moral virtue.

However, we recognize that our goal is not to turn our patients into
careless, denying, and pollyannish individuals. One hypochondriacal patient who had previously had cancer (but who had been worrying all his

life about cancer) responded well to cognitive-behavioral therapy. He had decreased his checking to a minimum. He then suggested that he might go a year without checking, against his oncologist's directions. I indicated to him that getting over obsessive checking was not the same thing as being careless about cancer. The goal was to become *prudent*, not *pollyannish*. He followed through with regularly scheduled checkups (as his oncologist requested) and avoided reassurance seeking and checking in between these checkups.

DISTINGUISHING OBLIGATION FROM SERIOUSNESS OF POSSIBLE OUTCOMES

Many obsessives believe they have a greater obligation to do something simply because they can imagine a very serious outcome. For example, a patient who had no history of high-risk behavior felt that he was personally responsible for getting repeated HIV tests even though four had proven negative during the last 2 years. His reasoning was: "You can die from AIDS. Therefore, I should do everything I can to check it out." When confronted with the very low probability of having four false negatives—and reminded that his risk of HIV was close to zero—he responded, "But what if you're the one in 10 million who has false results?" Simply imagining a horrible outcome (dying from AIDS) seemed to confer a personal responsibility to do everything imaginable to check it out.

Obligations regarding negligence are related to the degree of potential harm. For example, the U.S. Food and Drug Administration (FDA) requires stringent tests for all new drugs before they can be marketed, since the potential for harm can be high. However, as with most things in real life, the FDA and other agencies calculate the risk–reward ratios—that is, what are the probabilities and seriousness of potential negative outcomes versus what are the probabilities and magnitude of potential positive outcomes. The risk–reward ratios are calculated in terms of *probabilities and outcomes.*

In contrast, obsessive patients characterized by ideas of *absolute responsibility* believe that they are obligated to act despite the *probabilities* involved. This is illustrated by the illogical but psychologically compelling and familiar statement, "But what if I am *that one?*" This statement is illogical because it ignores the entire issue of group comparisons and probabilities and treats all events as *equally risky*—that is, there are no events for which you cannot be that one. By trying to reduce risk to zero the obsessive patient becomes immobilized.

MODIFYING RESISTANCE BASED
ON INDIVIDUAL RESPONSIBILITY

Individuals who resist change because they believe they are being moral are not convinced by arguments that moral statements are irrational or not empirically based. All-out attacks on should statements by therapists often backfire: the patient may think the therapist is a shallow, even hypocritical, person who has no moral code. In fact, I believe should statements and moral codes are essential to human relationships—we expect people to keep their promises, to show self-control, to avoid harming innocent people, and to respect the rights and human dignity of others. (Indeed, these are the guidelines for the ethical rules of the American Psychological Association.)

If the patient's ideal self-image is based on the view that she is a moral and ethical person, then a psychology of amorality will alienate that patient. I have found that many patients who read the popular books on therapy are offended by the amoral, glib, and dismissive attitude about morality depicted in them. The approach my colleagues and I have found helpful is to try to guide the patient to differentiate between reasonable or good moral rules and rules that do not stand up to a test of a good moral rule. Rather than eradicating should statements, we attempt to develop guidelines for good should statements. Rather than suggest to the patient that she should not care about infringements of moral rules, we attempt to guide the patient to a proportionate and problem-solving response. By doing so, the patient's moral view is respected, her need for moral guidelines is validated, and she is able to develop realistic moral rules.

Taxonomy of Shoulds

The first step is to elicit the should statements, rules, or musts that guide the patient. Examples of these statements are "I should never be negligent" and "If I recognize that there is something that I could do to reduce possible harm, then I am obligated to do it." Other should statements include "I should be perfect," "I should be certain," "I should never do anything that I could regret." Ellis (1985) has outlined numerous shoulds that are typical of depressed, anxious, and angry patients. This taxonomy of shoulds can include imperatives about self ("I should be perfect [superior, always kind, always sure, never hostile, etc.]"), others ("They should be fair [appreciative, rational, reasonable, etc.]"), and events that impact on the self ("Things should work out my way," "I should never get sick," "The subway should never get stuck"). Moreover, the patient may have shoulds about specific relationships ("My husband should always pay attention to me"; "Our sex life should always be great"; "We should never have arguments") (see Baucom & Epstein, 1990; Baucom, 1987).

Identifying Possible Causes and Outcomes

As I indicated above, there are many possible causes of an event—including actual behavior, omissions of behavior, and other events. The overly responsible obsessive or depressive patient characteristically attributes the only relevant cause to himself. In examining his moral reasoning, the therapist should encourage the patient to consider many possible factors other than the self that contribute to an outcome. First, the therapist needs to identify the outcome under consideration—for example, in the case of the journalist, his fear that the landlord would get upset and get divorced. There are two outcomes: upset and divorced. The first question, then, is, "Have these outcomes actually occurred?" The second question is, "Are there other possible—perhaps benign—outcomes?" It is possible that the landlord could address the housing violations, become a better landlord, or pay a fine that would lead to better conditions for the tenants in his building? It is also possible that the journalist's article could encourage other landlords to fulfill their responsibilities. Interestingly, obsessives do not consider other possible benign or positive outcomes.

The error in the journalist's causal analysis is that it suggests the article could be a sufficient and necessary cause of the landlord's divorce. This implies, for the obsessive journalist, a singularity of effectiveness—that his article would be sufficient to end a marriage that was a solid relationship.

Indeed, as indicated in Figure 7.1, it is far more plausible that, should the landlord's marriage end, it would end due to numerous factors—factors that supersede the critical article. The obsessive patient appears to ignore the other possible causes, any one of which is more likely to be determinative of the outcome. Indeed, the other causes of the outcome considered (divorce) are much more likely to be "sufficient causes."

The obsessive resists change because he confuses prior event with sufficient and necessary causes. Also, he ignores the difference between a prior event and a proximate cause. And, finally, he singles out a single behavior on his own part, and ignores the multicausal determination of most real outcomes, and the transitivity of causes.

This patient was able to identify the following as possible causes of the anticipated outcome: the landlord's negligence in the building, the

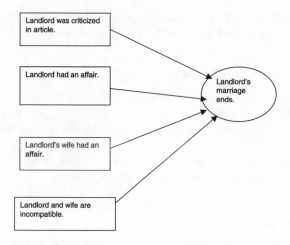

FIGURE 7.1. Possible causes of divorce.

poor condition of the building before the landlord took possession, the landlord's refusal to respond to tenants' requests, the laws that apply to the landlord, the landlord's temper and tendency to blame other people, and the possibility that the landlord has a shaky marriage.

A third question to ask is, "What are the natural consequences of the landlord's behavior?" This is similar to the question, "What is the natural consequence of going outside without an umbrella when it is pouring rain?" The patient was able to recognize that a natural consequence of violating the law is that tenants get angry, hire lawyers, and contact the press, and the landlord gets a bad public reputation. These factors were seen as more contributory or proximate causes of the anticipated outcome.

Validation of Moral Rules

It is generally counterproductive to invalidate the patient's belief in the need for moral rules or should statements. A more useful approach is to validate the general principle of moral rules: "I agree with you that it is important for all of us to act responsibly. Being responsible is something to be proud of and something that is central to who you are. Your standards and expectations for yourself are that you should always be responsible. You feel frustrated and self-critical when you do not act responsibly. Probably, if everyone acted responsibly, the world would be a better place." This foregoing statement indicates to the patient that the therapist understands the necessity for moral rules. However, the next step is to develop guidelines for "good" moral rules (see Table 7.2).

Application of Guidelines

A highly self-critical woman, suffering from major depression, claimed she should not enjoy herself because she was depressed. Her view was that she was not productive when she was depressed, and therefore she should not have pleasurable experiences. We examined her moral rule: "You should not have pleasure if you are not productive." The first test of the rule was to examine its universal application:

> "Would you say that everyone who is not productive should not have any pleasure?"
> "Would you say that someone whose productivity has decreased because of her depression should also be deprived of pleasure?"
> "What kind of world would it be if we decided that we would deprive people of pleasure because they were sick, depressed, or less productive?"

This test of universal application proved to be the most effective challenge for her.

The second challenge that proved to be effective was to examine whether her moral rule advanced human dignity. "Would the value and dignity of human existence be advanced if we applied this rule to you and everyone else?" Again, this challenge was effective since she recognized that depriving depressed people of pleasure would diminish human dignity.

TABLE 7.2. Guidelines for Moral Rules

Guideline	Example
Universal application	Would you make this a rule for everyone?
Capacity differs from should	Would you hold someone responsible for doing what he or she cannot do?
Reasonable expectation	Is it reasonable to expect people to do what almost no one does?
Proportionality	Are you able to make a distinction between smaller and larger consequences?
Human dignity	Does this rule advance human dignity?

Another application of these tests for moral rules was employed with a married man who had angry and violent obsessions, but who never acted them out. He attempted to neutralize these obsessions, which only maintained his belief that they needed to be controlled. He reported guilt over his thoughts, confessing that "I shouldn't have these thoughts." We examined this belief by distinguishing between "could" and "should"—that is, it is illogical to claim that someone should do something if they are unable to do it.

THERAPIST: You said that you should not have these obsessions. What can you do to eliminate them for good?

PATIENT: I can't think of anything. I've tried everything. I've tried to reassure myself, I've tried to stop thinking, I've prayed. I was in therapy for 2 years with someone else but it didn't help.

THERAPIST: So you're saying that you tried to stop but you are unable. You can't.

PATIENT: That's right.

THERAPIST: Do you think that you should be able to do things that you can't do?

PATIENT: No. But I want to stop and I can't.

THERAPIST: Should you be able to be a professional basketball player simply because you would like to be?

PATIENT: I couldn't do that. I'm not tall enough.

THERAPIST: Should you be taller than you are?

PATIENT: I don't have any control over my height.

THERAPIST: It's the same thing with your obsessions. You don't have any control over them even though you wished you did. You are not responsible for doing things that you can't do.

Examination of Intention

The obsessive considers the omission of an action that could prevent a negative outcome as equivalent to irresponsibility and negligence. However, responsibility is related to intention: if I lock my door once and check it, my intention is to assure my safety. By not checking it twice, I do not thereby intend to be negligent or to get burglarized. My intention may be to get over my checking through response prevention. However, the obsessive reasons differently: "If I have the thought that I could check, and thereby decrease the risk of being robbed, and I do not check, then I am being negligent. The thought of checking makes me responsible for checking." But what is the intention in not checking? Is it to be negligent?

THERAPIST: When other people do not check the third and fourth time, is it because they intend to be robbed?

PATIENT: No. It probably doesn't occur to them to check.

THERAPIST: But if it occurred to them, if they thought "Maybe I didn't check well enough," but then they don't check, do they intend to be robbed?

PATIENT: No. They just thought they had checked enough.

THERAPIST: So their intention was not to get robbed, but rather to avoid being compulsive about it.

PATIENT: I guess that's right.

Another factor affecting intention is *reasonable foresight*. I emphasize *reasonable* here, because the obsessive believes in *possible foresight*—that is, is it at all possible to imagine a negative outcome? But suppose we apply this to opening a door.

THERAPIST: You said it is possible that you could have cancer and that this slight discoloration is a sign of cancer.

PATIENT: I know that it's unlikely, as we said, but it is possible.

THERAPIST: So you're saying you can imagine the cancer occurring and you had thought of it beforehand and done nothing?

PATIENT: Yes.

THERAPIST: And that would make you think you were negligent or irresponsible?

PATIENT: Yes.

THERAPIST: So your thought seems to be, "If I can imagine a negative outcome that I could have prevented then I am responsible if it occurs"?

PATIENT: Yes. Now that I think about the possibility of cancer, I have to do what I can to prevent it.

THERAPIST: So imagining the possibility is the key to it? Then you're responsible?

PATIENT: That's how I feel a lot of the time.

THERAPIST: Can you imagine opening a door and *accidentally* hitting someone with it?

PATIENT: Sure. I can see that happening.

THERAPIST: Should you not open doors?

PATIENT: Well, it's very unlikely. But I can be really careful.

THERAPIST: But even if you are careful, it's possible you could overlook something and not see someone coming through the door really quickly and hit him.

PATIENT: That's possible, I guess, but I don't worry about that.

THERAPIST: Can you imagine getting into your car and driving along the street and not seeing another car come out of the alley and hitting you?

PATIENT: Yes.

THERAPIST: Should you not get into your car because you can imagine that something bad could happen?

PATIENT: I wouldn't be able to function if I just stopped doing things because I could imagine a bad outcome.

THERAPIST: But that's your moral rule about responsibility and negligence. You need to make a distinction between what you can *imagine* happening and what is *plausible or likely* to happen. Since you had your skin checked last month for cancer, and it was OK, you have to ask yourself what is *plausible or likely*, not simply what you could *imagine*. You could imagine anything at any time.

PATIENT: What is plausible is that I don't have cancer.

Building Acceptance of Limitation

With many obsessives, it is enough to have them engage in exposure with response prevention. But for others, whose worries are about unlikely events that could happen in the future, the conditions of exposure may seem unclear. This process involves four interventions: (1) identifying the feared thought; (2) examining the costs and benefits of accepting the feared thought; (3) reviewing the feared fantasy of the thought; and (4) practicing, through flooding, exposure to this thought.

Borrowing from Salkovskis and Kirk (1997), I have found it helpful to encourage patients to identify the thought about limitations that they have difficulty accepting. These thoughts include the following:

"No matter what I do I can never know for sure."
"It is always possible that I can do something that will harm myself or others."

"No matter what I do, it's possible I can regret it."
"There are many things beyond my control that can affect me and
   other people."

I find it useful to have the patient identify the thought that he "refuses to give up"—that is, the thought that drives his obsessions, worries, and compulsions. For example, the patient might obsess, "It is always possible that I could contaminate myself." By focusing on the
feared thought, we are engaging in *cognitive exposure*—that is, the patient's exposure to the thought that he is trying to neutralize.

Comments on Religious Resistance

Some patients resist change because they believe their excessive guilt is
demanded by their religious beliefs. However, it is usually the case that
the patient's depressive and anxious guilt has been the schema through
which religious beliefs have been assimilated. Thus, the Jewish patient,
who believes that he is following Mosaic and Talmudic teaching, may
conclude that any sexual feelings or sensations are a sign of his moral
depravity. In one such case, I indicated to the patient that moral decisions are always made in the context of temptation—as illustrated by the
importance of temptation throughout the Bible (Kierkegaard, 1843/
1954a, 1843/1954b). One does not make a moral choice unless there are
alternatives, one of which is "forbidden." Thus, according to Judaism,
the experience of sexual sensation is not immoral, it is the action that is
prohibited. The moral choice is deciding not to commit the action when
tempted to do so.

   Christian patients sometimes present with similar misinterpreta-
tions of religious belief. For example, a Catholic patient believed he was
morally unworthy because he had been hostile toward his wife. He indicated he was not following the teachings of Christ. I asked him to read
the Book of Mark from the New Testament, in order to examine what
Christ did teach. I asked him to focus specifically on the importance
Christ placed on forgiveness of those who showed sorrow for their mistakes. The question for him, as a Catholic, was to ask himself, if Christ
could forgive him if he was sorry, why could he not forgive himself? Indeed, in the next session we practiced a role play with an empty chair.
He played two parts: his acknowledgment that his hostility was wrong
and his giving himself forgiveness. In fact, this was helpful to him because it corrected his maladaptive schema about his religion: that Christians should condemn themselves for their mistakes. He developed a new
schema, consistent with his religious tradition: that Christians feel sorry
for their mistakes and forgive themselves.

SUMMARY

In this chapter I have reviewed several aspects of moral resistance. Some cognitive therapists make the mistake of attacking any should statement the patient may offer, as if the patient "should" be compelled to abandon any code of conduct. For many patients, this wholesale attack on shoulds appears naive and facile and only increases their resistance to change. However, we can address maladaptive shoulds by examining the differences between prior events, causes, proximate causes, and moral responsibility. We can distinguish contributory negligence or factors that may offset the degree of responsibility of the individual. We can illustrate the importance of mitigating factors, examine the importance of the double standard, and redirect the patient from self-condemnation to self-correction and personal forgiveness. Finally, we can help the patient develop an understanding of "rational shoulds," either by appealing to a Kantian categorical imperative or by invoking a rationalist utilitarianism (Hare, 1981).

8

Victim Resistance

> No one but you could gain admittance through this door,
> since this door was intended for you. I am now going to
> shut it.
>
> —KAFKA, *The Trial*

A JUST WORLD AND DESERVINGNESS
"Bad Things Happen to Bad People"

One question for any moral system is, "Why should I bother following these moral rules?" A strict utilitarian model would suggest that situational ethics can determine the correct choice. From the perspective of the individual choosing between alternatives, he might conclude that, if he can get away with it and it feels good, then it is worth doing. Much of Western religious belief is based on the view that "justice" or "righteousness" will eventually be realized and rewarded. Jewish religion emphasizes the belief that the covenant (sacred agreement) between God and the Jewish people will result in God's protection of the descendents of the children of Israel (Heschel, 1997). Thus, even though the individual may suffer in his current life, he is told that if he follows Mosaic Law, his progeny will be protected and saved. Consequently, justice and righteousness during this lifetime will be rewarded in the lives of one's descendents or one's people. Christian doctrine promises to reward righteousness in the "life to come"—in life after death (Pelikan, 1999). This religious belief system promises that the current world may not be just, but that justice will be forthcoming for those who are truly just and righteous. Thus both systems promise rewards for acting in a moral way.

Whereas Judeo-Christian doctrines recognize that justice may not characterize the current life (or world), many people do believe in a

160

"just" world. According to this model, the "naive" person believes that good things happen to good people and bad things happen to bad people (Lerner & Miller, 1978). For example, when people are told that someone who was sitting in a car was hit by another car, they have a tendency to devalue the individual who was hit by the car (Lerner & Miller, 1978). This devaluing renders the "accident" a "just event," implying that bad things generally happen to bad people.

The psychological advantage of this belief is that it allows us to maintain the illusion that if we act correctly, we will not suffer. The idea of "accidents" that happen to innocent, or even honest, people, implies that anyone can be a victim at any time. However, by labeling the innocent victim as "deserving" of harm, we protect ourselves from the unwanted and uncomfortable recognition that terrible things can happen to anyone.

However, if bad things only happen to "bad people," then the depressed individual may conclude that his depression is a sign of his moral failing: "I'm suffering because I must be bad." For example, a woman believed that her depression was evidence of her failure as a human being, suggesting to her that she had done something wrong. The therapist asked her, "What is the advantage of believing that your depression is a sign of your failure?" She answered, "If I can figure out what I do that is wrong, then I can change it and avoid this in the future." Thus her strategy was to condemn herself, while preserving her belief that the world is just, and that if she could figure out her mistakes she could avoid suffering in the future. Of course, the irony here is that her self-condemnation perpetuated her depression, which added further "evidence" that she was a moral failure. Some resistant patients believe that they "deserve" to suffer. One woman who self-mutilated by cutting her wrists indicated that she did not deserve to be happy. She believed that she had to suffer for her mistakes. She indicated that an advantage of self-punishment was that it reminded her not to make the same mistakes again.

Viewing depression as a sign of moral failure is an example of a *categorical error*. In this case, the patient had confused moral categories with medical or psychological categories. But she did this with the hope that she could at least "rescue" her belief in a just world. Piaget (1934) refers to this belief as *imminent justice*—that is, that justice will follow from every bad action and that negative consequences occur because the person has done something wrong. These "just world beliefs" are depicted in Figure 8.1.

The therapist who directly challenges these moral rules is viewed as "tempting" the patient into a life of further mistakes. One patient said, "You are trying to take away my standards! All you want me to do is be

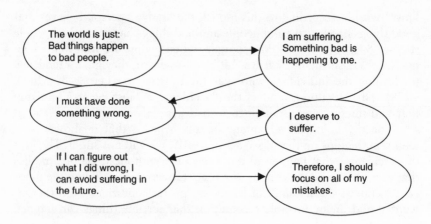

FIGURE 8.1. Just world beliefs.

selfish and say that 'Everything is OK.' " Thus, for this patient, getting help through therapy was a "self-indulgent" mistake. In fact, she not only viewed "feeling good" as something she did not "deserve," she believed that feeling good would lead her to making further mistakes. Indeed, she feared that if she began to enjoy herself, then she would become obnoxious and arrogant toward others, thereby alienating whatever little support she had.

"Good Things Happen to Good People"

A belief in the just world also takes the form of entitlement to being rewarded for being a good person. If the world is "just," and I am a "good person," then I should be "rewarded." I should be rewarded because I have done the right things that lead me to *deserve* the reward: "I work hard. My boss should appreciate me" or "I'm a good employee. I should get a promotion." The assumption underlying this is that the world should be fair and people should be rewarded for their good character, hard work, and their merit. This sense of "doing and deserving" also underlies the complaints of individuals who believe that bad things should never happen to them: "I've been a decent person. It's not fair that I lost my job."

Patients who believe their "good qualities" should be rewarded often resist making change toward more "strategic" behavior. For example, an executive who was passed over for a promotion a couple of years earlier complained that he was not likely to get a promotion this year. Rather than developing alliances with people who could help him, he made passive–aggressive complaints about his boss. When the therapist suggested he might try to become more rewarding toward his boss, he responded: "I shouldn't have to do that. I've been a good employee."

The patient who believes his good qualities should be recognized, appreciated, and rewarded expects to be treated fairly in all relationships, often regardless of evidence to the contrary. For example, a man took a job in an office where he was told by other employees that things were not run fairly and that the boss was someone who played favorites. Rather than think and act strategically, he approached his job with the assumption that he would be the exception to the rule. He adopted the role of innocent victim, complaining and resenting the unfair treatment. When his therapist suggested that he might take a more strategic approach to his boss and coworkers, he responded by saying, "Some of the others get away with things, why shouldn't I?" From his perspective, attempts on his part to be more strategic equated with condoning the unfairness in the office.

I will discuss the victim role in more detail later. In Figure 8.2, I outline the various responses to the "recognition" that "bad things happen to bad people" and "bad things happen to everyone."

VICTIM RESISTANCE AND STRATEGIC THINKING

These three responses to the recognition that "something bad is happening to me" illustrate the contrast between moral resistance and strategic responses. The assumption guiding cognitive therapy is that the individual obtains an advantage by recognizing that bad things happen to everyone and that consequences may occur independent of merit. Thus, if someone takes advantage of you, you may acknowledge that "this should not have happened." However, you can "accept the given"—that is, "Given that X has happened, what can I do to improve my situation?" The proactive strategic response in cognitive therapy leads to an exploration of available flexible responses that can lead to problem solving and rewards, while minimizing costs. To borrow a phrase from microeconomic theory, the individual looks toward *future utility*, rather than remain committed to protest of the past. From the perspective of the proactive strategic individual, the world is neither just nor unjust—it simply *is what it is*.

Contrast this proactive strategic response with the response of the individual who believes that bad things only happen to bad people— therefore "I must be bad." From this perspective, deservingness is deter-

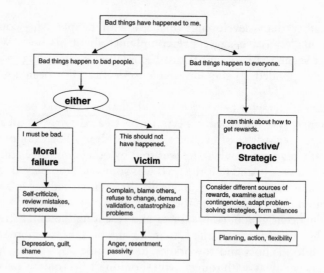

FIGURE 8.2. Self-blame, victim scripts, and proactive strategies.

mined by outcome. The assumption is that the world is just, so if something bad has happened to you, it must be due to your failure.

Contemporary, New Age beliefs that there is a "cancer personality" (Temoshak & Dreher, 1992) reflect this belief that some people have a particular "failing" or "flaw" which, if corrected, could prevent the occurrence of this dreaded disease. Other magical beliefs—such as "If something bad has happened, it must be for a purpose"—also reflect this search for justice in a morally neutral natural world. Religious beliefs, such as "God behaves in mysterious ways," are an attempt to find justice and relief in the tragedies of everyday life.

Paralleling this belief that "I must have failed at something, that's why I'm suffering" is the belief of the moral victim: "This shouldn't have happened to me, because I did not deserve it." The schema is one of "fairness"—"It's not fair!" I shall examine the victim script in more detail later; here I will only point out that the victim resists problem solving and considering his own role in the problem because to do so implies to him that "it was OK that this happened."

In this chapter, I examine how resistance to change may be predicated on utilizing excuses to avoid being judged by others (or by the self). Next, I examine how the victim role is developed and maintained and why the patient views the problem-solving approach in cognitive therapy as further evidence of victimization. Finally, I examine some interventions and conceptualizations that may assist the therapist and the patient in compartmentalizing the victim role and moving the patient toward more proactive behavior.

THE LOGIC OF EXCUSES

Most individuals will attempt to construe events so as to minimize their fault or blame. If one can minimize individual blame, then one *saves face*. In evaluating our own "blame," we may attempt to mitigate our responsibility by pointing to our lack of malicious intention, our lack of foresight, the duress affecting us, the lack of alternatives available, and the normalcy of our action. Furthermore, we can mitigate blame by mitigating the consequences—for example, by indicating that the consequences were minimal and transitory. We appeal to these excuses, justifications, and mitigating explanations in order to save face and in order to maintain or repair relationships.

Reliance on excuses may be problematic in therapy for a number of reasons. Excuses may become a "way of life," such that the individual is more invested in justifying his situation than in changing it. The more we use an explanation for our behavior, the more we believe our explanation. Furthermore, attempts by the therapist to challenge excuses are often interpreted by the patient as attempts to blame the patient. Since the excuse giver views his behavior primarily through the moral mode— that is, "someone has to be blamed"—attempts to modify excuse generation may lead to escalation of excuse generating and demands for validation.

Perhaps the clearest examples of this reliance on excuses occurs in couple therapy. Often, each partner relies on excuses for his or her behavior. The spouse explains and justifies his or her behavior by reference to a number of factors. These include the poor behavior of the other spouse, pressures at work, claims that one's own behavior is normal, justifications based on securing agreement from others (friends, other therapists) who agree with the spouse giving the excuse, and reference to the lack of reward provided by the other spouse. The underlying interpersonal goal is to justify behavior rather than to change it.

Judging Responsibility and Generating Excuses

In judging individual action, we generally consider a number of factors. First, we consider the *outcome*—that is, whether it is positive or negative—and the magnitude of the outcome. In general, we do not worry about "judging" an outcome that produces no change. The greater the negativity of the outcome, the more likely that the individual will assign blameworthiness (Weiner, 1995). Second, we consider *whether the cause is personal or impersonal*. For example, our judgments of severe outcomes are more severe if we conclude that the outcome was caused by an individual rather than an "impersonal factor" (such as a hurricane). A third factor that we consider is whether the individual had personal control, specifically, whether he or she *intent*, that is intended the outcome. Based on this consideration, we infer the degree to which the person "intended" the outcome to occur. Our inference of "guilty intention" is based on whether the individual was "constrained" by other factors. For example, we would consider the individual to be less blameworthy if we knew that he had been provoked or that she was suffering from an epileptic seizure. These constraining or limiting conditions imply that they were not free to act otherwise, and therefore their intentions were not malicious.

Fourth, our judgments of responsibility for an action are affected by the degree to which the other is viewed as a *unique cause* for that outcome—especially if there is a large magnitude for the negative outcome. We view others as less culpable if we believe they had constraints on their behavior or if they had diminished capacity to act in a different way. For example, if the individual had been provoked into saying something negative about us, then we would hold him to be less blameworthy. Moreover, we attempt to determine the extent to which the individual intended the outcome—for example, did he foresee that what he said would have such a negative effect on us (Hart, 1968)?

Fifth, we are also likely to judge someone more severely if we believe that he consistently acts in a negative way, since his *consistency of transgression* implies that he personally intends a negative outcome or that he does not care about us (i.e., negligence) (see Jones & Davis, 1966; Kelley, 1971). With consistency in the other's behavior, we are less likely to conclude "it was the situation," and thereby let him off the hook. Someone who is consistently late, especially after we have told her that this tardiness bothers us, is often judged as not caring about our needs. *The repeat offender is more offensive.*

We might judge someone to be the personal cause and to be responsible, but we may judge her as less blameworthy—that is, we are less likely to want to punish her—if we conclude that she accepts personal responsibility and shows remorse. If she offers restitution, all the better. Talk is cheap, so we may view the apology as less convincing than an apology *and restitution*.

The foregoing comments highlight the moral reasoning or judgments of individuals who view change in terms of a moral mode of thinking. Individuals who offer excuses for their behavior attempt to utilize aspects of causal and responsibility attribution. Excuses can take the form of denying consistency, claiming that it was distinctive for one person, suggesting limited capacity, denying intention, suggesting that there was lack of foresight, or invoking claims that one's options were limited.

Judging Intention and Offering Excuses

For example, if the wife in couple therapy believes that her husband deliberately withholds affection from her, she will be more likely to be angry and more likely to retaliate. Her "moral judgment" might consist of the following:

Magnitude of outcome: "It's terrible that I'm not getting affection. I absolutely need it!"

Personal cause versus impersonal cause: "This is something that he is doing—personally."

Constraints on freedom of action: "There's no reason why he's doing this. I do everything for him."

Inference of malicious intention: "He's intentionally withholding affection from me in order to punish me."

Consistency of transgression: "He's always withholding affection from me."

Acceptance of personal responsibility: "He doesn't recognize his responsibility."

Expressed remorse: "He doesn't care about my feelings when he does this."

Restitution: "He's not even willing to do anything to make up for this."

However, the husband might be able to escape this opprobrium if he recognizes that the way out is to enter the moral mode momentarily and respond to each of the inferences and demands:"

Magnitude of outcome: "It's terrible that I haven't been showing you affection."

Personal cause versus impersonal cause: "It's something that I should make more of an effort to do."

Constraints on freedom of action: "I should be more affectionate, but I've been so pressured and worried about work that I've been withdrawing into myself."

Inference of malicious intention: "I never wanted to hurt your feelings. You are important to me."

Consistency of transgression: "I know that this has been true recently, but I have been very affectionate at other times."

Acceptance of personal responsibility: "I know that I'm responsible for hurting your feelings and I also know that I am responsible for making things better."

Expressed remorse: "I feel so bad knowing that you are upset."

Restitution: "Let me do what I can to make things better. Perhaps we can go out for a special dinner tonight and have a romantic evening."

Giving Effective Excuses

The husband, confronted by his wife's anger and criticism, may be motivated to offer a set of explanations and justifications for his behavior. Indeed, he may anticipate the need for these excuses before a conflict arises, and be motivated to provide evidence of these explanations before she complains. His excuses and mitigations might take the following form:

Minimization of outcome: "It has only been the last few days that I've been like that. I'm sure that it hasn't been that hurtful" (This approach is not likely to work, since it is invalidating.)

Appeal to impersonal, external causes: "I was under such pressure at work that I was unable to pay attention to you."

Reference to constraints on personal behavior: "I have been so sick with this low-grade fever that I wasn't able to respond."

Mitigation of malicious intention: "Oh, I certainly didn't want to hurt your feelings. That wasn't my intention."

Reference to lack of consistency of transgression: "I know I wasn't responding well recently, but I think you could say that I generally respond well."

Expressed remorse for outcome, but denial of responsibility: "I'm really sorry that your feelings were hurt, but I don't think it was entirely my doing."

The reader can see that these excuses may make the excuse giver feel less blameworthy, but that they are unlikely to reduce the dissatisfaction of the person listening to them (Leahy, 1978; Weiner, 1974, 1985, 1995). The individual listening to these excuses probably would conclude that the excuse giver is simply trying to avoid responsibility and, since he is not taking responsibility for the problem, that he will likely engage in the same behavior again. However, the degree to which the "receiver" of the excuses believes the story determines the degree of mitigation of anger: more belief, less anger and vice versa. Ironically, the most effective response for the guilty party after a transgression is an apology, presumably because it indicates that the guilty party cares more about the harm done than in saving face. Moreover, if the person truly feels remorse, then he will refrain from transgressing in the future. Unfortunately, excuse givers fail to recognize this reality and often exit interactions feeling self-justified but having alienated others.

Modifying Reliance on Excuses

The therapist confronting moral resistance is often skating on thin ice and may be on the brink of plunging into a disaster. Simply saying to the patient, "You're making excuses for your behavior! Take responsibility!," will usually result in increased patient resistance and a new excuse: "My therapist is a judgmental jerk who doesn't understand me!" Denying the validity of the patient's excuses will only lead to magnification of these excuses and increased externalization of blame, since the excuse giver is committed to justifying her behavior. The therapeutic strategy that may work best is to acknowledge the validity of the patient's explanation (the excuse), and then to focus on how improvement can be obtained.

CONTRASTING THE FOCUS ON PAST CAUSES
WITH FUTURE BENEFITS

Consider the couple who enters therapy with the following litany of excuses. The wife explains her lack of affection for and attention to the husband by pointing to his absorption in his work and constant criticism of her behavior. The husband explains his work absorption by referring to his wife's lack of affection, for which he feels fully justified in criticizing her. To play on a famous phrase, "Both are right and both deserve penalties."

Attempts to determine who is the chicken and who is the egg will benefit no one. As the patients attempt to enlist the therapist as the judge between their competing complaints, therapy begins to resemble arbitration between litigants seeking damages. However, there are no damages to be rewarded and, as the cross-complaining and self-justifying excuses escalate, therapy decompensates.

The therapist can attempt to break this impasse by distinguishing between explanations and change. *Explanations* (or justifications, in this case) focus on past causes of past behavior. Since the past cause and the past behavior are now uncontrollable, this focus renders both parties helpless in their dispute. No amount of excuse generation or counter-defensive moves will improve the current and future situations. Pointing to the past will not help this unhappy couple obtain future benefits. (Of course, the future benefit that the complaining spouse seeks is apology from and self-criticism of the other spouse: "Yes, I now admit that I was a total idiot." However, since the other spouse is seeking the same satisfaction, both are trapped in eliciting proof as to who is more to blame.)

Refocusing attention toward the process of change—and away from explanations of past causes and their justifications—is essential. For example, consider the patient who goes to the doctor's office complaining of the symptoms of pneumonia. Which would be a more useful strategy: to search for the source of the illness or to administer antibiotics? Of course, eventually determining the source of an outbreak of pneumonia would be of great social value, but the treatment of this individual patient must focus on future utility (a cure) to be obtained by the use of antibiotics. In marital therapy, the therapist must determine if the goal of the patient is to *fix the blame or to fix the problem*.

The therapist can refocus the patient on problem solving and change by using some of the following statements he or she discusses with the patient:

> "It may be interesting and important at another time to determine who is more to blame, but right now we might be more effective if we could determine how to make things better in the future."
>
> "Although both of you raise legitimate points and both of you share important parts of the truth, we need to work on how new behaviors and ways of communicating can make things better in the future."
>
> "Of course we all know that the past determined the present situation. But we cannot change the past, we can only hope to change the future."
>
> "My experience has been that couples who improve substantially by changing their behavior and their communication are less concerned with why things happened in the past."
>
> "In fact, if you change your behavior and communication—and things improve—you may even have different ideas about what actually happened in the past."
>
> "When we think and talk about things, we might always ask ourselves and our partner, 'OK, how do you think we can make it work better in the future?' "

The Victim Script

A major impediment to change in therapy is that the patient often views himself entirely as an innocent victim. Certainly, patients who have been abused psychologically or physically suffer from the traumatic effects of their injuries. My focus here is not on the victims of trauma, but rather on the many patients who view ordinary negative life events as a sign that they are innocent victims. These life events include being treated "unfairly" by a family member (especially a spouse), a boss, doctors and other therapists, or someone else. I shall outline some of the major perceptions and assumptions of the victim role, examine the underlying "hidden agenda," illustrate how the victim selects a specific "schema-consistent" interpersonal world, and indicate how the therapist can modify this resistant role.

Typical automatic thoughts underlying the role of the victim include: "Don't blame me!" "You wouldn't believe what happened to me today!" "Why did you do that to me?" "Why does this always happen to me?" "My husband is always criticizing me." "I just can't stand it." "My father never listened to me."

Patients focused on their role of victim complain about bad things that happen *to them*. They usually deny their own role in the problem—although they may indicate that they were naive or not assertive and as a consequence, they suffered. The questionnaire shown in Figure 8.3 may be useful for examining the beliefs of the patient trapped in the victim role.

This questionnaire is for illustrative purposes and is not meant to suggest any norms for diagnosis. However, as examination of these questions suggests, the victim externalizes blame, believes in entitlement to special treatment, demands validation, demands that others should be

---

Answer the following questions as accurately as possible. Think of how you feel when things are not going well for you. There are no right or wrong answers. Answer Yes or No to each question.

1. People take advantage of me.
2. I deserve better treatment.
3. I can't get what I want because of other people.
4. Other people should change before I have to change.
5. My childhood experiences have prevented me from being happy.
6. I want other people to appreciate how badly I feel.
7. I wish I could get revenge on someone.
8. I complain about my problems.
9. People should be willing to listen to my complaints.
10. Terrible things have happened to me.
11. My problems are worse than other people's problems.
12. If you hurt me, I'll hurt you.
13. The world is very unfair.
14. I shouldn't have to put up with the things that happen to me.
15. I don't have any good choices.

FIGURE 8.3. Victim questionnaire.

punished for his problems, and expects that others should fix the problem. The victim personalizes the things that happen to him, acting as if events conspired to undermine him. Victims argue that they are innocent and that others are guilty. They often use therapy as a place to achieve catharsis for their complaints and as an opportunity to enlist the therapist as an ally and judge who will side with the patient against all those who have caused his suffering.

In Table 8.1, I have listed the typical dimensions of the role of victim. In contrast to the patient who resists therapy because of "moral concerns" regarding his "responsibility," the person in the victim role denies his responsibility and blames others. These two aspects of moral resistance contrast the focus on one's own "guilt" with the focus on retribution.

DIMENSIONS OF THE VICTIM ROLE

Catastrophizes the Problem

Victims insist that their problems are "awful." Typical victim statements include: "I can't believe that this happened to me," "I can't stand it," and "This is ruining my life." The victim appears to alternate between tearfulness and rage. Some individuals who are committed to this role will present with multiple physical complaints, visiting one doctor after another, each of whom fails to meet their needs. These "help providers" are then cast in the role of abusers who further victimize the patient.

TABLE 8.1. Dimensions of the Victim Role

Catastrophizes the problem.
Accuses others of personally causing problems.
Believes others acted freely with malicious intention.
Denies own role in the problem.
Insists that this happens to the self, uniquely.
Rejects problem solving.
Claims that the self is unable to solve the problem.
Rejects alternative interpretations.
Demands from others:
   Validation
   Sympathy
   Special treatment
   Others solve the self's problems
   Compensation

Accuses Others of Personally Causing the Problem

The victim attributes his failure to be successful to the malice, negligence, or incompetence of others. Distress in the marital relationship is attributed to the other spouse who has character defects and malicious intentions. Former therapists are blamed for not "solving the problem." Moreover, these failures on the part of others are viewed as personally directed toward the victim.

Believes Others Acted Freely, with Malicious Intention

In the case in which the other person actually is negligent or does not meet the victim's needs, the victim tends to focus on specific malicious intention directed at the victim. The employee who is not "recognized" for her achievements at work ignores the fact that most employees in her company are not recognized for their achievements.

Denies Own Role in the Problem

Since his focus is on ascribing all blame to the other, the victim fails to recognize, or acknowledge, his own role in the problem. The man who lends money consistently to people who do not pay back their debts fails to acknowledge that he had volunteered to lend the money, and that he had the choice not to. The woman who is involved with a married man, and then complains that he does not see her on weekends, focuses on his narcissism rather than also acknowledging her own self-destructiveness.

Insists That This Happens to the Self, Uniquely

Unlike many of us who may attempt to normalize our problems, the victim attempts to demonstrate that his problem is unique. Indeed, he personalizes his problem to the exclusion of recognizing that others have similar problems. His sense of the personal uniqueness of his problem leads the victim to demand special attention and privileges from others.

Rejects Problem Solving

Since the victim seeks validation and retribution, he rejects opportunities to solve his problem. Indeed, the therapist's attempts to move him toward a problem-solving mode are resisted, since he interprets them as an indication that he is to blame for the problem. These problem-solving alternatives are also rejected by the victim on the grounds that if he focuses on solving the problem, he is acknowledging that it was OK that he was victimized.

Claims That the Self Is Unable to Solve the Problem

As a result of this rejection of the legitimacy of solving the problem, the victim claims that he cannot solve the problem. He argues that he is helpless and that only the perpetrator of the problem—the other individual who is viewed as oppressive—can solve it.

Rejects Alternative Interpretations

The victim rejects any explanations that do not confirm his belief that something terrible happened to him and it was caused by someone else. Attempts to find alternative interpretations may result in the victim escalating his claims of injury and result in supporting his view that the therapist is unable to understand and validate his suffering and his rights to special treatment and compensation.

Demands from Others

> *Validation*: The therapist and others must understand that the victim's perspective is veridical and that the victim's suffering is realistic.
>
> *Sympathy*: The therapist and others must feel authentically badly about the suffering that the victim has experienced.
>
> *Special treatment*: The therapist and others should give special attention to the unique needs of the victim, including extending extra time, effort, and financial considerations to him.
>
> *Others should solve the self's problems*: The victim believes that he should not have to solve his own problems, but rather that others should address these problems. Others must change so that the victim can enjoy life once again.
>
> *Compensation*: Not only must others change, but the individuals who have caused these problems must compensate the victim.

Moral Superiority of the Victim Role

One important implication of the victim's claim to innocence and his assignment of guilt to others is that he can view himself as morally superior. In a typical scenario in marital therapy, the husband goads the wife into a hysterical emotional display and then glances at me, the male therapist, with the twinkle in his eye, suggesting "Do you see what I have to put up with?" The spouse who provokes his or her partner, and then sits back and watches, often feels a sense of emotional distance from and superiority to that partner. This form of activity serves the function of dis-

tracting both spouses from the husband's lack of affection and communication to focus on the "wife's problems with her anger."

Frank and Betty came to see me for marital therapy. Betty was often
extremely angry and depressed, but Frank would always say that "I'd do
anything to make her happy." As I watched the two of them interact in
sessions, I noticed that he would often ridicule her or ignore her when
she was talking about issues that she was very sensitive about. She
would then turn against him in a rage and he would sit back and watch,
and almost gloat, over "her problem." I pointed this out to them.

THERAPIST: You seem to sit back and watch Betty get angry. Do you
think you have anything to do with her anger?

FRANK: I guess I don't tell her what she wants to hear.

THERAPIST: When you think of saying something to her, but you choose
not to, what goes through your mind?

FRANK: I think, "What's the use? She'll just get angry."

THERAPIST: Would it be fair to say, then, that you often feel helpless with
Betty?

FRANK: Yeah, I guess that's true.

THERAPIST: What do you think about yourself when you feel helpless?

FRANK: I feel like a failure.

THERAPIST: Why not tell Betty that you often feel helpless and like a failure when you're talking with her because you just don't know what
to say that will work?

Frank followed my instructions in the session and later at home
with Betty. He found that as long as he stayed with descriptions of his
own feelings of helplessness their conversations were far less likely to
end in hostility. What Frank had been doing was to rely on ridicule, ignoring or avoiding Betty, to avoid hostile interactions at the moment.
This often gave him a sense of moral superiority because she was acting
out her anger. However, inevitably the hostility would escalate. By giving
up his moral superiority and acknowledging his feelings of helplessness
in that situation, Frank gained greater power to hear and accept Betty's
feelings.

Entitlement

Victims usually have an underlying belief that they are entitled to something better than they are getting. They continually refer to their *needs*

rather than to their *preferences*. A stockbroker on Wall Street complained bitterly that he "only made $100,000," and that he *deserved* at least $200,000. Similarly, a divorced woman complained about the lack of "available men." When I asked her to describe her criteria of acceptability, she indicated that the man had to be able to "take care of her," specifically he had "to make at least $250,000 a year." She indicated that she needed, and deserved, an apartment in the city and a home in the country: "I grew up in a nice household. We had a lot. My friends have a lot. I deserve this!"

The argument that "I deserve better" is based on the assumption that *"because I want more, I deserve more and need more."* Further, the assumption is that *"the other person should provide it."* Susan and Mike had just gotten married. They moved out to the suburbs near her parents. Susan had grown up in a wealthy and materialistic family, while Mike had grown up in a family with more modest means. Susan would continually badger Mike because he wasn't making enough money (even though he made $70,000—which was quite good given his training and opportunities). She felt deprived because he didn't provide her with *what she needed*. I suggested that if she believed that she needed these other things, then she might consider getting a job and earning the money to purchase them. She found this to be a surprising and undesirable suggestion.

Another entitlement assumption is that *"I should never be taken advantage of."* Victims are continually scanning the environment for evidence that they are being taken advantage of. Harriet came to see me complaining of a variety of physical and psychological symptoms. As she recounted the many doctors she had consulted, she indicated that she had lost faith in medical science because doctors never helped her: "They just want my money." Although the doctors failed to find any systemic problems with her that could account for her symptoms, and although they told her this, she still blamed them for "taking advantage" of her. She failed to recognize that *she* had consulted these doctors even *after* other doctors had indicated that her problems had no physical cause.

A secondary assumption is that *"If people take advantage of me, it is intolerable and awful."* Allison and Charles were getting into arguments that often resulted in Allison hitting Charles. She claimed that he would ignore her and that this was evidence that he was taking her for granted, didn't care about her feelings, and was taking advantage of her. I asked her what made her so angry when she felt taken advantage of. "It means that I could be destroyed, I could get hurt." This was an interesting conclusion for her because it obviously was related to a serious injury she had sustained as a child due to her parents' negligence. She believed that she had to make sure that no one would ever ignore her "needs" because her fear was that she would be rendered helpless and vulnerable to annihilation.

The assumption that many victims hold is that if people take advantage of them, then they should punish them—and *any punishment is justified*. In the case of Allison and Charles, Allison believed that "I need to make him feel as bad as I do so that he will hear my feelings." This is the search for *validation at any price*. Her fear is that "if he doesn't hear my feelings, then he will continue to not meet my needs and he won't be able to protect me." The consequence is that "I will be destroyed."

The Sickest One Wins

A typical interaction in marital therapy is that one spouse (say, the husband) blames the other spouse (the wife), who then retaliates with proof of greater injury suffered or greater burdens experienced. It is a game of who has suffered more. I call this *the battle of the doormats*.

HUSBAND: Why do you always nag me? Just tell me once and leave it at that.

WIFE: You know I have to spend the whole day with the kids, trying to take care of the house. You can go to work and not have to deal with any of this.

In this interaction the husband begins with a *complaint rather than a solution*. Most interactions that begin with "Why" usually are invitations to a prosecutor–defendant script. In the example above, the husband is simply registering a punitive criticism of the wife, attempting to demonstrate that he is unhappy. In response, the wife exchanges her own complaint, attempting to show her husband that she is suffering more than he is.

Consider the following exchange between an elderly mother and her adult daughter:

MOTHER: I don't understand why you think I haven't been fair with you. Do you realize that I'm an old woman—that my health is bad?

DAUGHTER: What are you talking about? I had cancer!

MOTHER: Yes. And I visited you. Thank God you're OK. But these criticisms of yours are too much for me.

DAUGHTER: Don't you realize how hard it's been for me to raise my two daughters on my own?

In this interaction the mother tries to establish that her daughter's criticisms are invalid because of her own greater vulnerability due to advanced age and poor health. After all, who could be annoyed with an old woman who is in poor health? The daughter brings up her cancer (which had been completely cured years ago) as evidence of her greater suffering. They go on with an exchange of *who has suffered more*. This family's drama could be called "the sickest one wins."

In these exchanges there are no rules that would prohibit a family member from bringing up "injuries" from the past. For example, two sisters (who are in their 40s) argue about "fairness" in the family.

FIRST SISTER: Our parents always preferred you to me.

SECOND SISTER: How can you say that? Dad spent more time with you when we were children.

FIRST SISTER: But when I was 10, he wasn't home for my birthday!

The second sister has used this sort of evidence of "unequal time spent with sisters" as the reason why she feels so bitter now. The first sister complains now that mother spends more time with the other sister. Not to be outdone in the suffering contest, the second sister explains to the therapist:

SECOND SISTER: You know, my sister complains that Mom and I spend so much time together having a great time. But it just isn't so. When Mom came over to my place last week, we ordered in Chinese food. *And it wasn't that good.*

THERAPIST: You seem to be arguing that since you didn't have such a good dinner, that you and your sister are even.

MODIFYING THE VICTIM ROLE

The clinician may have several personal responses to patients locked in the victim role. First, the therapist may endorse the victim role of the patient, believing that the patient is a sorrowful and helpless individual who has been permanently injured. The consequence may be that the therapist and the patient utilize therapy as a bonding experience involving catharsis and validation. Second, the therapist may be excessively task oriented, and may feel frustrated and annoyed with the patient's apparent endless complaining. This may result in the patient feeling that the therapist is one more person who does not understand or care. Third, the therapist may blame the patient, labeling him as a "whiner" who does not want to change. Each of these responses will fail to help the patient.

The clinician's approach to the victim script must take into consideration the fact that the victim may view any attempts at changing his behavior or feelings as further victimization. Consequently, the approach that I advocate is that the therapist first validate the victim script and then suggest further growth beyond the script to a strategic perspective. These interventions are described below.

Validation of Suffering

The therapist can attempt to find the truth in the patient's belief that he has been treated unfairly. The therapist may use empathic statements, identify the pain and suffering and the unfairness of the patient's experience, and indicate that he or she understands that the patient feels alone with his suffering.

Normalization of Response

Although the victim may be invested in claiming that his victimization makes him unique, I have found it helpful to join with the victim by saying that "most people would feel badly if this happened to them." I also suggest that many people would feel that they were treated unfairly and would want the other person to suffer. I suggest that desires for vindication and retaliation are part of being a human being: "When people hurt us, we often want to punish them." I also indicate that, when we feel victimized, we often feel alone in our experience and want other people to understand how bad it is for us.

Joining the Victim Script

To extend our therapeutic alliance, I examine with the patient the different feelings that follow from feeling like a victim—feelings such as anger, depression, humiliation, helplessness, and fear of being hurt again. These sessions, in which the therapist joins with the victim script, may be emotionally upsetting for the patient, for he will be focusing more on his suffering, feelings of helplessness, and sense of unfairness. However, the patient must first form a therapeutic alliance with the therapist before the therapist can be an agent of change. It often feels quite "natural" to me to join with the patient's victim "resistance" since there is often considerable "truth" in the patient's belief that he was treated unfairly and harmed: "That must have made you feel very angry," "It's amazing that she said that to you!," and "You were really treated unfairly."

Evaluating the Victim Script

The therapist can assist the patient in evaluating the meaning of being a victim. The therapist can introduce this questioning in a nonpejorative fashion: "Whenever we feel taken advantage of or victimized, we have certain thoughts and feelings about it. Each of us responds in our own personal way to these experiences. There is no right or wrong way to respond. What strikes me about the way you are feeling is that it has such a powerful effect on you. It really means something to you—something that we need to discover." The therapist can then delve further by using the following techniques.

COST AND BENEFITS OF THE VICTIM SCRIPT

"No one wants to be victimized. When it happens to us, we often find ourselves preoccupied with the victim role and the feeling of being treated unfairly. Part of you wants to change the way you feel, but another part of you knows that your feelings are real and important. But let's look at what the costs and benefits are of your *feeling stuck in being a victim.*" The therapist and patient can collaborate on examining the possible "benefits" of being a victim: "I don't have to change, I can feel sorry for myself, I can blame other people and punish them, I can make other people solve my problems, I can get attention from others, I can avoid other responsibilities, and I can feel morally superior." The costs of being a victim include feeling angry, depressed, helpless, and trapped. Most times the patient will not identify significant "benefits" of being a victim, responding "I don't want to be a victim. I just am!!! This is not something that I chose. It happened to me." The therapist needs to communicate that the patient is not being blamed for being a victim. Rather, they are examining together what it would mean to move beyond these feelings.

IMPLICATIONS OF FEELING LIKE A VICTIM

Part of the resistance to change is that feeling like a victim has activated specific thoughts, assumptions, and schemas. The therapist can examine these through the use of vertical descent, evaluating underlying assumptions and personal schemas.

Vertical Descent. The vertical descent procedure can be used to find the meaning of these events: "I was treated unfairly at work. This means I'm a loser." Other vertical descents have included "My boss yelled at me. This proves that I am worthless" or "The doctor did a terrible job.

He victimized me. Therefore I can't trust any doctors. I will be hurt. No one cares about me. I'm all alone."

Underlying Assumptions. Each of us responds differently when we are victimized. Patients trapped in a victim script may have a set of conditional rules and assumptions they utilize. These may include: "I should never be treated unfairly. It's awful if I'm treated unfairly. I have to punish people that treat me badly. If I let this happen to me, it must mean that I deserve this. I've got to get other people to see that I am right and that the other person is wrong." A recurrent assumption among victims is the belief that, if they have been taken advantage of, then they are "losers" who are "powerless." The victim sees himself as the person who is "acted upon" rather than as the person who acts. This assumption can be the target of an intervention that directs the patient toward a strategy of being Machiavellian rather than the victim of someone else's power.

Schematic Implications. The patient with a schema of personal defectiveness and unworthiness views her victimization as evidence of her personal inadequacies. The obsessive–compulsive, priding himself on his rationality, views his victimization either as evidence of his lack of rational ability (making poor choices) or as further evidence that other people do not have moral standards of conduct. The narcissist views his victimization as a challenge to his special status, resulting in humiliation. The individual with a schema of inability to take care of basic needs views his victimization of a possible threat to his biological integrity. These personal schemas are made clear in the patient's typical transference experiences, such that the obsessive, with his demands concerning rules and fairness, will demand that the therapist adhere to his moral guidelines and recognize that "this really was unfair." The patient with feelings of unworthiness may view the therapist's attempts to modify the patient's victim role as an indication that the therapist really thinks the patient is unworthy. Consequently, the therapist should take an "alternating" or "dialectical" approach, balancing "testing" schemas with validating some of the truth of the patient's perceptions and feelings.

MODIFYING COGNITIVE BIASES

Therapy can focus on testing the rigidity and validity of these apparent cognitive biases, balancing validation with testing: "We will examine these thoughts, for I know that there is probably some very important truth in each of your thoughts. However, sometimes, when we have been taken advantage of, we respond in an extreme manner. Let's look at whether these thoughts may be overly extreme and if there is a middle ground for you."

The patient who claims "No men can be trusted" can examine the costs and benefits of this belief along with information that conflicts with this gross overgeneralization. In addition, the meaning of "trust" as an all-or-nothing thought may be addressed, with the therapist exploring this concept along a continuum, rather than as a dichotomized perfect quality. Similarly, catastrophic automatic thoughts—for example, "It's terrible that I was taken advantage of"—can also be explained by having the patient examine all the behaviors and opportunities that she still has available to her.

Many victims hold to the underlying assumption that they must be "losers" or "idiots" for having allowed themselves to be treated unfairly. They may overcompensate by blaming and punishing, in order to "prove" that they are not foolish and that they will not be taken advantage of again. For example, the wife whose husband has been unfaithful may claim that she is a "fool" because she has been betrayed. The therapist can examine this arbitrary inference by asking whether she would think that another woman is a fool if she had been betrayed or injured. Victims often hold secondary assumptions, or conditional rules, such as, "If I have been betrayed, then I should always be angry about it and punish the other person." The therapist can indicate that the victim is holding onto the injury by continuing to focus on the injury and not on its cure. Thus, one can recognize the legitimacy of being betrayed—and the anger that naturally follows—but also recognize that pursuing positive rewards for the self in the future (such as work and relationships) is the cure for this anger. The therapist can point out the advantage of moving away from being "enemy-focused" and moving toward focusing on "goals for yourself."

Early maladaptive schemas are often activated during the victim mode (see Beck et al., 1990, and Young, 1990, for a discussion of schemas). These maladaptive schemas—such as being unlovable, stupid, abandoned, out of control, or defective—are elicited during the therapy and can be submitted to schema-focused therapy. The patient can examine the extent to which she feels these schemas are relevant in other areas of her life. She may examine how she has compensated for her schema or avoided situations that might activate the schema (Young, 1990). The origins of the schema during early childhood or later may be examined, with the therapist then directing the patient's attention to the continued distortion in thinking resulting from the schema: "You seemed to generally think of yourself in terms of your schema. But what if you were to look back for evidence that you are lovable?" The many interventions for schema-focused therapy are discussed in Chapter 6, on schematic resistance. These are especially relevant to the victim script.

Traumatic images are sometimes part of the victim experience—even when the individual's life has not been threatened. The clinician can utilize "imagery rescripting" to modify the impact of these experiences (see Foa & Rothbaum, 1998; Smucker & Dancu, 1999). In imagery rescripting the patient describes a detailed image of the upsetting event. (In the present context, I am not referring to life-threatening or even earlier traumas—only to singularly upsetting events, about which the patient has anxious or frightening ruminations.) The detailed image is then used as a template for imagery modification. In the frightening image, the patient describes all her upsetting memories of a single event (either actual or imagined). The patient describes the upsetting outcome. The therapist then asks the patient to describe her automatic thoughts during the image: "I felt like I was totally helpless" or "He was so much bigger than me. I felt threatened. Like I couldn't move." The therapist can then suggest some more positive outcomes, stressing patient efficacy and power, and the defeat of submission of the victimizing figure: "I want you to imagine him as very small, wearing a little dress. He is tied in the chair. You are telling him what a loser he is." The patient and therapist, using an empty chair technique, can play out these assertive/aggressive images, with the patient always taking the role of the powerful and aggressive figure.

In addition to the foregoing, the patient's schemas of helplessness and victimization can be addressed through retrospective schema-focused therapy (Beck et al., 1990; Leahy, 1985, 1991; Young, 1990). The patient can identify individuals from childhood—for example, parents—who have taken advantage of the patient or harmed the patient. The patient can write an assertive, angry letter (which is generally not mailed) in which she details why the victimizing figure was wrong and why the patient is worthwhile. In addition, self-nurturing statements can be encouraged through gestalt techniques, such as writing self-nurturing, reparenting self-statements. The patient's communication to herself might include: "You are worthwhile and decent and this should never have happened to you. You treat other people well. You are strong and independent now. No one is going to mess around with you again. Because you won't let them!"

Compartmentalizing the Victim Script

The therapist needs to incorporate many of the techniques for handling validation resistance in helping the victim change her perspective.

I have found it useful to tell the patient that there are two steps in dealing with the problem. The first step is called "The Given": "Given the fact that you have been treated unfairly and that this should not have happened to you, let us examine your options for moving onto the next step. What should the next step be?" The therapist can indicate that, just as it is important to recognize how unfortunate and wrong the situation may be, it is also important to place it in the perspective of the patient's entire life. The therapist can suggest to the "victimized" patient, "We can place this experience in a compartment that you can always be aware of. But we need to recognize there is much more to your life than this compartment. Otherwise, you end up victimizing yourself." Further, the therapist can say, "This is an opportunity for you to take control of the experience by placing it in a compartment and then examining how you can avoid being controlled by the experience." I find it helpful to tell the patient, "There are two stages. The first stage is recognizing what has happened. And the second stage is what you are going to do next."

Distinguishing between Stage 1 and Stage 2

In order to accomplish this task of avoiding the pervasive experience of being a victim, the therapist can suggest: "Let's try to think of what the next stage in your life can be. We have to recognize that these things happened and that they should not have happened. But what will Stage 2 be?" The therapist can indicate to the patient that there are many options that they can pursue: they can continue to focus on the victim experience, examine what it means to the patient, examine how it relates to other experiences—including how it is different and similar to other experiences—and determine what options are still available. Stage 1 is the recognition of "The Given" and Stage 2 is an examination of options.

Strategy Does Not Invalidate Injury

It is essential that the therapist not invalidate the injury that the patient has suffered. The therapist can indicate, "Many times when we try to develop new strategies, we feel that our suffering from injuries is being cast aside and ignored. Your suffering and injuries will always remain a fact for you and you may always remember it. But developing some new strategies to make your life better does not mean that we accept and say that it was OK for this to happen to you."

In order to avoid the almost inevitable conflicts with the therapeutic alliance, the therapist should periodically ask the patient, "Sometimes when we look at what has happened, you might feel that I am being critical of you or not supporting you. Could you let me know if this happens?" This will indicate to the patient that it is understandable that the patient would feel this way when the therapist is examining her thoughts of being a victim. By temporarily abandoning the appearance of having an "intervention," the patient can recognize the authenticity of the therapist's response.

Adapting the Strategic Role as the Next Step

Developing a strategy of making life better means that both therapist and patient are saying, "I have suffered enough! It is time for me to make my life better and not allow these past events to control me." The therapist can indicate, "Developing a strategy for your life now requires that you decide what your goal is." Many victims take a reactive approach to their experience, as if the only response is to feel injured and diminished. The therapist suggests that the victim can determine what "purpose" she wishes to pursue—turning her from being reactive to being proactive.

This proactive strategy involves thinking about options in the following way:

1. "What do I want?"
2. "What do I have to do to get it?"
3. "Am I willing to do what needs to be done?"

This refocuses the victim from "What happened to me?" to "What do I want to achieve or experience in the future?"

Examining the Resistance of the Victim Role

The therapist can fully acknowledge, with the patient, that the victim role will continue to surface, resisting attempts to find strategies to make things better now and in the future. "The victim role will attempt to make itself heard by repeating the many complaints that we have already gone over and by focusing on how you have been unfairly hurt. The victim role will surface with claims that you should seek revenge. In fact, you may often feel that I am being callous and indifferent to the injuries that you have. Whenever we talk about change, your victim script will surface and think, 'He doesn't understand how bad it is for me.' But the reason that I am trying to help you change is that I think that you deserve to feel better. Feeling stuck in being a victim is not going to help you feel better."

The Strategic Role

IDENTIFYING POSSIBLE GOALS

The patient can be confronted with the possibility that he has several possible goals before him. The therapist can indicate that the patient has already established the goal of proving that he has been treated unfairly. No additional evidence is needed, the point is "clear." The next question is what other goals does the patient want to accomplish? "You can focus your energy on making your life better by pursuing new goals that are within your control." For example, the patient who feels victimized by a breakup in relationships can be directed toward pursuing the goal of better relationships in the future, including better friendships. The individual who is focused on being treated unfairly at work can be encouraged to identify the ability to be a "player" at work as a desirable goal. Being a "player" can be defined in Machiavellian terms as the "ability to analyze the situation and make it work for you." Or she can be directed toward the ability to create career options elsewhere. The important point is to distinguish between "attainable goals" and "unobtainable goals." It may not be possible to assure that other people treat you fairly, but it may be possible to control your reactions to others and to learn how to "play the game."

RECOGNITION OF CHOICE OF GOAL

The therapist can ask the patient if she believes that she has any "choices" when it comes to goals at this time. What are the advantages and disadvantages of believing that you have a choice? Many victims experience their condition as both an imperative ("I must be angry and hurt") and as a trap ("There's nothing that I can do to feel better"), leaving them in a reactive role: "If I do anything to 'move on,' then I will be saying it is OK that this happened to me." Thus, to think that she has a choice implies that she excuses her victimizer. The therapist can indicate that one can truly be a victim and still have choices: "If you were the victim of a hit-and-run accident, wouldn't you go to the hospital to get treatment?"

LEARNING HOW TO BE MACHIAVELLIAN

Many people who feel like they have been taken advantage of believe that they are powerless losers who have no control over events. Often they are consumed by anger and a desire to protest. For example, I had a woman patient who felt that she was a victim of being treated unfairly by her narcissistic boss. After I acknowledged that she was being treated unfairly, I confronted her with several choices: "You can protest, feel depressed, or become a 'player.' " The idea of being a "player" intrigued her. I indicated to her that being a player meant that she would analyze the "game" at work, learn how to play it, and try to become adept at manipulating her narcissistic boss. I reminded her of the movie *The Godfather*: "Keep your friends close, but keep your enemies closer." I suggested that the goal was not to defeat her enemy, but to "use him": "Let's imagine that you have a cat that you are playing with. You have a stick with a string on it. The cat chases the string. I see you as the person holding the stick and your boss as the person chasing the string." This analogy further intrigued her, since it provided her with a sense of control and superiority. We collaborated in our analysis of the boss as someone who simply needed validation and compliments. I indicated to her that she, like the Godfather, should be less concerned with what was right than with playing the game to win and to accomplish her goals. Her new goals would be to secure her job, gain greater power at work, and feel like she was manipulating the boss. In a sense, the boss was an unknowing "victim" of her strategy, which was driven less by revenge and more by a desire to establish control at work.

Much to her surprise, this strategy of being a Machiavellian, rather than a victim, provided her with an almost gleeful pleasure at manipulating someone who, she thought, controlled her. She was surprised at how needy her boss was for compliments, further suggesting to her that he was "weak" and transparent. Rather than feeling defeated, she began to feel that only she (and the therapist) really knew what was going on. She was "calling the shots."

SUMMARY

Throughout this chapter I have tried to stress the dialectical dilemma in which the therapist and patient are locked. The patient, who views herself as a victim, requires validation and acknowledgment of her own innocence and the other person's guilt. Life becomes a trial in which relationships are defendant, prosecutor, and judge. The therapist is viewed as either on the side of the patient or as the prosecutor of the patient. This dilemma in the communication between patient and therapist can be addressed directly in sessions.

Although it may seem that many victims are invested in maintaining their role, there is countervailing evidence that they are suffering and coming to therapy for help. Some victims may think that help is "taking sides": indeed, the therapist must demonstrate her loyalty to the patient by validating the suffering and unfairness. If the therapist is too confrontational, then the patient will escalate the demands and prosecute the therapist. I have suggested a number of therapeutic strategies that help the patient break the impasse of feeling like a passive victim. However, throughout this endeavor the clinician should be careful to avoid ruptures in the therapeutic alliance by being willing to coordinate the dialectics of change: validation for past injury and pursuit of future goals.

9

Risk Aversion
and Depressive Resistance

Consider the following two examples as indicative of the *depressive paradox*. First, unlike the nondepressed individual, the depressive is in a state of deprivation. One might logically expect that the depressive would be *more highly motivated* to achieve pleasure, since pleasure has greater utility for the depressed individual. For example, a starving man would be expected to work harder to achieve money than a wealthy man. However, the paradox is that, unlike the starving man, *the depressed person acts as if pleasure has little utility; indeed, he is less willing than the nondepressed person to work for increments in pleasure.* This is the first part of the paradox.

The second part of the paradox is that the depressed person does not operate as a rational consumer or decision maker. Given the knowledge that a behavioral pattern has not worked in the past, why would anyone (including the depressed individual) continue to invest in *losing patterns?* Even laboratory pigeons and rats know when to abandon a defeatist or unrewarding pattern.

How can this paradox of the apparent lack of the law of effect make sense? Do depressed people ignore consequences? Are they masochists? In this section I present the investment model of depression, and argue that the depressive's behavior and choices do make sense when viewed as a negative investment strategy where the goal is *to avoid further loss at all costs.*

The current model of resistance that I advance is an "economic model" which I refer to as the *investment model of resistance* (Leahy, 1996b, 1997a, 1997b, 1997c, 1999a, 1999b, 1999d). This model draws on the assumptions of the schematic model and the cognitive-consistency model. Resistant depressed patients guide their decisions, or *investments*, by utilizing their negative schemas and by emphasizing cognitive consistency. Thus the depressive, according to the schematic processing model, makes investments guided by his belief in scarcity, incompetence, and unworthiness, and attempts to compensate for his perceived inabilities. Furthermore, the depressed individual is guided by his need for cognitive consistency; consequently, his investments are based on a high need for internal consistency, predictability, control, and self-justification. These decisions are further inhibited by the impermeability of his negative constructs.

THE INVESTMENT MODEL
OF RESISTANCE AND DEPRESSION

The investment model of resistance addresses the following question: "How do resistant patients view the potential for costs and benefits in making decisions?" According to this rational model of behavior, individuals use rules in deciding among alternatives that present them with possible benefits and costs. I do not argue that individuals are rational in the sense that they are always objective and adaptive. Rather, I propose that, even when depressed, the individual uses rules for decision making which, if subjected to inspection, reveal themselves as internally consistent and regularized. Further, I propose that there is regularity to the "biases," "distortions," and "evaluations" that the depressive makes.

Whereas classic microeconomic models *assume a rational person* who will try to optimize gains and minimize losses—and who will weigh information accordingly—research on everyday decision making indicates that "normal" individuals use *heuristics*, or decision models, that ignore base rates; place undue emphasis on information that is recent, salient, and personally relevant; and overemploy irrelevant information when it is available (Kahneman & Tversky, 1979). Depressed individuals appear to be highly sensitive to these heuristics. Depressed individuals commonly ignore base rates when they equate possibilities with probabilities—that is, if it is *possible* that they may fail, then it appears *probable* to them that regardless of their own past performance or the likelihood of anyone succeeding, they will fail. In attributing the causes of failure, depressed individuals underestimate task difficulty (base rates) and overemphasize lack of ability (Abramson et al., 1978, 1989; Alloy et al., 1988). Similarly, they are rendered helpless by recent, salient, and personal "failure" on a task; such failure is equated with being a failure as an individual and is generalized to other tasks (Abramson et al., 1978,

1989; Alloy et al., 1988; Beck et al., 1979; Seligman, 1990). Finally, depressed individuals often search for or emphasize irrelevant information that is consistent with their negative schema. In clinical practice, the therapist is often impressed with the lengths to which a chronically depressed individual will go to find reasons *not to take action.*

The idea that economic concepts can be applied to everyday decision making has been advanced and developed by economist Gary Becker and his colleagues (Becker, 1976, 1991; Becker, Grossman, & Murphy, 1991; Bornstein & Chapman, 1995; Daniel, 1995; Tommasi & Ierulli, 1995). Becker and his colleagues have advanced theoretical models (which have been empirically tested) that propose that everyday decision making may be described in terms of economic models in which individuals calculate past, present, and future costs and benefits, calculate utility functions (such as marginal utility), utilize price–demand rules (higher prices yield less demand, less demand yields lower prices), human capital, and the effects of past "purchases" on future demand. Becker's model and work (for which he was awarded the Nobel Prize in Economics in 1992) has been successfully applied to analyzing individual decision making in the realms of discrimination, crime, addiction, marriage, fertility, and religious choice.

The investment model of depression follows in the tradition of economic models of human behavior. I view behavioral models, such as operant conditioning and associationist models, with their assumptions that choice behavior is often dictated by perception of trade-offs of rewards and costs as microeconomic models. In the case of associationist models, choices are also often determined by habits and past links between a behavior and a reward (or cost). My purpose in the present discussion is to offer a *cognitive model of depressive investment strategies and processes,* and specifically to examine how depression may be related to biases or distortions in perceiving rewards and costs.

The economic model recognizes that decision makers are not the rational humans assumed by classic microeconomic textbook writers. In fact, my emphasis is precisely on the biases in decision making that depressives employ. For example, classic microeconomic models assume that individuals will attempt to maximize gain and minimize loss—attempting, generally, to try to improve their position. The current model assumes that the depressive begins with a negative schema or bias in which he assumes that events will not work out and in which he underestimates his resources and/or his ability to cope. The depressive inhabits a world characterized by scarcity, when he practices a strategy intended to avoid depletion, devastation, and surprise.

In this chapter, I first outline a model that identifies the biases in information processes (e.g., selective focus on negatives, overvaluation of negatives, underestimation of positives, difficulty imagining positives, hindsight bias, overestimation of negative causality, regret orientation). These processes further reinforce the general pessimism of the depressive. Second, I examine how the depressive develops strategies to avoid further loss. These strategies include risk aversion, hedging, the fear of hope, avoidance of disappointment, and high stop-loss criteria. As a result of these strategies, whose goal is to minimize loss, the depressive is handicapped in pursuing gains. Given the depressive's negative assumptions and given his emphasis on protection against loss, his decision making (which appears resistant to the therapist) has an internal consistency and logic. Furthermore, these processes and strategies have a purpose to the depressive: *the avoidance of further loss.* The depressive is not responding randomly or even illogically when he resists change.

Minimization and Maximization Strategies

People differ in their efforts to either minimize loss or maximize gain. Depressed individuals focus their information search and decision making on minimizing loss, whereas optimistic and nondepressed individuals place much greater emphasis than the depressive on maximizing gains. Given certain assumptions, resources, past experiences, and perception of contingencies, one can imagine constructing situations in which most of us might take a minimization strategy. To the depressive, those conditions are chronic and permanent. The patient believes that behaviors that the therapist may view as "adaptive" will lead to unacceptable losses with low probability of gains.

Consider the following economic analogy: Smith (the depressed individual) believes he has only $1,000 in net assets. He is almost completely destitute. He is unemployed and he believes that it will be difficult for him to find a job. He is presented with the possibility that if he invests $800 he might be able to gain $400 (a possible 50% return). But he also might lose some or all of the $800. The probability of gaining is unknown, but it is not high. He is told that the most likely probability of gain is moderate. But he has lost on other investments in the past—especially recently. What is he likely to do? A rational individual in this situation might very well try to protect the little he has left—that is, he might pass on the opportunity to invest and attempt to conserve his resources. After all, he does not know when he will find a new job. Any loss in his resources could be devastating. Smith avoids a *maximization strategy.*

In contrast to the depressed Mr. Smith, consider the fortunate and optimistic Mr. Jones. Jones has just examined his financial portfolio and he sees that he has a $1,000,000 net worth. Furthermore, he is making a substantial income and he expects a bonus next month. He is presented with the opportunity to invest $8,000, with a moderate probability of making a 50% return. He believes that, even if he does not make a 50% profit, there is a good probability of making some profit. He has been making excellent profits on his investments recently. What is Mr. Jones likely to do? I would expect him to make the promising investment because (1) it offers the possibility of gain, and (2) if he loses it all, he has such substantial resources the loss will be insignificant. In fact, he might make the investment simply because he might consider it "fun to be a player." Jones takes a maximization strategy.

These two individuals are prototypes of the depressed and the nondepressed individual. The depressed individual lives in a phenomenal world in which he sees loss, depletion, and disaster as actual or likely events. He sees himself as having few resources, substantial liabilities, and bad luck. In making decisions, he resists "positive" change, because he lives according to a strategy that he believes will prevent further losses. He is reluctant to invest in achieving positives because he believes he cannot absorb the loss of his investment and he views any gains as having marginal value and low probability.

This protective strategy is maintained by a set of economic rules for decision making that ironically maintain the depression but which the depressive believes protect him against further loss. Thus, these "distortions" are actually viewed by the patient as *strategies of adaptation*. To the depressive, abandonment of these strategies opens him to potential losses that he cannot absorb and for which he would blame himself.

Protection against Loss

The economic model of resistance is based on two assumptions:

1. Depressed individuals utilize strategies they believe will help them avoid further losses and greater depression.
2. Ironically, these strategies lead to resistance to change, resulting in a maintenance of the depression.

This section outlines the processes of information search, evaluation, and perception of utility that resistant depressives may use. I wish to emphasize that the depressive does not *want* to be depressed—even though his strategies result in or maintain depression. Rather, these are processes and strategies whose purpose, to the depressive, will help him avoid further loss. The pages to follow describe two general areas of depressive investment strategies: loss/gain processes and processes that limit change.

LOSS/GAIN PROCESSES

In describing the loss and gain processes characteristic of depressive thinking, I have identified the areas of interest to the clinician working with resistant depressives. First, I discuss how depressed individuals engage in a *limited search* for information, guided by their negative schema. Second, I review the *loss orientation* that guides the depressive—for example, I indicate how depressives are primed for loss, assume scarcity and depletion, and get "stopped-out" easily. Third, I indicate that depressives place a considerably higher *evaluation on loss*, viewing losses as extreme, final, controllable in the past but uncontrollable in the future, and spreading to other domains. Fourth, I examine the depressive's *gain orientation*, in which gains are undervalued, they are viewed as short term, they are demanded immediately, and, ironically, they predict future losses. I examine the depressive's myopia when considering gains, such that this myopia leads the depressive to get trapped into relatively unrewarding contingencies.

DEPRESSED AND NONDEPRESSED PORTFOLIO THEORIES

Economic models of investment and finance suggest that individuals develop *portfolios*, or a selection of investment instruments, guided by their concerns regarding resources available to them for investments, future earning potential, risk tolerance, and time frame. For example, some individuals have many resources, a high earning potential, a high tolerance for risk, and view themselves as "in the market" for a long duration. Such an investor may be willing to tolerate some wide fluctuations, or volatility, in prices, because he can absorb losses, he can diversify his investments, and he can wait out reverses because of the duration of his investments. In contrast, the more desperate investor believes that he needs a "quick kill" in the market. He may have few resources available, may have little future earning capacity, and may only be in the market for a short duration. Consequently, high volatility conveys very high risk for him. He may want to stay out of the market until he is absolutely sure that he can reduce his risk.

In Tables 9.1 and 9.2, I outline the portfolio models of depressed and non-depressed individuals contemplating how to allocate or invest their resources. In the pages to follow, I describe in more detail how depressives view loss in terms of extremity, finality, controllability, hindsight, and generalization. I will indicate how depressives paradoxically *undervalue* gains, see gains as having low probability, view investments in the short term, and predict that gains will *self-correct* to losses. These

TABLE 9.1. Loss Orientation for Depression

Loss orientation	Depressed	Nondepressed
Extremity of loss	Extreme/devastating	Mild to moderate
Finality of loss	Final/nothing left	Temporary
Controllability of loss	Past: Controllable	Past: Mostly uncontrollable
	Future: Uncontrollable	Future: Controllable
Hindsight bias	Bias against self: Should have seen it coming	Bias in favor of self: Couldn't have seen it coming
Generalizability of loss	Spreads to other losses	Limited to specific situation

differences between depressed and nondepressed individuals constitute the economic process in resistance.

Because of the depressive's negative view of losses and gains (i.e., his pervasive pessimism) and because of his low estimation of his resources (present and future), he "builds" a risk-averse portfolio. He views the market as volatile and unpredictable, he tends to see himself as having only one "investment" (tunnel vision—"This is the only chance I have"), and he views himself in the short term in regard to the possibility of gains or recovering from loss. His portfolio is limited and risk-averse. Table 9.3 outlines these portfolio theories for depressed and non-depressed individuals.

In the following sections, I examine the limited search of depressive thinking, the high valuation of loss, and the devaluation of gains. The apparently self-defeating nature of the depressive portfolio will appear more "rational," given the assumptions guiding depressive investment

TABLE 9.2. Gain Orientation in Depression

Gain orientation	Depressed	Nondepressed
Value of gain	Undervalued	Highly valued
Probability	Low	Moderate to high
Time frame	Short-term gains/long-term losses	Short- and long-term gains
Sense of urgency	Immediate demand for gain	Ability to delay gain
"Weight" of gain	Gravity: Gains predict falls	Momentum: Gains keep rising
Investment attitude	Rejects investment	Pursues investment

TABLE 9.3. Portfolio Issues for Depressed and Nondepressed Individuals

Portfolio concern	Depressed	Nondepressed
Assets available	Few	Some/many
Future earning potential	Low	Moderate/high
Market variation	Volatile	Low/predictable
Risk orientation	Risk-averse	Risk-neutral/risk lover
Investment goal	Minimize risk	Maximize gain
Functional utility of gain	Low	Moderate/high
Replications of investment	None or few	Many
Duration of investment	Short term	Long term
Portfolio	Single investment (exposed)	Diversified investments

decisions. There is a logic of avoiding further loss that guides the depressive's process of decision making.

Loss and Gain in Depressive Investments

LIMITED SEARCH

In considering the alternatives for decisions to be made, the ideal process would be to consider all alternatives, gather information, weigh the costs and benefits of each course of action, evaluate one's hierarchy of needs or preferences, and examine how alternatives compare as possible solutions to the problem. The depressed individual engages in a limited search of alternatives, driven by the following limitations, which comprise the negative hueristics of depressive thinking. According to Simon (1979), the individual utilizes a "satisficing" search, considering alternatives until he finds one that satisfies ("satisfices" according to Simon) the criterion employed. Searches are not exhaustive, they are "purposive," and are discontinued once a choice is found that meets the purpose defined. The depressive searches for reasons not to change, or for reasons not to take a risk, and will continue a search until he finds that evidence. Once that evidence is found, he will discontinue the search.

COST AS DEFAULT

Consider the following analogy. You go to your favorite Italian restaurant, when the waiter presents you with the menu and the list of specials. You are confronted with approximately 40 choices for entrees. Do you examine each entree, weigh its costs and benefits, and then compare each entree, in series, with every other entree on the menu? Probably not. Most likely you might think like I do. I have a limited search rule: "Do they have red snapper?" "Do they have a seafood pasta dish?" If the answer is "Yes" to either of these two questions, the other choices on the menu immediately lose relevance. The "default" question is focused on red snapper or seafood pasta. Perhaps boring to some, but satisfying to me.

The advantage of this "search-default" approach is that decisions can be made quickly, risk can be avoided (since these dishes have brought pleasure in the past), and control can be exercised immediately. The disadvantages include loss of variety and novelty in one's diet and the possibility that another dish could provide even greater pleasure.

Depressive thinking is much like the impatient, habitual diner described above. The depressive is not interested in pursuing an exhaustive search of all alternatives, weighing the almost infinite number of costs and benefits through all the permutations, and then laboriously making a decision after he has examined every comparison. Rather, the depressive is guided by his negative schema about failure, loss, rejection, or depletion. His general consideration is "How will I lose?" Because the depressive's thinking is guided by his negative schematic processing, his first question is shaped by and for the schema: "How will my actions lead to failure and loss?" Consider the depressive who is thinking about a homework assignment of planning positive behavior over the next week. The first questions that he might ask himself are, "How will this behavior lead to rejection? How will I fail?" Since any behavior runs the risk of failure or rejection, the answer is invariably, "Yes, I might suffer a loss."

Rather than conduct an exhaustive search of possible costs *and* benefits, the depressive terminates his search once as soon as he identifies a cost. Since almost any action involves a possibility of some negatives, it is often difficult for the depressive to take action. Furthermore, since negatives (or effort or expense) often *precede* reward, the depressive might find it difficult to tolerate the frustration necessary to gain reinforcements.

The depressive's limited search often leads to impulsive decisions. For example, one might view suicidal behavior as a "solution" to the problem of depression. The depressive, whose "negative solutions" are higher in the hierarchy of solutions that are possible, may make the following information search: "I feel depressed. What can end my depression quickly? Suicide." Of course, suicide is a possible "solution" to depression, but anything beyond this limited search will yield other, more desirable, solutions: therapy, medication, activities, and spontaneous remission of symptoms. The goal of therapy is to expand the search beyond these limited alternatives—a technique referred to by Kelly (1955) as *constructive alternativism.*

Searching for Reasons Not to Change

Once the depressive has recognized that "I can lose," he then searches for reasons to bolster his decision to avoid risk. Similar to individuals guided by the cognitive-dissonance or cognitive-consistency models described in earlier chapters, the depressive is committed to not changing. The procrastinator may delay action until he has examined all the evidence that he can find *not to change,* placing considerable emphasis, at times, on information that appears irrelevant or only tangentially related to the question at hand.

For example, a woman who was thinking of remodeling her apartment asked herself, "Is it possible that I could make a mistake and then regret it?" Since the answer is, "Of course it is *possible,*" she was then motivated to come up with all the reasons why she should not remodel her apartment. Since these possible reasons are always available, this search led to further reinforcement that she could make a mistake, leading to further selective searching for reasons not to remodel, in an infinite "do loop" of self-confirming doubt.

Absence of Savings

The depressive search is not limited to the present situation. It also reflects his selective filter about past decisions. The depressive does not "record" his savings—that is, his past gains. He selectively records his "withdrawals"—that is, his losses. This results in his inability to reflect on past decisions that may have led to gains. Because of the schematic processing that limits memory of past positives, the depressive does not readily recall how he has succeeded in the past, nor does he recall or recognize the positives available in the present. Problem-solving models of depression and therapy, such as that advanced by D'Zurilla (1988) and his colleagues, view depression as a consequence of poor problem-solving skills. I agree with this model and suggest that one reason this may be the case is that the depressive fails to recall his past successes. The goal of therapy should be to increase the awareness of past and current success so that the patient's "investment portfolio" can be diversified and strengthened.

For example, I had a patient who had achieved considerable success in his business career and was a father of three children. He would continually focus on the possibility that he had made or would make a mistake. He offered many reasons why his actions might lead to mistakes. One day I surprised him by asking, "Now, can you tell me how do you explain how you have been so successful? What accounts for all of your successes?" The patient was taken aback, since his view was that all he did was make mistakes. It did not occur to him that his successes provided him with "credits" that could be used to bolster his self-esteem or that, if he made mistakes, his past successes implied that he could absorb the cost.

Underestimation of Resources or Potential Gains

As a consequence of his inability to "record gains," the depressive underestimates the resources available to achieve his goals (e.g., he underestimates his skill), his ability to "absorb" costs should they occur (e.g., he underestimates what he has left even if he does fail), and the possibility of improving his situation (e.g., he does not "search" for evidence of improvement).

Seligman and his colleagues (Abramson et al., 1978; Seligman, 1990) have argued that depressives' explanations for their successes focus on transient factors, such as luck or an easy task, while their explanations for their failures focus on internal stable factors, such as lack of ability. As a consequence of these negative attributions, the depressive not only fails to build self-esteem when he succeeds, but lowers his self-esteem each time he fails. Similarly, the lack of self-reward for positives further leads to his underestimation of his potential resources (Rehm, 1990).

For example, a woman who had just broken up with her partner began to think, "I'll be alone forever. I have nothing going for me. No one would want me." I asked her to examine the resources available to her, including her personal qualities, her past successes, and her support network. I made a list of all the qualities that she desired in a friend and then rated her on these qualities. To her surprise, *she* was the kind of person that she was looking for. Moreover, I examined many of the pleasurable activities that she could engage in by herself, with her friends, and with other men. As much as she had valued her ex-lover, she was able to recognize that she had dramatically underestimated the resources available to her.

Loss Orientation

The depressive's negative schemas focus on losses experienced or anticipated. Many of the depressive's cognitive biases—for example, negative fortune telling, overgeneralizing, mind reading, personalizing, and labeling—catalyze the emphasis on loss. Simple frustrations, minor life events, daily hassles, and random fluctuations unrelated to the self are interpreted as losses and failures. The depressive fears negative change (loss), even if this loss has been preceded by gains and even if the loss is balanced by other positives in his portfolio. For example, the depressive who may have achieved some success in his work and friendships will view a recent loss as if all other achievements and resources have no value. Losses are not offset by gains.

DEFINING "LOSS"

The depressed individual has a low threshold for defining loss or failure: any fluctuation from a positive (either actual, imagined, or anticipated) is defined as "loss" (or failure). Correspondingly, he has a high threshold or criterion for defining "gain." Definitions of loss are elastic toward over-inclusion and definitions of failure are impermeable and underinclusive.

For example, a female patient received some mildly critical feedback from her boss. This activated the train of thoughts that she had failed, she was a failure, and that she would lose her job. It further activated thoughts about other "failures" past and present. She rejected evidence of her successes at her current job and her many successes in overcoming other problems. She discounted any evidence of positive feedback from her boss. She had an overinclusive and impermeable construct of failure and she underincluded positives.

SCARCITY ASSUMPTIONS

The depressive views the world as providing few opportunities for rewards. The individual's phenomenal field of experience is viewed as sparse or empty. Consequently, instrumental action is considered futile since rewards are few and small. The depressive lives in a world that appears barren and empty to him—a world in which all the rewards are reaped by other people. For example, a depressed and angry man, envious of the successes of his sister, believed that his life was ruined because he did not inherit as much as he thought he would from his father's estate. He believed that his sister's success in her work deprived him of success. He would point to other individuals' success in relationships and finances and "explain" his lack of success in this way: "You see? They have everything, I have nothing." He argued that he was too old and not wealthy enough to enter into a relationship or pursue a career. Not only were rewards scarce, but they were rapidly evaporating.

The angry and envious depressive needs to be convinced by the therapist that there is plenty of room in the world for successful behavior.

The therapist should ask the depressive to imagine what an extremely optimistic person might do if confronted with the challenges the depressive faces: "What if a very optimistic man in his thirties were trying to find a relationship with a woman and he did not have tremendous wealth? How would he go about developing a relationship? Are there any people who are not wealthy who develop relationships? What do women find appealing about them? Are there any single women in this city who would like to meet a man?"

DEPLETION ASSUMPTIONS

Not only does the depressive believe that rewards are scarce, he believes that his resources either have been or will be depleted. He believes that if he takes action he will be depleted of energy or self-esteem. Rather than viewing energy as something that may actually increase when he takes action, the depressive views energy as a limited resource that can be quickly exhausted. Thus he must conserve his energy.

Ironically, many nondepressed individuals are characterized by *learned resourcefulness,* which I would define as the ability to derive satisfaction from the *exertion of effort in pursuing a goal* (Eisenberger, 1992; Eisenberger, Carlson, Guile, & Shapiro, 1979). Effort need not be viewed as a negative. In fact, effort can have a positive motivational connotation, such as challenge, competence, and the sense of overcoming obstacles. Furthermore, one might view behavioral activation (i.e., increasing behavioral output) as promoting *appetitive* drives: thus, once a behavioral sequence is activated, it propels the individual forward toward the completion of desired goals. A clear example of this is sexual arousal and sexual behavior: once arousal occurs, the individual is highly motivated to continue pursuing his goals. Sexual behavior is not depleting—rather, it leads to the satisfaction of an "appetite."

Another question that can be used with depressive people is to ask them what they will have left if they take action. "If you take the exam and don't do well, what can you still do in the life that is pleasurable?" Or, to challenge the view that energy will be depleted, the therapist might ask the patient, "What would happen if you exercised even though you are tired?" The patient might realize that, even in the unlikely event that his depletion theory is accurate, the only probable outcome is that he might become more tired.

Cost Cascades: The Linear Trends of Loss

For the depressive, losses are viewed as signifying more losses that may eventually lead to catastrophe. I call this imagined sequence a "cost cascade." The depressive does not view a loss as a "compartmentalized" event or as a random event; he views every individual loss as a "future predictor" of further accelerating losses. Moreover, the anxious depressive may subscribe to a *trapdoor theory* of loss, such that an unexpected loss might rapidly lead to catastrophe. Losses cascade downward, with each new loss promoting further losses in a rapidly accelerating sequence.

Because the anxious depressive views losses as cost cascades, even a simple, mild loss suggests considerable danger. A loss is not compartmentalized—or, according to attribution theory, a loss is not *specific or situational* (Abramson et al., 1978, 1989; Alloy et al., 1988). For the depressive, a loss predicts the unfolding of accelerating losses—a slippery slope of losses. The patient keeps asking, "Yes, but what if . . . ?," then demands absolute reassurance that nothing bad will happen. Since the therapist cannot guarantee absolute certainty, the patient treats the possibility of loss as if it is a probability.

For example, a woman whose supervisor criticized her work on one project concluded that she would be criticized for all of her work. This conclusion led to pessimistic thoughts about losing her job, her condominium, and all her assets. She quickly jumped to the (false) conclusion that some mild criticism at work conceivably could lead to economic disaster for her. She fantasized that she would become a streetperson.

The rapidity of cost cascading is sometimes not apparent to either the therapist or the patient. The patient appears so distraught over the loss that he has difficulty identifying what the implications of the loss might be. The therapist will find that the vertical descent procedure—that is, asking the patient, "If that is true, then what would happen next that would bother you?"—is a useful technique to examine cost cascading. The therapist can ask the patient to "freeze-frame" each point in the sequence of losses, examine the reasons why this loss would *not be likely* to occur, and examine how costs can be contained or even reversed.

High "Stop-Loss" Criteria

Since the depressive believes that *any* loss carries with it the potential for more imminent unacceptable losses, he "pulls out" (stops behaving) at the smallest loss: "I must stop further losses from happening immediately." Consequently, frustration leads to termination of invested behavior. The depressive gets "stopped out" of potential recovery from loss.

The depressive may approach positive behavior with the question, "What will be some signs that it is not working?" Since he selectively focuses on negatives and uses these negatives as a criterion for "stopping out" (quitting), he will withdraw from situations that provide even small amounts of frustration. This "stop-loss" strategy underlies the frequently observed helplessness of depressed people who terminate behavior when they fail. In contrast, nondepressed individuals may persist after failure (Abramson et al., 1978, 1989; Alloy et al., 1988; Beck, 1976; Beck et al., 1979; Dweck, 1975; Dweck & Goetz, 1978; Peterson et al., 1993).

Some depressives utilize a *straddling strategy*—that is, they have one foot in, one foot out. Rather than commit to a behavior (or, in some cases, to a relationship), the straddler only offers a small investment. He holds himself back until he can see for sure that it will work. For example, a single woman who complained of a lifelong history of almost no dates, indicated that when she met men at parties or dances, she would hold herself back, not smile, and not show much interest in them. If a man showed the slightest lack of interest, she would excuse herself and leave. Since she was driven by her negative schema of rejection, she would often mind read rejection when it was not there. She "straddled," in that she always allowed herself the option of a quick exit. The therapist encouraged her to look more carefully for any signs that the man was interested. She was told to reinforce those men who talked to her by smiling and showing an interest in anything they said. This effort dramatically improved her social life, resulting in a significant increase in dating experiences.

A problem for straddlers is that they seldom see themselves as *causing* the negative outcome through their straddling. They will often point to the fact that they have *tried* many of the techniques advocated by the therapist: "I have tried listening to my wife—it doesn't work" is the comment of a straddling husband. When the therapist examined exactly what he did—that is, he listened to his wife, but impatiently and critically—it was apparent that he was already pulling out of conversations with his wife even as they began.

Risk Aversion

Unlike optimistic "investors" who are in the "market" to maximize their gains, the depressive attempts to "minimize" losses. This minimization strategy, or risk aversion, means that the depressive will make only minimal "investments," which, of course, guarantee minimal payoffs. Ironically, the depressive justifies his risk aversion and minimization strategy, which results in a low frequency of positives, by pointing out that the few risks he has taken have not paid off. Often, his observations of evidence that things do not work out are based on his stop-loss strategy and straddling.

Short-Term Focus and Lack of Diversification

All investments or behaviors carry risks, direct costs, and opportunity costs. Even the optimistic investor recognizes that events may not work out as he hopes. The problem for the depressive is that he does not employ positively adaptive risk-management strategies. Optimists know that risk can be reduced by taking the long-term view (i.e., betting on duration) and diversifying one's portfolio.

Consider the following observation. Many people view the stock market as a risky investment. Stocks go up and down by the minute. The Dow Jones average can drop 100 points in a day. Even within a 1-year period, in the past, stocks have lost up to 65% of their value. However, if one stays in the market and holds securities for a long time, this volatility is dramatically reduced. The average variation is 2.5% per year over a 40-year period. Short-term variation is offset by long-term holdings. Duration offsets the risk of volatility. Unfortunately for the depressive, he is in the short-term trade. He focuses on every down-tick, every momentary loss. Consequently, the minute-to-minute perspective conveys high risk.

The patient can be encouraged to view events in a *long-term-duration perspective*. For example, the patient who is going through a divorce with his wife, and who is understandably upset now, can be asked how he will feel 1 month, 6 months, 1 year, and 5 years from now. Over the longer duration, he may be able to recover from his loss and move on to enjoy other rewards. The "duration" perspective can help the patient decenter from his emotional reasoning during the present to consider the "protection" offered over the long term.

Another risk-management strategy is *diversification*. For example, rather than invest everything in high-risk high-tech stocks (as an example), one might decide to hold a variety of lower risk dividend-paying instruments—such as bonds, treasury notes, and CDs—and even money-market funds. By analogy, the depressed person believes that he has only one investment: the one he recently lost. Therefore, he views his portfolio as wiped out. The therapist might assist the patient by inquiring about a variety of sources of rewards. For example, a patient who had been doing well in his business experienced a financial setback. His thinking reflected the cost cascading I mentioned above: "I'm going to be wiped out financially." The therapist asked the patient about other financial resources, past and present, and other sources of rewards. These included savings, real estate, and future earnings (for his financial diversification), a good marriage, friends, health, and his children. He could see himself enjoying many of the benefits of living in the city, and many relationships with friends that he valued. Consequently, a temporary downturn in one area could be offset by benefits to be derived elsewhere.

Ironically, depressed people, with their risk intolerance, are most in need of a diversified portfolio, but they are often the least likely to actually arrange their lives in a diversified way. They may get too focused on a single friend, too focused on a partner, or too obsessed with their work. Research by Brown and Harris (1978) on women who experienced negative life events demonstrated that the women who were most likely to cope well with the loss of their husband were the women who had productive work and a supportive social network. These *protections* against loss—which I view as diversification strategies—are less often found in the very individuals who need them the most: the depressed.

Evaluation of Loss and Cost

In addition to his schematic bias toward loss—that is, his predisposition to search for losses—the depressive gives high value to loss and views one loss as the beginning of a series of losses. A single loss may be viewed as extreme, regrettable, and predictive of the spread to other losses in other domains. To the depressive, losses are not simple inconveniences. Rather, they are interpreted as salient, personally relevant, morally significant, and predictive of further losses in other domains. Ironically, because losses are so overvalued, the depressive will *avoid loss at all costs*. Since the opportunity costs may be greater than the loss, the depressive pays too high a price for loss aversion.

Extremity of Loss

Depressives view losses as extremely negative—they are polarized. There are few gradations or qualifiers in thinking of a loss: it is "terrible," "devastating," and "unbearable." Losses are viewed as depleting, leaving few resources with which one might cope. Because he overvalues loss, he demands an even higher probability and greater magnitude of gain. The depressed patient has difficulty placing a loss in perspective. For example, a woman was concerned over a conflict she was having with her supervisor at work. Although most of the feedback she had received at work was positive, the conflict undermined her self-esteem and led her to believe that her job was on the line. When the therapist asked her to use the "continuum" techniques—that is, rate negative events along a continuum from 0 to 100% negative, she was only able to identify the extremes of the continuum. Rather than view negatives as qualified—"somewhat negative" or "inconvenient"—depressives usually view all negatives as "awful."

This tendency to view losses or negatives as extreme is similar to "danger" alarms that characterize anxious individuals. Once he labels an event as "dangerous," the anxious individual responds with a variety of physiological and cognitive responses that might assist in flight, fight, or freeze responses (Barlow, 1988; Beck et al., 1985; Marks, 1987). Examples of these "danger" responses include rapid heartbeat, increased respiratory output, narrowly focused vision, hypersensitivity to sound, and cognitive appraisals ("It's dangerous, looming, coming at me. I can't stand this, I've got to get out of here"). The depressive response to loss also has this exaggerated or dichotomized quality. The therapist needs to assist the depressed patient in placing the loss in perspective, utilizing the continuum technique, examining the alternatives still available, and helping the patient recognize his ability to do damage control.

Finality of Loss

The depressive views losses as a final point—as the termination of behavior and possibilities. Unlike the gambler who may have more credit to play, there are no further "replications" of the game. For the depressive, the game is over and he has lost—to him, everything.

The finality of loss is the highlight of *learned helplessness* (Abramson et al., 1978; Seligman, 1990; Peterson et al., 1993). Carol Dweck (1975; Dweck & Goetz, 1978) has shown that children who give up responding following failure (i.e., "helpless children") believe that further responding is useless since they lack the ability to solve the problem. According to the attributional model, the helpless individual believes that loss is final because he attributes the loss to a stable, internal factor (lack of ability), generalizes this to other behaviors and tasks, and exaggerates the importance of the task (Abramson et al., 1978, 1989; Alloy et al., 1988; Dweck, 1975; Dweck & Goetz, 1978). Abramson and her colleagues have further expanded this model into the *hopelessness model* of depression according to which the depressed individual expects either further loss or, at best, no improvement.

For example, the patient described above believed that the conflict with her supervisor predicted that their relationship was ruined and that she would lose her job. She believed there was nothing that she could do about it. However, when she recognized that she had a long history of positive behavior (and interactions) at work (her "savings" or "credit"), that she had other projects on which she could do well, and that she could ask her supervisor for ideas about how she could improve her performance, she felt more hopeful.

Similarly, individuals experiencing the loss of a relationship (e.g., through divorce or breakups) may view their loss as extreme and final.

One patient, whose Beck Depression Inventory was 53, came to therapy complaining about the end of her marriage. Her automatic thoughts were "I can never be happy without him" and "I'll never find anyone else." To her, her loss was extreme and final. The therapist helped her recognize that the end of the marriage was not the loss of an extremely positive relationship (since there were significant negatives associated with this marriage) and that there would be new opportunities that could present themselves to her now that she was divorced. As she examined the fact that she would be more free to pursue her own education, see more of her friends, and have something to offer in new relationships, her depression began to lift. (See Riskind, Sarampote, & Mercier, 1996, for a discussion of "optimism therapy" as an antidote to hopelessness.) By presenting this patient with the idea that the loss was less extreme than she believed, and that opportunities for pleasure were still available to her, the therapist assisted her in the belief that there were more "replications" of the game to be played.

Controllability of Loss

Past losses are viewed as potentially controllable by the self-critical depressive (e.g., "I should have known better"). However, many depressives view future events as beyond their control ("I won't be able to find someone"). Consequently, the only control that they can manifest is the refusal to engage in "pointless behavior"—for example, "trying to find someone."

Ironically, self-critical depressives believe that they should have been able to control prior losses but that they cannot control future losses. This *asymmetry of controllability* enhances their difficulty in making decisions. Since he blames himself for what he *should and could have done* but believes he has little or no control over *what he still can do*, the depressive risks being frozen out of opportunities to change while he still criticizes himself for what he has previously done. For example, consider the divorced woman described above. She blamed herself for the divorce ("I wasn't a good wife," "I should have been able to make him happy"), but she believed that she could not have any control over any future relationships ("I won't be able to find anyone else," "If I do, I'll mess it up"). Consequently, she was initially reluctant to take any action to improve her current situation.

The therapist can address the issue of "controllability" of the past by diversifying the causes of "failure." For example, in the case of the woman just discussed, the therapist can ask did the marriage end because both of them initially made the wrong choice? He can ask did it end because both she and her husband did a bad job of communicating, solving problems, and rewarding each other? (See the discussion in Chapter 7.) To what extent do they share responsibility? Furthermore, the patient can be asked what she can learn from past mistakes. In this case, can she learn to make better choices in partners, improve communication and assertion, be less dependent on her husband, and be more rewarding?

The asymmetry in controllability is due to the patient's belief that he has a *stable disposition* to fail or even that he has "bad luck." Consequently, he sees no possibility of variation in his behavior or ability to improve. His belief is that he failed and will continue to fail because he is incompetent. These rigid dispositional beliefs can be challenged by helping the patient recognize the variability of his behaviors across time and situations. For example, the woman just described believed that she was not good at having a relationship. This was challenged by indicating that she had many friends who all attested to her ability to be a good friend. Furthermore, the therapist could argue that, given her husband's nonproductive behavior in the marriage, it would be hard to see how any woman would have been able to have a good relationship with him. Finally, her belief that she would not be able to control positives in the future could be addressed with planned interpersonal events in which she enjoyed the company of her friends and placed herself in the position to meet new people. This was further enhanced by indicating to her that relationships may be improved by *skill acquisition*—that is, by learning how to reward, communicate, problem solve, and assert. This could help her change from a self-critical mode to a learning mode.

Hindsight Bias

The depressive does not view losses as the cost of doing business in the real world. After the loss has occurred, he may select bits of information that he believes he could have used to avert the loss. Consequently, he blames himself because, with hindsight, he can see how "simple" it would have been to avoid failure. The resistant patient may believe that his hindsight is evidence of what he *should have known* when he made his decision. Since foresight seldom matches hindsight, he is often frozen out of making decisions because he lacks the information requisite for perfect decision making.

Hindsight bias for nondepressed people is often self-serving and ego-enhancing (Hastie, 1981). Nondepressed people review their decisions with the "advantage of hindsight," such that they believe that they saw patterns or evidence that they in fact did not see. In contrast, depressed individuals have a hindsight disadvantage, such that they believe they *should* have seen information that they did not see. Rather than viewing decision making as "making the best decision under the circumstances," the depressed person believes that he should be omniscient and always make the best decision that will produce the best outcome.

Regret Orientation

Once decisions are made, the depressive evaluates their outcome from the perspective of regrets—for example, "I should have known better." Thus, the patient mobilizes his defenses against making decisions, lest he open himself to a flood of regrets and self-criticisms. The therapist may assist the patient with regrets by examining the costs and benefits of regrets versus the costs and benefits of *self-correction*. Even if the patient made mistakes in the past, hopefulness can be achieved by focusing on what he can learn and change in the present. The therapist can address this issue directly by asking the patient, "What problems do you need to solve *now?*" For example, the divorced woman had to solve the following problems: reduce her hopelessness, self-criticism, and regret; find positives in her life today; develop both short-term and long-term plans; develop her support network; and engage in pleasurable activities.

Spreading Activation of Loss

For the depressive, once a loss occurs, its "meaning" pervades other areas of the patient's life. Loss is overgeneralized beyond the immediate situation or theme to encompass the view that other areas of the patient's life are also vulnerable. Thus, loss at work may be overgeneralized to loss in relationships and in health. This may be a consequence of the depressive's pessimistic view of what the world "really is"—that is, it is *negative*. Losses are viewed as *confirmatory of general pessimism*. Perhaps the depressive generalizes his current loss to other situations because he believes that by "learning negativity" he will be able to avoid other "foolish mistakes."

The therapist might view this as an overprotective strategy in which the patient's belief that he is "failing" is tested in other domains. Presumably, if there is a central error in functioning, then it might be useful to hesitate in making other decisions lest the error be repeated. Unfortunately, most depressed people incorrectly overgeneralize. Where applicable, they use this as an opportunity to self-criticize rather than to self-correct.

The divorced woman overgeneralized her loss to other aspects of her life: "I'm doing poorly at work," "I don't feel well physically," and "I'm a burden on my friends." She was instructed to increase the positives that she would "perform" for her friends, decrease complaining and ruminating around friends, examine the evidence for and against the idea that she was doing poorly at work, and to see a physician for an examination. This was helpful in compartmentalizing the *limited liability* of her loss.

Past Behavior Affects Perception of Future Prices

The depressed individual has developed a habit of avoiding positive behavior. Because he is experiencing short-term rewards for avoidance and not receiving rewards for the positive behavior, his avoidant behavior will increase his perception that the positive behavior, on subsequent occasions, will yield little reward. Inertial inhibition accumulates—it becomes more difficult to exert energy and to devote resources toward the positive.

These past negative behaviors increase his perception that he has a stable negative trait, which increases his estimation of the cost or price of future positive behavior. This is because he believes that individuals such as himself who have stable deficiencies will have to pay a higher premium or price for positives, thereby adding to his hopelessness about future gains.

Consider the following example. A married depressed man, who had avoided sex with his wife for over 2 years, would think that sex with his wife would not be enjoyable and that he did not feel comfortable about pursuing sex. Each time that he chose to avoid sex he observed a decrease in his anxiety, but this decrease was followed by longer term depression. Avoidance was rewarded by anxiety reduction. As he began to reflect on his behavior, he developed stable attributions about himself, his wife, and his relationship: "I don't have any desire," "She's a nag," and "The marriage can never work out—I can never have a normal sex life." Rather than the avoidance leading to a buildup of desire ("pent-up demand"), it actually led to a decrease in desire and greater anxious inhibition ("increased price estimation"). Moreover, he indicated that he believed that if he had sex with his wife and it was not enjoyable, then he would have to get a divorce—a decision that he felt unready to make. The "price" (emotionally) of future sex became higher the longer the avoidance continued.

Because his past behavior (avoidance) led to an *increase* in the perception of future price, or cost, he would be expected to avoid indefinitely. The therapist indicated to him that sexual desire decreases the less sexual behavior is reinforced—that is, sexual desire is not a hydraulic system like hunger. The therapist proposed that his past avoidance became the rationale for future avoidance and that it would be "normal" to expect that initiating sex would provoke discomfort. The question posed was, "Are you willing to invest in longer term sexual behavior until it *becomes* pleasurable?" This conceptualization and strategy was helpful in breaking his resistance to pursuing sex with his wife which, indeed, at first was less enjoyable but which became more enjoyable later.

Gain Orientation

One can recognize the importance of losses and not be depressed or hopeless if losses are offset by the quest for gains. Resistant depressives, however, do not employ a maximization strategy. Thus, gains achieved or gains anticipated do not provide a counterbalancing optimism in the depressive's balance sheet. In fact, many depressives view gains with suspicion, lest they lead them into a "false optimism" in which further "investments" will lead to greater exposure and loss. Just as the depressive may guard against loss, *he may also guard against gains.*

Undervaluation of Gains

Because of the depressive's negative bias, he views his potential or actual gains as either neutral or of minor positivity—a gain is, at best, a small improvement of little significance. Depressed individuals have a high *threshold* for perceiving gains—that is, they are underinclusive of gains. Even if a gain is perceived as a gain, its improvement over the current situation is viewed as minimal. In addition, the depressed patient does not value himself or his behavior in producing the gain (Rehm, 1977, 1990). As I indicate below in "managing expectations," the depressed patient discounts his gains.

Many chronically depressed patients have difficulty imagining positive outcomes or goals. In fact, if anything, their goals are usually framed as *the absence of a negative.* For example, the depressed patient will say that he hopes to become "less depressed" or "less self-critical" rather than to become "happy" or "self-confident." When gains do occur, they are given perfunctory attention. A single male patient who wanted to improve his social life was given the homework assignment of saying "hello" to 10 women over the week. When he returned to his next session, indicating that he had greeted 10 women, he did not seem pleased with his performance. On inquiry, he indicated that he had not asked any of them out.

Since gains are undervalued, shaping of desirable behavior in chronically depressed patients is often impaired. Even when their behavior does improve, the ability for them to perceive the improvement is limited, as is their ability or willingness to self-reward. Consequently, it is difficult for them to build on past successes (just as it is easy for them to build on past negatives). It is important to administer the Beck Depression Inventory (BDI) each session with chronically depressed patients because improvements are seldom spontaneously noticed. For example, the patient whose BDI decreases from 35 to 25 (i.e., he becomes less depressed) might say "I'm still depressed," rather than noting how much *less* depressed he has become.

Low Probability of Gains

Potential gains are perceived as having little likelihood of occurring. As indicated above, the "threshold" for perceiving gain is high—that is, it is difficult to see a gain even when it exists. Since the depressive believes that gains are improbable, his motivation to invest in progress is minimized. Cognitive therapy with depressed individuals typically confronts this pessimism early on in treatment. The patient is asked to schedule specific behaviors between sessions, and then is asked *to predict* the pleasure and mastery he will experience. For example, a chronically depressed man was asked to plan some activities and to list them on the Activity Schedule. He predicted that he would be unlikely to achieve any pleasure from these activities—predicting "0" pleasure—but that he would be willing to carry out the experiment as part of his commitment to therapy. At the following session, he indicated that he was surprised that he acquired some pleasure (i.e., ratings of "3" and "4" out of a possible "10"). The therapist asked him if he tended to predict that positives will not occur:

PATIENT: Yes. I never think that anything will work out.

THERAPIST: Does that affect what you will or will not do?

PATIENT: Well, I won't try anything.

THERAPIST: So if you don't try anything, then that guarantees that nothing will work?

PATIENT: Yes, that's true.

THERAPIST: And, then, you use that to support your belief that nothing will work?

PATIENT: Yes. I guess you could say that.

THERAPIST: So it sounds like you're saying that you have a self-fulfilling prophecy.

Short-Term Gains/Long-Term Losses

Depressives perceive gains as having only short-term value and not leading to any further gains. Consequently, the depressive "sells out" once a short-term gain is achieved, since he believes that he cannot amass any further benefits. Gains are viewed as having only marginal utility—that is, gains have diminishing returns since their hedonic (pleasure) value is underestimated and their costs are overestimated. In contrast to his belief that costs will cascade into a linear trend of devastating, uncontrollable losses, the depressive believes that gains are short term and compartmentalized. The depressive seldom "pushes forward" for more gains. To acquire further gains appears, to the depressive, to be unrealistically optimistic and not worth the added risk, effort, or cost. For example, a depressed man who was trying to develop a social life would make small efforts with women. When he obtained positive responses, he actually decreased his behavioral output. His belief was that further responding would lead to no improvement and that the small gains were insignificant anyway. In contrast, when his behavior led to negative consequences, he would generalize to the future and claim "Nothing will ever work anyway."

Immediate Demand for Gain

The depressive believes that "acceptable" gain must be achieved immediately. He cannot delay his gratification. The depressive "trades" on gains, that is, he expects a rapid turnover, or repayment, for his investments. He rapidly experiences frustrations if gain is not immediate and salient. (Given his high threshold for defining gains, he seldom sees the gains even when they are there.) If the gain is not achieved quickly, he gives up. The inability of the depressive to delay gratification is the hallmark of low frustration tolerance. I view this demand of immediate gratification as a function of the depressive's greater need for some reward and his negative schema that the world is characterized by scarcity or depletion. Consequently, to the depressive, receiving a small reward now has greater personal utility than waiting for a larger reward that may never come (see Schwartz & Lacey, 1982, for an operant model of delay of gratification). The "logic" of the pessimist is "Why invest in something big that will never happen? I can use the small reward now!"

Another reason the depressive demands immediate gain is that he views costs as extreme and depleting. In contrast to the *resourcefulness* of some individuals who actually derive greater motivation from exerting greater effort, the depressive views effort as depleting. Given his myopia, he cannot see the advantage of exerting more effort for the "possibility" of a reward later.

Contingency Traps and Myopia

As a consequence of the demand for immediate payoff, depressed individuals get "trapped" by the immediate consequences of their action.

They have difficulty seeing beyond the immediate moment (*myopia*), and therefore focus on the momentary reward (or lack of reward). For example, if a behavior will lead to an immediate small reward (or reduction of an aversive experience), the depressive will fall into habitual responding to achieve that small reward and not examine alternatives for bigger rewards that may be available. Once a contingency (i.e., behavior leading to a reward) is established, he has difficulty giving up responding to that contingency. In operant models of behavior, I refer to this as *contingency traps*.

Thus, in learned helplessness, the individual may feel anxious about continuing to respond when he has just failed. Termination of responding immediately leads to reduction of anxiety and effort. This reduction of anxiety is rewarding, and thereby leads to a contingency trap—that is, "*If frustrated, give up responding to reduce frustration.*" This contingency rule is then applied to other situations that are frustrating, expanding the individual's domain of helplessness. I refer to this as the myopia or contingency trap. One can view this as the "consumer" ignores the effects of current consumption on future utility because choices are determined by rewards in the present. This economic approach has been applied to models of addictive behavior (Becker et al., 1991; Grossman, 1995). The addict's myopia (focusing on the current pleasure) ignores alternatives available in the present and the long-term costs—that is, he demonstrates both contingency traps and myopia.

The therapist must recognize that the habitual avoidance and escape patterns of the resistant depressive individual provide short-term rewards and that these patterns are long-established and rewarded habits. It is axiomatic in learning theory that the most effective reward is the one delivered immediately. To escape from myopia and contingency traps, the patient must be assisted in examining the current alternatives and the long-term costs of each alternative. Expanding the "duration" of investment and the replications of behavior needed to get a reward mitigates against this myopia. The therapist can indicate to the patient that a considerable amount of behavior over a longer period of time will be necessary in order to achieve results. Analogies to physical training are helpful. One would not expect to achieve results by going to the gym once. Costs are *front-loaded*, results come later.

"Gravity of Gains"

For the depressive, actual gains are perceived as carrying their own limitations: "What goes up must come down." The depressive fears rising expectations because he views them as unrealistic. They confer the risk of overinvestment of resources. Since loss, depletion, and scarcity are considered "the real state of the world," the depressive may become anxious if gains occur, since they are viewed as aberrant. The world "self-corrects" toward the negative norm—that is, gains are viewed as predictive of further *losses*.

Manic optimism is the opposite of thinking of gravity of gains. The manic believes that small improvements predict future unlimited gains (Newman, Leahy, Beck, Reilly-Harrington, & Gyulai, 2001; Leahy & Beck, 1988). Thus, the cognitive theory of mania is the mirror image of the cognitive theory of depression—except in mania, distortions are un-realistically positive (Leahy, 2000a). The depressed view of gains is that they cannot be trusted. The depressed individual has a *regression to the mean* theory of gains: they will eventually self-correct to the negative.

An example of gravity of gains is in the anxiety that accompanies improvement. As the depression scores fall on the BDI, some chronically depressed patients become anxious. One patient who had numerous epi-sodes of depression superimposed on his chronic dysthymic disorder claimed that his recent improvements in cognitive therapy led to his anx-ious thought: "I'm just waiting for the next shoe to drop." Another chronically depressed woman, whose improvement was due to a combi-nation of medication and cognitive therapy, said that she felt uncomfort-able about the prospect that her BDI could fall below 15. Her concern was that she would become unrealistically optimistic and face future dis-appointments. Since she believed that improvements represented aberra-tions from the norm, her belief was that things would inevitably get worse. Consequently, holding onto some of her pessimism seemed self-protective.

The therapist must be sensitive not to sound like Dr. Pangloss in Voltaire's *Candide, or Optimism* (Leahy, 2000d). The therapist should recognize that the chronically depressed patient has experienced many negative life events—or so it seems to him—and that to suddenly portray the world as *"the best of all possible worlds"* will appear naive (as, in-deed, it is). The patient may be told that cognitive therapy is the power of realistic thinking, not the power of positive thinking, and that one must always be prepared to handle downturns. I find it useful to help the patient recognize that he has taken a too conservative, self-protective strategy regarding gains and that a more moderate, optimizing strategy can be useful.

MANAGING EXPECTATIONS

Because the depressive anticipates that change will lead to further expo-sure to loss, he is exquisitely sensitive to the risk of overextending himself. He wishes to keep his exposure to possible damage to a minimum. If he begins to expect more from himself (or if others expect more from him), he might be encouraged to risk more. Consequently, he must manage any positive expectations lest they "deceive" him into taking a positive position. The following processes are involved in managing expectations.

1. *Improvement widens the risk.* Each step forward is viewed as implying greater risk. If he succeeds on one task, he may risk exposure to more significant tasks where he might lose more (e.g., he might be publicly humiliated). Each improvement opens a door into a wider arena in which failure seems more devastating.

2. *Discounting gains.* The depressive will minimize potential or actual gains, viewing them as nonpredictive of further gains. By discounting actual or future gains, he maintains his "conservative strategy" of not getting his hopes up too far.

3. *Fear of hope.* Although he complains about his hopelessness, he also views hope itself as a risk. "Hoping" might lead him into "naive" risks, resulting in disappointment and greater loss. As he begins to feel more hopeful, his anxiety may increase, since hope may take him into greater exposure to further loss. The depressive views pessimism as "risk management" (Leahy 2000d).

4. *Rejection of encouragement.* Others may attempt to lift his spirits by indicating that things are not as bad as he thinks or that events may change. Since this runs the risk of raising his expectations—and exposing him to possible future disappointment—he may become more resistant the more positive his friends or therapist may be.

5. *Lowering others' expectations.* It is not enough to keep one's own expectations low: he must attempt to convince others to have low expectations of him. If others expect more from him, then he runs two risks: first, he might succumb to their optimism, become hopeful, and expose himself more; and second, he might fail to live up to others' expectations and thereby humiliate himself.

Commitment to Stability

Since change may lead to further loss, the depressive is highly committed to maintaining the status quo. As much as he might complain about the current situation, he fears even more further losses. As his life appears more constrained, negative, and hopeless, he feels a greater need to predict and control events and to maintain some consistency in his life.

1. *Negative predictions are self-fulfilling.* The depressive is almost always able to find some evidence that confirms his negative prediction.

Since he either avoids risk or "stops out" early, there is substantial evidence to support his view that nothing will work.

2. *If I am surprised, it will be by positives.* The depressive's emphasis on avoiding negative surprises—since negatives that are unexpected are "signals" of cost cascades—gives him a higher commitment to pessimism as a way of assuring that he will not suffer a sudden loss. The depressive is willing to accept the costs of pessimism, with the possible benefit of being surprised by a positive.

Competence in Negativity

Since most people wish to have some domains in which they are competent, the depressive turns to the one area in which he feels he has some negativity—specifically, proving that he has a right to his depression. By viewing his depression as "realistic" and intractable, he places himself in a position of "negative power." Thus, he can always have the "last word"—that is, he can always reject help.

1. *Sadder but wiser.* The depressive believes that his negativity is evidence of his greater "wisdom" about the true nature of his world—he knows, better than the therapist, that nothing will work. He may believe that he has failed in other areas of his life, but he is secretly proud of the "fact" that he is sadder but wiser.

2. *Psychic victories are victories.* By proving that he is correct about his negativity and that the therapist is pollyannish in his optimism, the depressive believes that he has achieved some "victory"—he has proven the therapist wrong. Even though this may add to his sense of hopelessness, he at least feels some momentary superiority to the "naive therapist." By engaging help givers in "debates" in which others try to convince him to change, but he can reject their advice, he places himself in the "superior" position of the judge who decides "what makes sense to me." Since he can always reject advice, he can always win these debates.

3. *Optimism conveys risk, but negativity implies protection.* Optimism invites the depressive into a world of achievement in which he expects failure. However, he believes that he can be competent in protecting himself with a negative, minimization strategy. He believes that he made mistakes in the past, but he can master the techniques of negativity.

4. *Positives are beyond control, but negativity is always controlled.* The depressive may have given up on the hope that he will achieve positives—these are beyond his control. However, he believes that he can control his negative predictions—after all, he is the one who makes the predictions.

SUPPORT FOR THE INVESTMENT MODEL

I have proposed that depressed individuals utilize a negatively biased "portfolio theory" in considering their options (Leahy, 1997a, 1997b, 1999c). A *portfolio theory* is the individual's perception of his resources, diversification, maximization/minimization, potential for regret, hedonic utility for gains and losses, and risk tolerance. The portfolio theory of depression, based on investment models of decision making, proposes that individual variation in risk tolerance is related to the depressed individual's assumptions of scarcity and depletion, regret orientation, criteria for defining losses and gains, rules for quitting, and information demands prior to making decisions. This model proposes that depressed individuals are risk-averse and tend to place less emphasis on maximizing gains and more emphasis on minimizing losses.

In a recent study (Leahy, 1999b) several hypotheses derived from the portfolio model of depression were tested. One hundred fifty-five clinic patients were administered the Beck Depression Inventory and a 6-point, 25-item questionnaire that assessed a variety of dimensions of decision making derived from the portfolio-theory model. Correlations were calculated among all items and for depression scores. The depressive portfolio theory, which is risk-averse, was largely supported. More depressed patients utilized a "negative portfolio theory," which was based on assumptions that current and future resources are scarce, outcomes are unpredictable and uncontrollable, there is a low utility for gains, and a high disutility for losses. Depressed individuals were more inclined to blame themselves for failures and less likely to internalize success. They generalized negatives, stopped-out early, had a high criterion for defining gains and a marginal criterion for defining losses, and had a greater demand for consensus building before taking action. Depression was negatively associated with the goal of maximizing gains. Independent of depression, there was strong confirmation for the portfolio model of risk, which largely paralleled the findings for depression and portfolio concerns indicated above. Risk aversion was associated with almost all of the decision dimensions correlated with depression and with greater demands for information and with utilizing waiting as a strategy.

Contrary to the portfolio model, depression was unrelated to claiming that one attempted to "minimize loss." This may be due to the fact that depressed and nondepressed individuals may interpret this question differently. Support for the portfolio model of loss aversion was reflected by the fact that depressed patients stopped out earlier, waited longer, required more information, and were risk aversive.

SUMMARY

I view the investment model as a cognitive-operant model of depression. Leading learning theorists have long been employing "cognitive" terms, such as *expectancy* or *matching*, in order to more adequately describe the behavioral regularity of organisms ranging from pigeons to humans (Schwartz, 1986; Schwartz & Lacey, 1982). The investment model of depression has the advantage of explaining the apparent resistance of chronically depressed individuals and indicates how the therapist may conceptualize and intervene with these patients.

Given the negative information search, emphasis and overvaluation of loss, and the discounting or negativity of gain, the depressive often utilizes a strategy that minimizes change. Depressives utilize three strategies in limiting change. First is *commitment to stability*. Depressives, driven by their need for cognitive consistency (prediction and control), often find that their negative predictions are self-fulfilling. One might ask, "Why abandon a theory that has proven to be correct?" Further, depressives are committed to stability (even though it is negative) because of their fear of disappointment. A second concern is their belief in *competence in negativity*. Many depressives view themselves as "sadder but wiser" and they believe that negativity in perception is the one thing that they can control (since they believe that they cannot control positives). Depressives believe that optimism conveys risk and that the one "victory" that they can have is in defending their negative position in therapy. A third strategy is to *manage expectations*. Depressives often believe that improvement widens risk, that hope may be dangerous or foolhardy, and that they must work at lowering their expectations and that of others. In the next chapter, I examine the self-limiting strategies used by depressives to avoid further loss of resources and self-esteem and the interpersonal processes that result from resistant strategies.

10

Self-Handicapping

HIDDEN AGENDAS

Paul and Vickie, friends of mine, sail in the Virgin Islands. They told me about an incident they had experienced at sea. A couple sent out a distress call: "We are trapped in the Bermuda Triangle. We can't get out! We sail 20 yards in one direction and then stop. We sail 20 yards in another direction, but we can't go any farther. We're trapped in the Triangle!" Paul and Vickie sailed to the place where the other boat was "trapped." As they approached it, Paul could see the worry on the faces of the man and woman. But Paul set them at ease by saying, "You're not caught in the Bermuda Triangle, you just forgot to lift your anchor."

Hidden agendas are these "Bermuda Triangles" that trap people. The individual seems to make some progress only to feel thwarted that he cannot go any further. He focuses on what is "in front of him"—the things he thinks are blocking his progress. Indeed, he points to the effort he has made to make changes, only to be prevented from achieving his goals. The hidden agenda, though, is like the anchor we do not see. Like other anchors, it is supposed to keep us safe. It keeps us from drifting out to sea or from overturning in a storm. But if we forget to lift it, we will find ourselves making limited moves—often to sabotage ourselves in the process.

In this chapter, I describe some common hidden agendas that are self-limiting and often self-defeating. A variety of purposes are served by these hidden agendas, but I will focus on three common goals. The first is to avoid evaluation of the self under optimal conditions. In order to accomplish this "self-camouflage," the individual manipulates attribution processes and data. The second purpose served is to avoid risk of greater loss or sudden unexpected and uncontrollable loss. The patient hedges, straddles, and provides minimal compliance. The third purpose served by hidden agendas is to avoid further progress that may lead to greater exposure and greater public humiliation. One can think of this as "one step forward, two steps backward."

ATTRIBUTION MANEUVERS
AND SELF-HANDICAPPING

Explanations of Personal Causality

One of the most influential models of the last 30 years is attribution theory. There are several variations of attribution theory, but they all pertain to how we explain the causes of personal behavior or outcomes related to personal behavior. Heider (1958) was interested in "naive psychology"—that is, how individuals come to understand and explain psychological phenomena in everyday life, such as intention, motivation, and personality characteristics—the forerunner of what became known as "social cognition."

H. H. Kelley carried Heider's model of naive psychology to the next stage. Kelley's (1971) attribution theory proposes that individuals use an analysis-of-variance model to explain whether someone's behavior is due to the person or to the situation. According to this model, people are more likely to make a personal attribution when the individual's behavior is distinctive, consistent, and not in consensus with others (Kelley, 1971). For example, imagine someone I know goes to the movie *Titanic*. I ask her after the movie, "Did you like the movie?" She indicates that she did not like the movie. If I had not seen the movie myself before, I might consider her response in terms of whether she likes most movies, but not this movie—that is, Is her response distinctive for this movie? If it is distinctive, I would be more likely to think the movie in question is not very good. I might also ask, "How do others respond to this movie?"—that is, What is the consensus? If almost everyone else I know likes the movie, I might think there is something unusual about her that she does not like the movie. Perhaps it is a good movie, but she does not like romantic spectacles. I might also evaluate whether she would have the same response if she saw the movie again—that is, How consistent is her evaluation of the movie? If she consistently watches the movie and consistently does not like the movie, it may indicate something about her: she *really* dislikes the movie. According to Kelly's *covariation principle*, we tend to attribute outcomes to factors that uniquely covary with that outcome.

Another attribution model is based on how we determine whether someone's achievement or failure is due to him or her or to other factors. Weiner (1985) proposed that we can explain success or failure along two orthogonal dimensions: internal/external or stable/unstable (see Figure 10.1). If I succeed at something, I can attribute my success to my ability or to my effort (both internal) or to the easiness of the task or to my good luck (both external). My effort and my luck can change (each is unstable). For example, if I explain my success by referring to my ability, then I will take pride in the outcome and tend to generalize this ability to new tasks. In contrast, if I attribute my success to the fact that it was an easy task at which anyone would succeed, then I will not feel pride and I might even be apprehensive about other tasks.

Related conceptually to the attribution cube is Kelley's (1971) multiple causal scheme model. According to this model, we often do not have available or we do not examine the range of "covariation" information, but rather rely on simple "presence/absence" information. Kelley proposed that individuals utilize discounting and augmentation principles. The *discounting principle* states that if two causes are present that could plausibly account for an outcome, we tend to discount one of these causes in favor of the other. For example, if Susan goes to see the movie *Titanic* and says that she does not like the movie—*and* we learn that someone has offered her $100 to tell us this—we are likely to discount her not liking the movie by referring to the bribe. The bribe is viewed as a *sufficient* condition to explain her report to us. The bribe is viewed as a "facilitative" cause, since it adds to the likelihood of the outcome.

However, we can also consider inhibitory causes. For example, what if we learned that someone paid her $100 to say she *liked* the movie, but she reports that she did not like it? We then conclude that she *really disliked the movie*, since she had to overcome an inhibitory cause (the bribe) to produce her report. Thus, the presence of an inhibitory cause *augments* our attribution about Susan's real likes and dislikes.

Preserving Self-Esteem

Individuals who wish to preserve some self-esteem do not want to find out that their failure was due to lack of ability. Self-esteem can still be

	Internal	External
Stable	Ability	Task difficulty
Unstable	Effort	Luck

FIGURE 10.1. Weiner's attribution model.

protected by attributing failure to the task difficulty or by claiming that one did not exert effort. Or one can attribute one's failure to an "inhibitory" cause—such as drug or alcohol use—that can be interpreted as transitory (unstable) and not as reflecting one's true abilities or character. Moreover, by creating an inhibitory cause, such as lack of preparation, intoxication, or lateness, the individual can claim that whatever success he achieves is a true manifestation of genius. The desire to preserve these attribution possibilities often underlies resistance to change.

Individuals are generally motivated to enhance their self-esteem by preserving their image of themselves as reasonable, competent, and good people. When an individual considers taking an action that might result in success or failure, she often anticipates the "attribution position" that will result from her action. For example, "If I take the exam and fail, what will that say about me?" or "If I succeed, what will it say about me?" The foregoing attribution models are utilized *prior* to decisions to act in anticipation of how one can interpret unknown outcomes.

Peter is thinking of taking an exam. He has high expectations of himself—as do others. However, he is now in a college that is more competitive than the high school from which he came. His dilemma is the following: "If I study hard, it increases my chances of doing well. But if I study hard and do poorly, it means that I'm inferior to the other students here." Peter finds himself considering the *attribution cube:* Will my (potential) failure be attributed to my ability, lack of effort, task difficulty, or bad luck? No one will believe "bad luck," so he is stuck with the other possible explanations. If others do better than he does, he cannot attribute it to "task difficulty." He certainly does not want to conclude that he lacks the ability. So he can consider constructing events so that he could reasonably conclude, "He did not try very hard." Not trying very hard is something that can change: he can try harder in the future. Furthermore, if he does well on the exam, and does not try hard, he can conclude he is a genius. In other words, he has "overcome an inhibitory cause"—not trying—which then augments his tendency to attribute the outcome to his exceptional ability.

Peter may not feel completely protected by "not trying hard." He may pursue other inhibitory causes that get in the way of performing. These could include drinking, using drugs, staying up late, complaining about his depression and anxiety, or complaining about his chronic fatigue syndrome. As he escalates his inhibitory causes—or excuses—he decreases the chance that his failure will say anything about his "optimal potential" and it leaves open the possibility that his success—should it occur—will demonstrate his genius and heroic nature in overcoming the many handicaps that beset him.

Self-handicapping focuses on avoiding direct evaluation of one's ability or self. The strategy guiding self-handicapping is that individuals

(1) attempt to protect their self-esteem, (2) in conditions of uncertainty, (3) by obscuring evaluation by engaging in excuse generation, creating impediments to performance, or erecting barriers to attribution of ability (Arkin & Oleson, 1998; Berglas & Jones, 1978; Jones & Rhodewalt, 1982; Snyder, Higgins, & Stucky, 1983). Excuses include reference to (usually) preexisting conditions that inhibit performance: "I don't feel well. I'm coming down with something. And I have a big exam tomorrow." The excuse is a sufficient explanation for failure, thereby bypassing direct inferences of low ability should the individual fail. Some individuals create impediments to performance, also obscuring self-evaluation: "I know I have a big exam tomorrow, but I'm going to go out and get blasted tonight." Another example of self-handicapping includes creating barriers to attribution, such as not trying hard on a difficult exam, thereby clouding the issue of whether failure is due to lack of effort or to lack of ability.

Depressed individuals, already suffering from low self-esteem, may employ *attribution maneuvers* in order to prevent direct evaluation of their "optimal abilities." Thus, the individual may pursue unusual and low probability outcomes, since failure at these outcomes does not reflect true potential (i.e., anyone would have failed). Minimizing effort, quitting early, provoking others, and setting excessively high standards are other attribution strategies that allow the individual to avoid being measured by the standard by which others are measured. Thus, a depressed individual rejected the feasibility of making smaller steps toward success, since failure at any smaller step conferred greater implication of less ability, whereas failing at the "grand scheme" might only mean that he set his goals higher than others did.

Take the case of a college student who often compared himself to his father, who had achieved considerable fame as an intellectual. He appeared committed to drinking and playing pool, rather than to studying. Yet he took the most difficult courses he could. His self-handicapping attribution was that if he failed, he could attribute it to his independence from the "grind" of "meaningless courses," whereas if he succeeded his success proved he was a genius. Either way, there was no direct assessment of his true potential available. Both failure and success were within his "attribution control."

PROTECTIVE PERFECTIONISM

Another self-handicapping strategy is to demand perfection as a protection against viewing the self as average. If you fail at perfection—which is "extreme task difficulty"—then you obscure direct inferences about personal ability. (As Salvador Dali said, "Don't worry about perfection. You'll never achieve it anyway.") A severely depressed woman strongly resisted abandoning her demand for a perfect partner partly because of her belief that these perfectionistic standards maintained her self-esteem: "If I gave up my standard then I would be just like everyone else. Even though I don't have the perfect partner, I still have my standards." From her perspective, abandoning perfectionism would relegate her to a world of all-or-nothing nobodies. Once she abandoned her excessive ego ideal regarding a partner and a career, she was able to make significant changes that helped decrease her depression.

Similar to the attribution self-handicapping illustrated above, perfectionism allows the individual to avoid being measured on a normal curve. If he fails to be 100%, then the only conclusions that are warranted are that he is not perfect (which is not *informative* since it is not distinctive) and that he has high standards (which he considers admirable). The perfectionist avoids being measured on a standard scale in order to avoid determining his relative standard.

MODIFYING SELF-HANDICAPPING

The self-handicapping patient faces a dilemma: she wants to change so that she can feel less helpless, but she fears that change will place her in a position whereby failure can not be disattributed to other factors. Thus, she risks direct evaluation of true ability. Her second fear is that she will be too exposed to commitment, so that pulling back will be more difficult. She fears reaching the point of no return.

In the remainder of this chapter I discuss strategies for modifying self-handicapping or self-defeat. It is important when using these interventions that the therapist not blame the patient for her depression (or problem). The therapist should indicate to the patient that therapist and patient together can develop a curiosity about why it is difficult to change: "Are there ways that you have become too cautious?" or "Are you accidentally, unintentionally, getting in your own way?"

Agenda Setting

> *"What problem would you like help with today? Can you specify exactly what you want from this session?" When patient goes off-task, "How does this relate to your making progress on the problem you put on today's agenda? What are the costs and benefits of not working on this problem?"*

If the patient can avoid creating and sticking to an agenda, then lack of progress can be attributed to the therapist. For example, a patient who feared pursuing success at work and in relationships, and who refused to abandon her idealized view of what she needed in her life, continually resisted setting an agenda. When she did set an agenda, she quickly departed from it, bringing up complaints about how bad she felt. When the therapist asked her what the advantages were of not following an agenda, she answered, "I don't have to face my problems and I don't have to do anything." She indicated that she feared that once she started setting an agenda and following it, she would then be compelled to do things that she would fail at.

Identifying Patterns of Self-Defeat

> *"Have you noticed that you put a small amount of effort into things and then quit? This seems to be a pattern." "Is it possible that you have a vested interest in keeping yourself from moving forward in certain areas?"*

For example, the patient can recognize that she often provokes men in relationships, thereby leading to quick rejection. This led one patient to recognize that she was afraid of being rejected on a more intimate basis, so that being rejected early on gave her a sense of control. She also believed that she would be more devastated by rejection if she were more intimate. Thus, her provoking and self-defeating behavior conferred some protection over greater losses. However, she realized that this self-defeating strategy further reinforced her negative view of men, thereby making her more likely to be pessimistic in the future.

Examining Costs and Benefits of Self-Defeat

> *"Every pattern that we have has costs and benefits. What could be the costs and benefits to you of hedging [failing, provoking, hiding, etc.]?" "How would your life have been different if you never hedged [failed, provoked, hid, etc.]?"*

One patient who continually derogated himself when talking about his work noted that he hoped to "beat others to the punch" in derogating him. He also indicated that he did not want to appear "conceited," lest that lead to more rejection. The therapist asked, "If you don't say that your work is any good, then why would someone else think it is?" The patient examined how his life would have been different if he had not constantly derogated his own work. He believed that he would be much further along and his work would be more highly visible. Interestingly, this admission then led to his next fear: "But then I might fail in a really big way! At least, with what I'm doing, my failure is limited and somewhat private."

Monitoring Self-Defeat

"Let's keep track of when and how often you hedge (fail, provoke, hide, etc.)." "What situations or thoughts seem to trigger your self-defeat?"

Rather than engage in "competency tracking," the therapist instructs the patient in engaging in monitoring self-defeat. The advantage of making this a conscious target is that self-defeat operates more powerfully when it has a "clandestine" quality—that is, the patient is more undermined by self-defeat when the self-handicapping behaviors are not clearly in awareness. Thus, the therapist can say, "I'd like you to write down all examples of your self-defeating behavior." The therapist and patient can catalogue examples of this behavior, such as "making negative statements about yourself to others," "discounting compliments," "putting in some, but minimal, effort," "or "provoking another person." These targeted behaviors can then be examined for costs and benefits. The thoughts or situations that elicit self-defeat can also be identified using the self-monitoring. I have found that patients are more likely to engage in self-defeat when they have a combination of recently rising expectations accompanied by the belief that something negative is either happening or about to happen.

Examining the Negative Implications of Success

"Let's imagine that you succeeded at [something]. Perhaps this has some negative implications for you. What could they be? What would happen next? Higher expectations, more public failure, let yourself or others down, have to maintain success, not deserve success? How would you handle these consequences of success?"

The therapist should examine the patient's ambivalent feelings about success. Although the patient shows ostensible sadness over his lack of achievement or his inability to form a relationship, the therapist can direct the patient's attention to the fear of moving forward too much. For example, a patient who complained that he was trapped below a "glass ceiling" at his job, decreased his performance at work to the point where he might have been terminated. However, because of policy changes in his company, a new opportunity opened up where he would have been highly likely to get the job. His performance on the new job would be more obvious, since there were clear expectations of production. This led to procrastination and self-sabotage. The patient indicated that he feared getting the new job, since he believed that this would reveal how incompetent he really was. At least, he felt, on the current job, with his passive–aggressive behavior, he could always attribute his lack of success to lack of effort. Thus, there was no way to assess his true ability. Like many self-defeating personalities, he had an alternating dichotomous view of himself: that he was "incompetent" and that he had "special abilities."

Examining Fear of Self-Evaluation or Self-Exposure

"Sometimes we try to avoid finding out what we could do under the best of circumstances—that is, when we have put all our effort into something we might fear finding out that we are not as good as we think we are. Do you ever have that fear? Do you do things to make sure that you don't get a clear evaluation of yourself? What do you expect or demand of yourself? What would you think of yourself if you found out you were not as good (or as great) as you think you should be?"

Idealized views of the self and what one should accomplish often result in minimal effort in conditions in which performance could be an indication of "true potential." A student indicated that she was almost always late in handing her papers in, resulting in several "incompletes." She would do very little work on her papers—or on her preparation for exams—often distracting herself by talking on the phone, watching television, or sleeping late. Although she indicated that she thought the content of the courses she took was quite interesting, she would often spend an inordinate amount of time on reading that was unrelated to any evaluations or tests in these courses. She indicated that she always thought she had to be superior to everyone else in school, but that when she got to college she realized there were many other very intelligent people. Consequently, she reduced her effort in her courses, anticipating that she feared finding out that, if she exerted herself and got her papers done on time, they would not be exceptional. She claimed, "If I'm not special and superior, then I'm just like everyone else. And if I'm like everyone else, then I'm pretty worthless."

TACTICS OF SELF-LIMITATION

Table 10.1 lists typical "tactics" by which the resistant patient attempts to undermine the process of change in therapy (Leahy, 1997c, 1999e). Direct maneuvers include motivated negative cognition, devaluation of alternatives, and attempts to prove hopelessness. For example, a writer with considerable talent insisted that everything was "lousy" in his life (his apartment, his relationships, his writing), that any changes the therapist suggested were naive and stupid, and that hopelessness was the only reasonable alternative. This is an example of "motivated negative cognition." The therapist can recognize motivated negative cognition be-

TABLE 10.1. Self-Limitation Tactics

Tactic	Example
Motivated negative cognition	Argues vigorously for hopelessness, becomes angry or despondent when confronted with positive information.
Devaluation of alternatives	Views positive alternatives as naive, dangerous, or pointless.
Off-task distractions	Changes the subject in session to irrelevant discussion, trivializes the therapy session with complaints.
Readiness demands	Insists that he must feel like changing or be ready to change before he is willing to change. Focuses on his lack of motivation or discomfort.
Perfectionism procrastination	Demands a perfect solution before he is willing to try new behavior.
Proving hopelessness	Despite positive resources or progress, attempts to show that everything is hopeless.
Minimal compliance (hedging)	Complies with minimal effort in self-help and then concludes that therapy does not work.
Somatic and vegetative preoccupation	Frequent complaints and overfocus on how badly he feels physically or how exhausted he feels.
Blaming others	Focuses on how others are the cause of his problems—either currently or in the past.
Provoking therapist	Insults therapist, questions therapist's competence, or is sexually provocative.
Disattribution self-handicapping	Creates "barriers" to self-evaluation by self-sabotage (e.g., getting drunk), minimal effort, or taking on impossible tasks.
Hiding	Comes late to sessions, infrequent attendance, hypersomnia, and withdrawal.

cause the patient energetically argues the negative, often to the point of bringing up extraneous material completely unrelated to the topic at hand. By proving the negative and embracing hopelessness, the patient can rest assured within his cocoon of controllable safety. Once the writer was confronted with his investment in proving the negative, he was able to recognize that he was attempting to avoid more "public failure" and humiliation that he feared would occur once he completed his project.

Readiness demands are also central for resistant patients. These individuals utilize emotional reasoning to guide them in making a decision to change. They would rather talk about their problem than actually make a change. "I have to feel ready for a relationship" or "I have to feel ready to move out on my own" are examples of self-limitation that limit risk. They often view talking about their problem as the means whereby they may feel "ready" at some unforeseen point. The patient can be asked, "What would happen if you took this action and you were not ready?" or "Have you ever exercised when you were not ready to exercise?" Individuals focused on readiness can be told that motivation often comes after behavior rather than before it. Behavior is a "warm-up exercise" for motivation (Leahy, 2000d).

Some patients utilize *minimal compliance* (straddling) as a self-limitation tactic. They make a minimal effort and quit early. From the patient's perspective, straddling has a number of advantages. First, the patient can claim that she tried. Second, straddling allows her to "test the waters." If it is unpleasant, she can quit early and not run any further risks. Third, the patient can appear to please the therapist, but maintain her risk-management strategy. Some patients modify the agenda by focusing entirely on somatic and vegetative complaints: "My legs ache. I'm tired. I feel spaced out a lot." These preoccupations not only elicit sympathy from some—especially if the patient is a "doctor shopper"—but they also make her concerns immediate, concrete, and unrelated to self-esteem. The patient often operates with the assumption "If my problems are really medical, then there is nothing wrong with who I am."

Finally, a common method to resist change is "hiding"—simply not showing up. Many patients come late to sessions, attend infrequently, withdraw or become silent, or engage in "no-show" behavior. In many cases, this behavior reflects the patient's ambivalence about the value of therapy, but in some cases it may also reflect the patient's belief that therapy requires too much change. For example, one patient, contemplating separation from his wife, was fearful of separating but unmotivated to work on improving the marriage. He claimed that the therapy sessions were very helpful in making him confront his fears, but he often utilized hiding as a technique both in therapy and in his marriage.

MODIFYING RESISTANCE

The patient implicitly indicates his desire to change by coming to therapy, but he may also be unable to bring about this change. We can view the patient as locked in the classic *neurotic conflict*—that is, trying to achieve two goals simultaneously that appear to him to be self-contradictory. For example, the patient may want to feel less depressed, but fear that change will make him more depressed. In a sense, the patient's conflict is with himself and only incidentally with the therapist. The therapist's role is to help the patient *negotiate change within himself.* The patient should be encouraged to examine this *dialogue with himself*: the part that wants change and the part that resists. I have found that most "resistant" patients are fully aware of their resistance and that they sometimes find confrontation with this resistance refreshing. It "feels authentic," they may say, and it may help them address the confusing dialogue going on within themselves: "I want to change, but I am afraid that this will only make matters worse."

Table 10.2 identifies a number of interventions that may be used to modify resistance. As in *principled negotiation* (Fisher & Ury, 1981), the therapist mediates this negotiation by helping the patient identify his primary goal and examining, collaboratively, how subsequent behavior is related to the goal. For example, the patient's primary goal may be set in the initial treatment planning sessions: "What do you want to accomplish in our work in therapy?" The patient may indicate that his goal is to "feel less depressed" and "to get out of a bad relationship." These goals become the reference point for evaluating resistance. Later, as the patient resists change by attacking the therapist or not doing homework, the therapist should direct the patient's attention to the initial goals: "How will attacking me help you become less depressed?" or "How will not doing homework help you resolve this relationship problem?" The patient's resistance should be conceptualized as a "battle within the self" rather than as "a battle with the therapist"—that is, as conflict between the principle goals and the resistance.

Patients may resist by not setting an agenda. The therapist should refer back to the primary goal: "How will not setting an agenda help you overcome your depression?" or "What are the costs and benefits of not having an agenda?" One patient indicated that the cost of setting an agenda was that he would then be committed to change. If the therapist imposed an agenda, he reasoned, then he could reject the agenda as irrelevant—thereby avoiding change—or he could explore the agenda to see if it was "safe." The therapist can also directly identify patterns of self-defeat in other areas of the patient's life: "I have noticed that you do not have an agenda for our sessions. I wonder if this is a pattern that you

TABLE 10.2. Contrasting Success with Self-Handicapping

Tactic	Example
Examine reasons for and against success in the future	"Let's examine all the possible reasons why you might [or might not] have success in the future. Are any of these potentially within your control? What if you persisted at something for a long time?"
Recall previous successes	"You have had some success at some things in the past. What have you had even partial success at? How did you do that? What did you say to yourself? Can you apply any of that to your current problems?"
Externalize the self-defeat voice	"Let's practice arguing against the negative self-defeat voice. I'll be the negative voice, you argue against me." THERAPIST: It's too good to be true. You may as well quit now and not be a fool. PATIENT: I can make progress on some things. I'm not a bad person. I deserve some good things in life.
Experiment with success	"Let's set up some experiments with small amounts of success and see what it triggers for you. Do you become anxious, angry, sad, confused, regretful, etc? What are your automatic thoughts? How would you challenge them?"
Contract against self-defeat	"Would you be willing to put off sabotaging yourself until you speak with the therapist?"
Slow down success	"Rather than become demanding and impatient with success, would you be willing to experience success only in small doses and pull back momentarily from too much success?"
Lower the idealization of success	"Some people get too far ahead of themselves when they think of success—in fact, they think of perfection. Is this what you do? Do you get disillusioned? Would you be willing to consider progress, not perfection, as the goal? What are the costs and benefits of accepting progress rather than demanding or needing perfection?"
Write a success script	"Describe, from beginning to end, how you could succeed at something. At what points in the script do you feel anxious, angry, depressed, confused, etc.? What's going through your mind?"
Self-reward for success	"You have had mixed feelings about progress, so it's important to reward yourself when you experience positives. Make a list of ways of praising yourself when you pursue positives."

may have in other areas of your life. For example, do you find yourself 'reacting' to events rather than actively making them change?"

Straddling strategies can be identified and examined for costs and benefits. For example, a woman who would remain aloof and distrustful with men, even though she claimed she wanted a relationship, indicated that by holding back (straddling) she was able to "test out" the man's true intentions. It had not occurred to her that her aloofness was perceived as cold rejection by men that then led them to withdraw, thereby confirming her negative predictions about men. The therapist was able to convince her to temporarily abandon straddling and to focus on monitoring any positive attention from men. She was also instructed to reward positive attention. This offset the straddling, which then helped disconfirm (partially) her negative view of interacting with men.

Some individuals self-defeat because they fear that they cannot adapt to the "costs of success." These individuals believe that further movement forward may demand greater intimacy (and rejection), greater success (and a more precipitous fall to failure), and greater public recognition (and a higher risk of humiliation). Motivated negative cognition and vigorous arguments favoring hopelessness often reveal these fears of success. (I view this as a fear of the *consequences* of success, rather than a fear of success per se.) The therapist can examine these fears directly by asking the patient about the fears of greater demands, higher expectations, greater exposure, or greater disappointment, which might accompany greater success. The therapist may ask how the patient has handled success in the past. For example, one patient indicated that she did well on her graduate exams, leading to an increase in her hopes, only to be rejected by all the schools to which she applied (given her perfection, she had only applied to a few elite schools). Another woman indicated that she had become very close to a man she planned to marry but then he suddenly broke off the engagement. This resulted in her future relationship choices: she either chose men who were less successful than she was, thereby allowing her to devalue them as marital choices, or she would act out through infidelity when she was involved with men whom she viewed as plausible marital partners. Her ultimate fear was that she would end up in a marriage that would not work and that this would lead either to a man betraying her or to her sense of failure. By "self-sabotaging" she was able to achieve her goal of preventing "success" from moving forward into the risks of "ultimate betrayal and failure." As indicated, moving forward, for many of these people, may confer greater risk.

The patient may have fears of greater exposure. The writer mentioned earlier feared that once he completed his work, it would either be rejected by the publisher or it would result in his public humiliation once it was published. This individual utilized marijuana smoking as a self-handicapping excuse: "I'll get around to my writing once I get a handle on my smoking." His inflated ego ideal—of being a famous writer—resulted in his utilization of numerous self-defeating strategies: hypersomnia, conflicts with his partner, and fixing his apartment. Once these fears of self-evaluation were exposed, he was able to finish his writing.

The emphasis on minimization of loss as a strategy is central for many individuals resisting change. For example, the patient may only search for evidence of the possibility of failure. Once he finds this "evidence," he quits. This "stop-loss" approach may result in the patient saying, "I've tried all these things before, but they do not work." The patient has *really* tried straddling in order to minimize losses. The therapist can help the patient by asking him to self-contract for continued effort or longer duration in a situation (e.g., a relationship), before quitting is "allowed." Normalizing loss, rather than catastrophizing it, may also help the patient overcome the minimization strategy. For example, viewing loss as a learning experience, a normal step toward later rewards, the cost of "doing business," or as compartmentalized, may be helpful in allowing the patient to view experience and loss as investments in the future.

Some patients act like "binge eaters" when success occurs. They "jump" into relationships too quickly and too intensely and then are bitterly disappointed when these relationships do not work out. The therapist may introduce the idea of a "deprivation-hunger" model to highlight the increased demand for immediate and great success. The patient can examine the costs of demanding more success immediately—for example, the tendency to overcommit too early to problematic relationships, thereby confirming the belief that "relationships don't work out." In many cases the hunger-deprivation process may alienate others, thereby resulting in the self-fulfilling prophecies of the depressed patients. One analogy that is useful is that of "rappelling ropes" in climbing: short changes in height or descent are accompanied by readjustments to the safety ropes. I have found it helpful to have patients "slow down" success so that they do not get their hopes up too high or demand too much from others.

Many self-defeating individuals have been busy creating stories about their possible failures. Detailed narratives are helpful in assisting the patient in imagining success and making it plausible. In contrast, cognitive therapy homework may often appear too intellectual and dry—it may lack a "real-life feeling." Stories tend to be memorable, which may account for their popularity in all cultures for conveying important "lessons." The patient can be asked to write out brief (two-page) stories about specific details about how she can be successful in developing a relationship. For example, one woman found it helpful to write out a short story about meeting a man, going out on a date, getting to know each other, and developing a meaningful relationship. Even though she had been in relationships before, she indicated that this was a totally novel exercise for her since she seldom visualized things working out. Narratives are valuable as a way of "concretizing" the plans that the patient can imagine executing in solving a problem and achieving a goal. These narratives may also reveal the points when the patient becomes anxious or depressed: "I became anxious in my story when we talked about sex because then I realized that I thought he was just trying to use me." The patient's fears of this "exploitation" may be addressed by asking the patient, "What would it mean to you if all he wanted was sex?" One woman indicated that it meant that he was superior and she was worthless. Her anticipation of this exploitation often led her to provoke the man aggressively, and thereby avoid the risk of intimacy.

SUMMARY

Inhibition of movement is often very adaptive—such as the inhibition to sail in heavy winds or to cross a swaying bridge. The approach presented here allows both patient and therapist to collaborate in understanding the "value" of resistance and to explore the implications of change. By examining the negative self-verification of straddling, hedging, hiding, and provoking, the patient and therapist can reattribute "failure" to "too much risk management" rather than to personal and permanent inadequacies. Conceptualizing resistance as self-protective "adaptation" is considerably less pejorative for patients than to view them as "unmotivated." Resolving the internal conflict—between the self that seeks improvement and the self that fears loss—allows "resistant" patients to understand how getting in their own way has appeared to them necessary for self-protection.

PART III

*Cognitive Therapy
and Countertransference*

11

Evaluating the Countertransference

*I*n Donald Light's (1970) classic, *Becoming Psychiatrists*, the author describes the socialization process for the psychiatrist in medical school. The task for the psychiatrist, according to one resident, was to learn to go down the "path" with the patient, to see and experience the world from the patient's viewpoint, but then *be able to return*. The work of therapy is difficult, rewarding, and, for some, frightening. None of us is free from countertransference—nor should we be. To understand our own limitations, our own *resistance* to change, is to discover more about the patient and ourselves: as we learn about how the patient's behavior affects our own countertransference, we are also learning about how the patient affects others.

The therapist uses all of the automatic thought distortions in the countertransference: "This patient is resistant" (labeling); "He'll never get better" (fortune telling); "He's made no improvement" (all-or-nothing thinking); "It's all my fault the patient is still depressed" (personalizing); "I can't stand it when the patient whines" (catastrophizing); "The patient should do homework" (shoulds); and "My patients won't get better" (overgeneralizing).

There are numerous reasons why individuals are attracted to the profession of psychotherapist. Many clinicians would like to believe—or wish others to believe—that their primary or even sole motive is the desire to help other people. Indeed, altruistic motives rank quite high for many, if not most, therapists. Yet the role of "therapist" allows the individual to pursue other motives or needs too. These include the desire to be wanted and needed by another person, power and control, emotional

voyeurism, the desire to vicariously experience other lives or intense feelings, prestige, money, the need to "repair"or atone for damaged relationships of one's own, the need to be a "good" person or to be perceived as "good" by others, and the need to be admired. In some cases,
the focus on the patient's problems may allow the therapist to compartmentalize and avoid her own personal problems or may allow the therapist to displace her conflicts with others onto the patient. This list, of
course, is far from exhaustive. Moreover, any one therapist may have
multiple motives that are pursued in the profession (Pope & Vasquez,
1998; Schafer, 1954).

Some people are attracted to being cognitive-behavioral therapists
because it allows them a sense of competence, superiority, and apparent
efficacy. Many have read the popular books on cognitive-behavioral
therapy and approach their work with the assumption that they will be
able to "cure" their patients within 10 sessions. Some may even turn to
treatment manuals or books on techniques (Beck et al., 1979, 1990;
Leahy & Holland, 2000) with the idea that these "tools" will allow the
therapist to "fix" everything. This *illusion of competence* may allow the
therapist to unconsciously pursue other goals, such as the need to have
power or control, or the need to compartmentalize, intellectualize, and
isolate oneself from one's own problems.

When most of us first learned to do cognitive-behavioral therapy we
ignored the countertransference. Our underlying assumption was, "If
the transference doesn't touch you, don't touch the transference." Certainly, if we ignored the transference, we would ignore our own countertransference. Perhaps we were overly optimistic about the power of the
techniques, treatment plans, and "professionalism" that our approach
offered. Yet I have observed a substantial range of efficacy in how different therapists apply cognitive therapy. Some therapists have considerable
difficulty being assertive and utilizing interventions, while others are too
technique oriented. Some do reasonably well with borderline patients,
others feel consumed, mistreated, and defeated by them. Some therapists
have high dropout rates, others build a loyal following.

Success or failure is not reducible to intelligence or training. Some
therapists who publish many articles and books have narcissistic countertransference that leads to high dropout rates and hostile confronta-
tions that appear unnecessary—if not unethical. In fact, my own overly
optimistic views of cognitive therapy led me, early in my work, to overlook the deeper pathology of some of my patients and not to recognize
that a patient was on the verge of dropping out. My schemas were too
positive and too self-serving, making me feel good and leading me to believe that I was more competent than I really was. So initially I missed
the dynamics, fears, and self-protective strategies of some patients.

This led me to ask myself two very general and, I think, important questions:

1. What were some signs of the patient's pathology that I had missed?
2. What was it about me that made me miss them?

I have since found it useful to keep these questions in mind on a daily basis. Typical problems in the countertransference among people I have supervised include the following:

- Ambivalence about using techniques because of fears of alienating the patient
- Guilt or fear over the patient's anger
- Feelings of inferiority when working with narcissistic patients
- Discomfort if the patient is sexually attractive
- Inability to set limits on sexually provocative or hostile patients
- Overextending therapy sessions
- Lack of assertion in collecting fees or enforcing policies
- Inhibition in taking an adequate sexual history
- Anger at patients who make phone calls between sessions
- Catastrophizing the issue of hospitalizing a patient

Therapy is difficult work. You are not only applying techniques and conceptualizing problems, you are applying *yourself*. When patients present with issues such as abandonment, dependency, devaluation, demandingness, sexual preoccupations, abuse, betrayal, or exploitation of others, they may arouse your own feelings and vulnerabilities about these issues. Hiding behind the techniques of cognitive therapy or dismissing the patient with a label ("She's a borderline") will inadvertently sabotage the therapy. Perhaps some patients are exquisitely tuned to the countertransference in the therapist—perhaps they can "read" the therapist's vulnerabilities. But we cannot make the countertransference go away simply because we might wish it did not affect the treatment.

In truth, countertransference can be one of the most *useful* tools in helping patients—it can provide a window into the "real-world effects" that the patient has outside of therapy. If the patient is devaluing the therapist, then he is probably devaluing other people. This can be helpful in diagnosing his problem and helping the patient understand how his behavior may affect others. It may be used to develop the patient's understanding of what has led to this mode of interaction, provide the patient with a role model (i.e., the therapist) who does not devalue the patient, and help him to develop more effective ways of communicating and relating in therapy. There are two questions for us to consider. First, How can we evaluate the countertransference to help ourselves? And, second, How can we use the countertransference to help the patient? Let us turn to some guidelines.

GUIDELINES TO UNDERSTANDING
YOUR COUNTERTRANSFERENCE

• *It exists*. Despite the manualization of treatment and the emphasis on techniques and pharmacotherapy, countertransference does exist. Even if you think it does not exist for you, it does. Your claim that you do not have a countertransference may only illustrate how highly defended and unaware of it you are. Your belief that you are successful and your patients like you is no proof that you lack a countertransference and, in fact, may be part of your countertransference.

One therapist, who viewed himself as exceptionally rational, efficient, pragmatic, and unaffected by emotions, claimed that he did not have any countertransference. He was "just doing his job." He was contemptuous of the idea of countertransference: it was a useless vestige of "outmoded psychoanalytic thinking." However, his highly defended, intellectualized, and emotionally isolating style came across to patients as sterile, mechanical, condescending, and artificial. Some patients viewed him as knowledgeable about techniques. However, others viewed him as limited. When patients would fail to "comply" with his regimen, he simply dismissed them as "unmotivated." Consequently, his approach to patients was dramatically limited by his denial of his countertransference and his unwillingness to directly validate and empathize with his patients' strong emotions.

• *Examine the kinds of problems or kinds of patients that arouse strong feelings in you*. Your countertransference may not be strong with all patients, but it may be activated with certain kinds of patients—some of whom you may be avoiding. Imagine that I were now going to describe a patient that would really push your buttons, someone who would always make you angry, defensive, or anxious. What kinds of problems would that patient present? How would they communicate them to you in a way that would bother you?

Therapists often comment that what they find especially disturbing about borderline patients is their intense anger, neediness, lability, "manipulation," demandingness, and their tendency to "act out" by noncompliance, substance abuse, or parasuicidal and suicidal attempts.

These therapeutic problems affect the countertransference in a variety of ways (which I shall discuss later), but it is important to keep in mind that the therapeutic conflict is not only in the patient: it is in the clinician too.

• *Are there some patients or problems that bore you or some patients or problems you do not care about?* Some therapists claim they are bored with patients that complain or whine. But what is the countertransference issue for the therapist? One therapist indicated that complaining patients activated feelings in her of being helpless and feeling "trapped." Her attitude was "I've got to sit here and listen to this when I could be doing something more productive." Her schemas were those of demanding standards: the need to be productive and to have control. She experienced patients' complaints and demands as an infringement on her autonomy. We will examine later how one can modify boring interactions.

• *Are there some patients that "feel like friends"?* This may sound like an odd question—after all, what is so wrong with really liking a patient? The problem that may arise is that seeing a patient "like a friend" may keep you from seeing the "pathology" or problems that he or she has. It may make it more difficult for you to assert yourself with the patient. Thus therapy may focus more on agreeing with one another and less on the need for change. The patient may also see his relationship with the therapist as "friendship" and consequently may be reluctant to bring up certain issues. Moreover, for the therapist, there may be a risk of crossing into a dual role with the patient. Ask yourself, "How would I feel about bringing up difficult topics with this patient?"

• *What are your typical schemas or the conflicts in your interpersonal life?* In order to examine the countertransference, you should examine the kinds of life problems that you typically have. Are you someone who is concerned about rejection or abandonment? Then you should examine how these issues arise in your contact with patients. Are you someone who always has to be "right"? Then examine how you may be trying to defeat patients in debates, and thereby invalidate them. Are you someone who is afraid of failing, because you think that success or failure indicates how worthwhile you are? Then examine how you may be afraid of dealing with difficult patients or afraid of taking chances in therapy. None of us has a conflict-free life. Conflicts will either inhibit your ability to do therapy or they could, if processed appropriately, help you and the patient.

• *What is your worst nightmare or worst possible scenario in dealing with patients?* When I have asked therapists this question—using the vertical descent procedure ("What would happen next?")—I have received a variety of responses. These worst outcomes include the patient's suicide, being sued and discredited, or having a failing practice. Other "less-than-terrible" outcomes that are envisaged include being humiliated in front of peers, losing control with a patient, being physically attacked, getting fired, or losing referral sources. Are you worried that problems with patients will unravel into your worst fantasy? How likely is this to happen and how would you prevent it from happening?

For example, one therapist worried that if a patient dropped out of therapy because she was angry, then word would spread that the therapist was not competent. The final consequence would be that all referrals would drop out, he would have no income, and his family would think he was a failure.

COUNTERTRANSFERENCE SCHEMAS

Just as the patient's schemas will result in resistance, so also the therapist's individual schemas will affect the countertransference. For example, the therapist with a perfectionistic or "unyielding standards" schema may find that the patient's lack of responsiveness to therapy interferes with his own goals of being a perfect therapist. There are probably as many schemas as there are adjectives to describe people. A number of the most common therapist schemas are listed in Figure 11.1. Later in the chapter I examine the assumptions underlying each schema (see Table 11.1). Many therapists display more than one schema. Moreover, some patients are more likely to activate certain schemas than others. For example, borderline patients may be more likely than obsessive–compulsive patients to activate autonomy schemas in a therapist because the borderline patient is more likely to press the therapist's boundaries. A number of these more common therapist schemas are described below.

Demanding Standards

Perfectionistic or obsessive–compulsive therapists often view patients as irresponsible, self-indulgent, and lazy (see Beck et al., 1990; Shapiro, 1965). These rigid character types believe that the expression of emotion, or even uncertainty, is wasteful. They have difficulty expressing warmth and empathy toward the patient because of their insistence that the patient needs to "get down to business." Their emphasis on time efficiency may be helpful in maintaining focus in sessions, but often causes

In the "Rating" column below, indicate how you feel about this particular patient thus far in working with him or her. There are no right or wrong answers. Try to avoid giving answers that you think are desirable.

Rating scale: 1 = Very untrue, 2 = Somewhat untrue, 3 = Slightly untrue, 4 = Slightly true, 5 = Somewhat true, 6 = Very true

Assumptions	Rating
1. I have to cure all my patients.	____
2. I must always meet the highest standards.	____
3. My patients should do an excellent job.	____
4. We should never waste time.	____
5. I am entitled to be successful.	____
6. My patients should appreciate all that I do for them.	____
7. I shouldn't feel bored when doing therapy.	____
8. Patients try to humiliate me.	____
9. Conflicts are upsetting.	____
10. I shouldn't raise issues that will bother the patient.	____
11. If my patient is bothered with therapy, he or she might leave.	____
12. It's upsetting when patients terminate.	____
13. I might end up with no patients.	____
14. I feel controlled by the patient.	____
15. My movements, feelings, or what I say are limited.	____
16. I should be able to do or say what I wish.	____
17. Sometimes I wonder if I will lose myself in the relationship.	____
18. I have to control my surroundings or the people around me.	____
19. Some people are basically bad people.	____
20. People should be punished if they do wrong things.	____
21. I often feel provoked.	____
22. The patient is trying to get to me.	____
23. I have to guard against being taken advantage of or hurt.	____
24. You usually can't trust people.	____
25. I want to be liked by the patient.	____
26. If the patient isn't happy with me, then it means I'm doing something wrong.	____
27. It's important that I like the patient.	____
28. It bothers me if I don't like the patient.	____
29. We should get along—almost like friends.	____
30. I want to withhold thoughts and feelings from the patient.	____
31. I don't want to give them what they want.	____
32. I feel I am withdrawing emotionally during the session.	____
33. I feel I don't know what to do.	____
34. I fear I'll make mistakes.	____

FIGURE 11.1. Therapist's schema questionnaire.

(continued)

Assumptions	Rating
35. I wonder if I'm really competent.	____
36. Sometimes I feel like giving up.	____
37. The patient is blocking me from achieving my goals.	____
38. I feel like I'm wasting time.	____
39. I should be able to achieve my goals in sessions without the patient's interference.	____
40. I should meet the patients' needs.	____
41. I should make them feel better.	____
42. The patients' needs often take precedence over my needs.	____
43. I sometimes believe that I would do almost anything to meet their needs.	____
44. I feel frustrated when I'm with this patient because I can't express the way I really feel.	____
45. I find it hard to suppress my feelings.	____
46. I can't be myself.	____

FIGURE 11.1. (*continued from previous page*)

them to overlook or discount the patient's emotional turmoil. The perfectionistic, rigid character type places so much emphasis on "logic" and "rationality" that the patient may feel that therapy is simply an opportunity for the therapist to show that he or she is smarter than the patient.

For example, a number of years ago I was called on to supervise a beginning intern in cognitive-behavior therapy. The intern seemed to believe that therapy involved nothing more than showing the patient how stupid and irrational he or she was. In conducting role plays with this therapist, in which I played the role of patient, I felt barraged and belittled by the intern. When we explored the intern's assumptions, it became clear that he believed the patient "should not be irrational." He also believed he should try to impress me, the supervisor, with how smart he was. I asked the trainee, "Why should the patient be rational?" His response was, "Because being irrational won't help him." I pointed out that all of us are irrational sometimes and that the patient's irrationality may be why he came for treatment. I also suggested that the trainee examine whether demanding rationality from patients was an irrational assumption.

The perfectionistic therapist has unrealistic expectations of self and patient, usually expressed in *imperatives*:

Self: "I *should* be able to cure my patients"; "I *should* know everything about the patient's problems"; "The session *should* go according to my plans."

Patient: "The patient *should* do the homework"; "The patient *should* be more responsible."

The perfectionistic therapist may attempt to compensate for underlying feelings of incompetence and worthlessness by demanding perfect performance from self and patient. When the therapist examines his or her automatic thoughts, the following is a typical sequence of thoughts: "My patient is not getting better → I'm not doing my job → I'll be exposed as a fraud → I'm a failure → I can't accept any failure in myself." Therapists with perfectionistic standards may attempt to avoid their schema by refusing to take on difficult cases, or by assuming that the patient is correct—that is, that his or her depression is hopeless.

Conversely, the therapist may compensate for her perfectionism by demanding more and more from the patient. The patient may perceive this as evidence that he has failed the therapist and the therapy, since he cannot keep up with the therapist's demands. The demanding therapist, in her effort to constantly produce change, may not allow the patient to move forward at his own pace. The patient may get the impression that the therapist does not listen or that the demanding therapist is trying to control him. I have found myself in this role of demanding change when change was not occurring. I would heap one technique on after another, only to find that my patient did not "comply." Finally, recognizing my own schematic problem with an "avoidant" and "passive–aggressive" patient, I decided to practice the opposite of such demandingness.

THERAPIST: I have been demanding too much change from you. I've been trying to get you to do what I want you to do. I think that this has been frustrating for you.

PATIENT: That's right. You have to understand that I am extremely shy. I don't do things that easily.

THERAPIST: I agree with you. I've decided to step back from trying to change you. I have decided that for the next few sessions I will only try to understand you and not try to change you.

The patient found this new approach to be a relief. I did too. I realized that I could still do therapy without demanding change from patients. The patient began describing some changes (asking a woman out) that he wanted to make. Knowing my own proclivity for demanding change and his style of demanding autonomy from my control, I simply relinquished change to him.

THERAPIST: I think that it's up to you what you do about asking her out. I don't want to get into trying to change you. I think you need to think this through for yourself.

PATIENT: What do you think I should do?

THERAPIST: Are there any cognitive therapy techniques that we have used in the past that you might want to assign to yourself?

Abandonment

Therapists concerned about abandonment issues are often worried that if they confront the patient, then the patient will leave therapy. Any premature termination of therapy is interpreted as a personal rejection of the therapist. As Bowlby (1969, 1973, 1980) has indicated, anxiety about attachment issues may take many different forms, which we might see reflected in the countertransference—for example, in clinging by the therapist, excessive caretaking of the patient, or even avoidance of entering into a meaningful therapeutic relationship. The *clinging* therapist has difficulty in letting the patient leave therapy—or even ending sessions. For example, the clinging therapist may extend session time, provide free therapy over the phone, and protest vigorously and defensively when the patient wants to leave therapy. *Excessive caretaking* by the therapist takes the form of trying to protect the patient from any difficulties and taking on the patient's problems as the therapist's own to solve.

Attachment avoidance is one strategy that the therapist may use to avoid threats of abandonment: if the therapist never allows the patient or the self to become attached, then abandonment is not an issue. *Attachment-avoidant* therapists seem to trivialize therapy, often focusing more on superficial techniques (such as biofeedback) than on more meaningful personal issues. The attachment-avoidant therapist may see the patient as simply a collection of symptoms or as a "very sick person."

The therapist who is concerned with abandonment often personalizes the patient's lateness, nonpayment of bills, failure to show up for a session, or lack of interest in therapy. Abandonment-oriented therapists will often compromise their professionalism in order to keep patients interested and involved in the therapeutic relationship. For example, therapists who view the patient's resistance as personal rejection and threat of abandonment may extend sessions beyond the customary time limit, not collect fees, avoid confronting the patient's irrational thoughts and self-destructive behavior, and engage in excessive between-sessions phone contact with the patient.

Exceptional fear of patients leaving therapy may lead the therapist to avoid difficult topics with patients, trivialize the sessions, and refrain from using anxiety-provoking interventions, such as exposure techniques. Among those I have trained, the therapist who is most afraid of losing a patient is the one most likely to lose patients. Very few people want to go to a therapist who seems desperate for patients.

The therapist who is overly concerned with abandonment by patients should examine the purpose of therapy. Is the patient coming in to therapy because the therapist needs patients? Does the patient really believe that everything that is said in therapy will be pleasant and soothing? Patients seeking help will be more likely to come back when they think that the therapist is helping them change. Therapists who are overly concerned about abandonment can think of very successful therapists that they know. Do these therapists always please patients? Do they ever say things that may be unpleasant for the patient to hear? Do they use exposure techniques? Do they set limits? And, even if they are very successful, do they still have patients that leave treatment prematurely?

One assumption is that patients who are really upset are more likely to leave therapy. Indeed, one can make an opposing argument, claiming that patients with intense emotions are in greater need of therapy. Therapists who are overly concerned about abandonment may be especially adept at validating the needs of patients—an ability that may help bond the patient in therapy. However, structuring the therapy with the patient—setting agendas, eliciting and challenging negative thoughts, providing homework assignments—is the key element in effective cognitive therapy. The therapist who believes that only validating the patient will effect change soon learns that the patient can go elsewhere for these needs.

The narcissistic patient may intimidate the therapist who fears abandonment—especially if the patient is highly achieving. These narcissistic and highly achieving patients are exquisitely tuned to the vulnerabilities of dependent individuals. They may attempt to exploit the therapist's fears by threatening to leave treatment by showing up late, or by devaluing the therapist. The therapist may express his vulnerability by extending special privileges or, alternatively, may become defensive. In either case, the narcissistic patient gains confirmation for his pathology—that is, "I can be treated as special" or "I can't trust people with my feelings." The therapist should avoid extending special privileges, but can elicit thoughts and feelings from the patient about the limitations established in treatment: "It seems that you were upset last week when I did not extend the session time. I wonder what your thoughts were when we completed the session?" This inquiry may lead the narcissistic patient to confess his feelings of inadequacy or rejection—for example, "I didn't feel as important as the other patients that you see" or

"I didn't feel that you cared about me." These statements can then lead to admissions of more general feelings that the self is less important than others, and the feelings of envy involved with this, and to feelings that the patient seldom obtains understanding and support. The therapist can then examine the kinds of feelings and behaviors that follow when these thoughts occur—for example, does the patient then devalue others or distance himself?

Special, Superior Person

The narcissistic therapist views therapy as an opportunity to "shine," to show off his or her special talents. Therapy with the resistant patient may begin with grandiose hopes, expressed by the therapist, that the patient has finally found the "right therapist": "Now your problems will be solved." The therapist's investment in her own image of being a special, superior therapist may result in her joining with the chronically depressed patient to vilify all the other therapists who have "failed" the patient. Or the narcissistic therapist may feel envious of other relationships that the patient has—for example, with friends, spouse, or another therapist.

The narcissistic therapist feels entitled to having the cooperation and adulation of the patient. This may result in the therapist encouraging boundary violations by the patient or, in some cases, the therapist herself may initiate these boundary violations. To the narcissistic therapist, boundaries, like other rules, do not apply to special people like herself. As the therapeutic relationship unfolds—if the patient does not make rapid progress—the narcissistic therapist may grow bored with, angry at, or punitive toward the patient. The patient's "failure" to improve is inconsistent with the therapist's belief in her special talents, raising uncomfortable doubts for the therapist. Rather than empathize with the patient's understandable frustration with lack of progress, the therapist may turn on the patient, blaming the patient for a lack of desire to improve or, in a paranoid construction, may view the patient's inability to change as a personal affront or attack on the therapist.

Narcissistic therapists utilize the three defenses that Kernberg (1975, 1978) has described: idealization, devaluation, and distancing. In order to bolster her own self-esteem, the narcissistic therapist may idealize the patient as extraordinarily successful and attractive, basking in the reflection of the patient's glamour. Alternatively, the narcissistic therapist may idealize the cognitive-therapy model, and herself as an expert, viewing the therapy, in her hands, as the panacea—which it is not. The initial satisfaction of this idealization acts as a compensation for feelings of envy that the therapist may experience or feelings of helplessness, which becomes apparent once the therapy departs from the idealization.

As the patient fails to live up to the idealization—or the therapist recognizes that he is not as wonderful as she assumed he was—the narcissistic therapist may begin to devalue the patient. The patient's resistance becomes a "failing" on the part of the patient, rather than a window into his vulnerabilities and strategies of coping. The patient is labeled as a "borderline," "narcissist," or just plain "pain in the ass," who "doesn't want to get better." The narcissistic therapist may engage in attempts to humiliate the patient by ridiculing his thinking or situation, further leading to protests by the patient, which are then interpreted by the therapist as proof that the patient cannot be helped by anyone.

The alternative to devaluation—-or what often comes after—is distancing from the patient. The patient who has "failed" the narcissist therapist may find that the therapist seems bored, does not return calls, shows little empathy and expresses very little interest in the patient's life. Usually the patient has decided to terminate the therapy by this time, further supporting the narcissist therapist's view that the patient was not serious about changing. These profound empathic failures of the narcissistic therapist may have lasting negative effects on the patient, who may view this failed therapeutic relationship as proof that no one understands him or can be trusted.

Unfortunately, the nature of therapy appeals to the narcissist. She can feel superior to the patient, who is in the role of someone who is needy and who has little power in the relationship. Patients may idealize the therapist, fueling her narcissism. The cognitive-behavioral model may appeal to an individual who wishes to avoid empathy, reject any moral obligations, and delude herself with the idea that she has a fix on a panacea. Yet, if the narcissist is able to acquire fame, her narcissism may continue unabated as the therapist gains referrals and support for her illusion that she really is effective.

This is not to say that the narcissistic therapist is *not* effective. Her style may appeal to other narcissists, obsessive–compulsives, and dependent patients who are not too demanding. Yet the narcissist may wish to examine the limitations that this schema of "being special" may have in achieving the goal of being a better therapist. Despite my own training in the techniques of cognitive therapy, and my own overconfidence at times, I recognize that the greatest insights come from patients, not from therapists. Like Socrates, we gain our understanding of what is true by asking the right questions, which reveal the vastness of our ignorance.

To modify the narcissistic perspective, one needs to ask one question: "What would your life be like if you had to walk in the shoes of this patient?" It is facile to dismiss a patient by attaching a label—"She's a borderline" or "He's a paranoid"—but it is something quite different to imagine what your life would be like to have these problems. Who among us has not experienced despair, fear, loneliness, humiliation, or distrust? Was it so simple to modify one's own experience—even with cognitive therapy tools in hand? By recognizing the limitations of the cognitive-behavioral model in your own life, you may gain some understanding of how difficult it really is in the patient's life.

Some cognitive therapists sound like Pangloss, in Voltaire's *Candide*, who always claimed that "this is the best of all possible worlds." Predicaments and dilemmas that are real and losses that feel overwhelming to almost anyone are viewed by the glib narcissist as "simple problems with obvious solutions." One serious consequence of the therapist's narcissism is that she provides the patient with little authentic validation.

The narcissistic therapist wishes to feel "on top" of the situation, yet reality often means that we are helpless, but sympathetic, witnesses to the tragedies of life. A patient that I had been seeing for quite some time told me that his 22-year-old son had died suddenly, for no apparent reason, while sitting on a bus next to his grandmother. The patient was in a state of desperation. For that moment I knew that I was totally helpless, in fact, in awe of the situation he was in. My only response was to say, "My God. This is the most horrible thing that has ever happened to you. I cannot imagine how you can ever be consoled." That moment of our mutual helplessness, the feeling of sadness that we both felt, established our bond and helped him, at least for a moment. I was not a special person, nor was he. We shared our bewilderment: both of us were sad, both recognizing our helplessness, both not knowing what to say.

Ironically, the confidence and sense of superiority of the narcissistic therapist results in a superficial therapy—a sense that it is shallow, not special, not meaningful. In contrast, to empathically understand the patient's construction of reality, and the patient's reasons for resisting, may give the therapy special significance for both patient and therapist.

Need for Approval

The "people-pleasing" therapist, who wishes to make the patient feel good regardless of what is going on, is averse to any expression of anger or disappointment by the patient. These "pleasing" therapists may be highly skilled in showing empathy for the patient and, by virtue of this empathy, certainly help the patient to feel valued and understood. Yet this may conflict with perceiving the angry emotions of the patient. For example, a "pleasing" therapist, whose warmth and empathy were much appreciated by many patients, had difficulty recognizing that borderline patients were very angry. She would "underdiagnose" patients because she feared labeling them in a negative way and thereby alienating them. Another therapist found it difficult to make the decision to hospitalize a suicidal patient because of her concern that the patient would get angry with her.

The pleasing therapist will avoid raising questions about the patient's substance abuse, anger, resistance, and self-defeat. These topics are viewed as too disturbing to the patient, and therefore as not appropriate. The therapist and patient may continue in a "chumship" that goes unchallenged by either party until the patient eventually recognizes that he or she is getting nowhere and leaves treatment.

Therapists with a high need for approval may inadvertently communicate the idea that the therapist approves of or does not care about the more negative behavior of the patient. Patients may act out by missing sessions, showing up late, or not doing homework, but the high-need-for-approval therapist, who does not want to cause a "conflict," communicates the idea that acting-out behavior is acceptable. The therapist may find that the patient's anger is difficult to tolerate. When a borderline patient abruptly walked out of the session, her therapist followed after her into the waiting room in tears: "She is furious with me! I really screwed up. She won't come back!"

The therapist concluded that the patient's anger was intolerable, awful, catastrophic, and would necessarily end treatment. In fact, it was part of the modus operandi of this particular patient, who would intimidate people (including her past and present therapist) with this kind of behavior. The therapist personalized the patient's behavior and viewed the patient's disapproval as a sign of her own failing. His assumption was, "If the patient is angry at me, it means that I failed."

Excessive Self-Sacrifice

Many people became therapists because of their codependent personalities. Many therapists find vicarious meaning in feeling needed by patients. The self-defeating or masochistic therapist may feel unworthy of being assertive with the patient—especially if the patient seems to be worse off than the therapist. These self-sacrificing therapists may hold to an implicit contract: "I will do everything for you as long as you don't leave me." Some of these therapists will not collect fees, lest the patient think that the therapist is too greedy and uncaring.

There are a variety of negative consequences for such excessive self-sacrifice. First, the nonassertive therapist becomes a very poor role model for the patient. Second, he may blur professional boundaries, confusing the patient as to whether the therapist is a friend or a professional, available at all times. Third, excessive self-sacrifice makes it difficult for the therapist to encourage the patient to engage in unpleasant exposure. Fourth, self-sacrificing reluctance to collect fees suggests to the patient that the therapist may question the value of the service. It may even make some patients apprehensive that they will eventually be presented with a huge bill. Finally, extending sessions beyond their normal time limits may suggest to the patient that other boundary violations may be permitted—such as sexual intimacy or demands on the therapist.

For example, a therapist marked by doubts of his competence to provide adequate treatment for patients was extremely reluctant to engage phobic patients in exposure to fear hierarchies. He disliked making anyone feel uncomfortable. He would extend sessions beyond the allotted time frame and he allowed his patients to be late in paying for appointments. Rather than charging the standard fee, he would often express his own doubts that the patient could afford the fee and spontaneously offer to lower the fee. His attempts to please the patient and sacrifice his own interests resulted in a high dropout rate.

THERAPIST 1: If you were a physician, and the patient needed a shot of morphine, would you be reluctant to give it to him because the injection might hurt?

THERAPIST 2: Probably not.

THERAPIST 1: And if the patient needed surgery, would you refuse to operate?

THERAPIST 2: Not if I thought it would help them.

THERAPIST 1: Often, in therapy, patients must engage in behavior that raises their discomfort in order for them to get better—very much like the patient receiving an injection or experiencing surgery. Very much like when you or I go to the dentist. Patients return to therapy and refer their friends to you because you help them change, not because you refuse to challenge them.

Autonomy

For the therapist with an overdeveloped sense of autonomy, the patient's emotional expression, unpredictability, lateness for appointments, refusal to do what is asked, and, especially, emergency phone calls or demands for extra attention will cause conflict. For example, a therapist complained of an emergency phone call.

THERAPIST 1: Let's look at your automatic thoughts here. "This phone call bothered me because I thought . . . ?"

THERAPIST 2: She will take over my whole life.

THERAPIST 1: And then what will happen?

THERAPIST 2: And then I won't have any life of my own.

Although the therapist was doing very good work with this challenging patient, his own anger might have gotten in the way of empathizing and supporting the patient during this time. The therapist was able to recognize that he, himself, was overgeneralizing and catastrophizing—indeed, this was the first time since the patient had begun therapy that she had made an emergency phone call. In fact, the emergency contact could be construed as an example of the respect that the patient had for the therapist, since she had turned to him during a time of need. Moreover, the view that a therapist should never be called unless it is a life-or-death emergency was challenged.

THERAPIST 1: If you were an internist, would you expect that your patients would call only in a life-or-death emergency?

THERAPIST 2: No. They would call about their medications or about medical problems that were not life-threatening.

THERAPIST 1: Perhaps you could reexamine your expectations about what it means to have patients in clinical practice. Perhaps it might be more realistic to expect that every once in a while you will have a phone call after normal hours with a patient in a crisis. If you built that into your expectation, then you might be less upset about it.

EXAMINING THERAPIST SCHEMAS

Table 11.1 lists some common maladaptive schemas that many therapists may ascribe to. First, examine the table and ask yourself if any of these schemas or assumptions apply to you. Second, ask yourself if there are certain patients who seem to elicit one schema rather than another. In examining your response to the questionnaire, note if you score "5" or "6" for any of the schemas listed. For example, take "goal inhibition"—many cognitive-behavioral therapists are quite instrumental in their orientation. They expect to change the patient rapidly. But the patient may not change—in fact, the patient may refuse to do any homework. One therapist indicated that she felt very frustrated that the patient was not complying. Her (the therapist's) automatic thoughts were: "She's not changing. She's blocking me from getting my work done. I'm

TABLE 11.1. Therapist's Schema Questionnaire: Guide

Schema	Assumptions
Demanding standards	"I have to cure all my patients. I must always meet the highest standards. My patients should do an excellent job. We should never waste time."
Special, superior person	"I am entitled to be successful. My patients should appreciate all that I do for them. I shouldn't feel bored when doing therapy. Patients try to humiliate me."
Rejection-sensitive	"Conflicts are upsetting. I shouldn't raise issues that will bother the patient."
Abandonment	"If my patient is bothered with therapy, he or she might leave. It's upsetting when patients terminate. I might end up with no patients."
Autonomy	"I feel controlled by the patient. My movements, feelings, or what I say are limited. I should be able to do or say what I wish. Sometimes I wonder if I will lose myself in the relationship."
Control	"I have to control my surroundings or the people around me."
Judgmental	"Some people are basically bad people. People should be punished if they do wrong things."
Persecution	"I often feel provoked. The patient is trying to get to me. I have to guard against being taken advantage of or hurt. You usually can't trust people."
Need for approval	"I want to be liked by the patient. If the patient isn't happy with me, then it means I'm doing something wrong."
Need to like others	"It's important that I like the patient. It bothers me if I don't like a patient. We should get along—almost like friends."
Withholding	"I want to withhold thoughts and feelings from my patients. I don't want to give them what they want. I feel I am withdrawing emotionally during sessions."
Helplessness	"I feel I don't know what to do. I fear I'll make mistakes. I wonder if I'm really competent. Sometimes I feel like giving up."
Goal inhibition	"The patient is blocking me from achieving my goals. I feel like I'm wasting time. I should be able to achieve my goals in sessions without the patient's interference."
Excessive self-sacrifice	"I should meet my patients' needs. I should make them feel better. The patients' needs often take precedence over my needs. I sometimes believe that I would do almost anything to meet their needs."
Emotional inhibition	"I feel frustrated when I'm with this patient because I can't express the way I really feel. I find it hard to suppress my feelings. I can't be myself."

wasting my time." Doing a vertical descent on this led to the following: "I shouldn't be wasting my time. If I keep wasting my time with this patient, my life will be wasted."

Interestingly, this was a very effective therapist, who showed considerable empathy and assertiveness with very challenging patients. However, she found herself frustrated with some noncompliant patients. I examined her demanding standards and overfocus on goal attainment: "Are there any effective things that you have done with this patient? With other patients? How much time do you spend working with this patient? Is it a small percentage of the time that you spend working with other patients or doing other work? Are you overgeneralizing? Do all therapists show 100% effectiveness? Should you be better that everyone? Why or why not?"

I suggested that the therapist develop a position of curiosity rather than a demanding position regarding the lack of goal attainment. Perhaps she could examine whether the patient had a fear of moving forward. Perhaps the patient had a hidden agenda of remaining sick or of keeping herself from finding out what her own limitations would be when she was well. By shifting from the demand that everything needed to be changed to an inquisitive, observer role, the therapy began to progress and the therapist felt less frustrated.

THERAPIST–PATIENT SCHEMA CONFLICT

We all know that we can work better with some patients than with others. Conversely, a patient who seems very frustrating to us will work well with a colleague. There are several dimensions of resistance: validation, moral, schematic self-consistency, and risk aversion. The therapist's personal schematic issues in the countertransference will determine how well she works with each of these dimensions of resistance.

For example, the therapist whose schemas are those of *demanding standards*, *special person*, or *autonomy* may be frustrated with the patient who needs or demands validation. If the therapist believes that she and the patient should be pursuing specific goals, consistent rationality, and homework compliance, then the patient who wants validation may "fail" to live up to the therapist's demanding standards. The consequence is that the therapist may push the patient further or criticize the patient, thereby further invalidating the patient.

Similarly, the therapist who views herself as a special person will have difficulty validating the patient. The therapist may view the patient's need for validation as "beneath her" and may feel dissatisfied that the patient does not gratify the therapist's need to be successful. Thinking of herself as a special person, the therapist may have considerable difficulty imagining herself confronted with the predicaments that the patient describes.

The therapist whose schema is that of autonomy may find it difficult to tolerate the patient needing validation, since this may be viewed as infringing on the therapist's boundaries. Similarly, the autonomous therapist will become anxious and angry when the patient with strong attachment needs requests extra time or extra care from the therapist. By arbitrarily and defensively setting boundaries, the therapist may invalidate the patient and arouse even greater anxiety about attachment needs. This may result in escalation of the patient's validation and attachment demands, further resulting in the therapist setting limits and rejecting the patient.

Autonomous therapists often have constricted affect, or, at least, low tolerance for strong emotional content and expression. Their overemphasis on rationality and productivity makes it difficult for them to tolerate and appreciate the need for some patients to "find their feelings." Consequently, the autonomous and overly rational therapist, overfocused on "productivity and efficiency," may become a "ruthless agenda setter." Therapy becomes formulaic and driven by "treatment plans" that appear sterile, dismissive, and irrelevant to the patient who has high needs for validation and attachment.

Therapists who have difficulties with validation and abandonment patients may themselves find comfort in understanding what their problem is. First, these therapists should be challenged to develop a case conceptualization of why the patient has such strong needs for validation. Second, the therapist can examine why she has such a strong need for autonomy. The therapist may ask herself, "Were my parents overprotective and demanding?," "Were my needs for validation frustrated?," or "Am I jumping to conclusions about all of my boundaries being lost with this patient?" Third, the therapist can consistently and intentionally practice active listening skills (Stuart, 1980), using rephrasing, empathizing, validation, and inquiry—and see what happens. Does the therapist lose all boundaries if she intentionally validates the patient? Do both therapist and patient feel that the session was a waste, or is there some improvement? Fourth, the therapist can discuss with the patient the "dialectic" (Linehan, 1993), the need to move between the extreme of total validation and the extreme of total problem solving and rationality. They can negotiate to set aside some time each session for validation and some for problem solving.

SUMMARY

It is essential that we keep in mind that the patient is not simply responding to a technique, a treatment plan, or "cognitive-behavioral therapy." The patient is responding to a particular therapist—another person—who may take the model of cognitive-behavioral therapy and use it to frustrate the patient further. In fact, it is important to recognize that what most therapists are doing when they are doing cognitive-behavioral therapy is *not* cognitive-behavioral therapy; rather, they are relating to another person.

12

Using the Countertransference

*T*herapists often talk about "difficult patients"—and, in fact, I am writing here about "resistant" patients. But it might be more accurate to describe these individuals as "people who do not comply with the therapist's agenda." For example, the cognitive-behavioral therapist might think of a patient who is emoting about how bad everything is as someone who is "not engaging in problem solving," whereas the psychoanalytic therapist might view the problem-solving patient as resisting through intellectualization and isolation. When the patient does not comply with our (the therapist's) agenda, our own assumptions, schemas, and adaptations are elicited.

In this chapter I examine how we may use the countertransference to understand how the patient is affecting other people. I will focus, initially, on narcissistic patients, a group that many therapists find especially difficult to work with. However, by utilizing the countertransference—by recognizing how it feels when the patient devalues, idealizes, and distances himself—we come to understand both how the patient affects others and how the patient has been affected by these same experiences. What has been done to the patient the patient will very likely do to us. Further, I will examine how the therapist must utilize his countertransference to work with excessively dependent, demanding, and abusive patients.

COUNTERTRANSFERENCE WITH
NARCISSISTIC PATIENTS

The narcissistic individual often relates to the therapist with alternating behavior. Initially, the patient may idealize the therapist, even tend to "merge" with her during the "honeymoon" phase of treatment. During the idealization phase of treatment, the patient may flatter the therapist, favorably compare the therapist with others who have failed, buy the therapist gifts, and ask to borrow the therapist's books, since these are viewed as valued objects (and as representative of the therapist's uniqueness in the patient's life). Later, after the therapist fails to live up to the patient's idealization and demands, the patient may distance himself from the therapist by coming to sessions late, refusing to comply with homework, or not coming to sessions at all. Moreover, the therapist may find herself being devalued and criticized, with the patient threatening to quit therapy.

During the course of treatment, the narcissistic patient will describe examples of his exploitation of others, his lack of empathy, his sense of entitlement to special treatment, and his idealization of himself as superior. The therapist may find herself "disgusted by" or "not caring about" the narcissist who is unfaithful to his wife, visits prostitutes, treats people like servile objects, demands special arrangements, and brags about his many accomplishments. Alternatively, the therapist may be impressed, charmed, or intimidated by the patient's confidence, success, poise, or indifference to convention. The therapist may find the patient's initial idealization of the therapist very appealing, sexually arousing, or reassuring.

Eliciting the Therapist's Automatic Thoughts and Assumptions

Although the therapist may believe that the narcissist's behavior would elicit the same response from any other therapist, I have found that there are a range of responses that therapists have—not all negative. Even though many therapists may respond negatively to narcissists, there is a wide range of content in the responses. For example, consider the emotional responses as illustrative of a range of the therapist's automatic thoughts and assumptions. Imagine that we ask different therapists why it would bother him or her if a patient is selfish, devaluing, or unreasonable.

- Anger: "They're selfish," "They devalue," "They don't appreciate anything you do." *Therapist responses: "People shouldn't be selfish," "People should be fair," "They make me doubt myself."*
- Anxiety: "I'm worried that they'll criticize me," "They might leave treatment." *"When they criticize me, maybe they're right—I'm not that good a therapist." "If they leave treatment, it's because I didn't do a good job."*

- Inadequacy: "I feel unable to handle them," "They make me feel inferior." *"I should be able to handle them," "I should never be inferior to anyone," "If someone is more successful than I am, then I'm a failure."*
- Indifference: "I find myself bored with them," "I secretly hope that they'll drop out of treatment." *"I can't stand listening to them. They're selfish. I'm not going to let them affect me."*

The therapist may have a range of automatic thought distortions with the narcissist: "He's looking down on me" (mind reading), "He's a selfish bastard" (labeling), "He never cares about anyone" (all-or-nothing thinking), "He'll never change" (fortune telling), "He's doing this to me because of who I am" (personalizing), "This is intolerable" (catastrophizing), and "I can't help my patients" (overgeneralizing).

The therapist's underlying assumptions and rules are activated. These include:

- "People should always be fair. If they're not fair, then they are bad people and they should be punished. I should punish them. I should disown them."
- "If a patient is angry at me, then it is my fault. Patients should never be upset with me. It's a sign of my inadequacy."
- "The patients' feelings are my responsibility. If they are upset with me, then I can't stand it. I have to change the way they feel."
- "When patients are upset, I have to make them feel better. I have to give them what they need."
- "My needs are not important if the patient needs me. I should always put my needs and rights second to the patient."
- "The patient should never press my boundaries. It's awful when patients press boundaries. I have to create greater barriers whenever this happens or I'll be eaten alive."

Considering the Consequences of These Assumptions

The therapist who believes that the patient should be fair will judge the patient, feel disgust about his or her behavior, and criticize the patient. The narcissistic patient, exquisitely tuned to any criticism, will view this as evidence that people cannot be trusted. Consequently, the patient will criticize the therapist and leave treatment.

The therapist who believes that patients should never get angry with him will find that therapy with narcissists is unbearably difficult. If the therapist believes that the patient's anger is indicative of the therapist's inadequacy, then the therapist will avoid confronting or challenging the patient's thinking and behavior. The patient may then recognize that his own anger can be used to intimidate the therapist, which will then encourage the patient to act out even more. The patient may conclude that the therapist is weak and incompetent and that he, himself, is entitled to his acting-out behavior.

If the therapist believes that the patient's feelings are his (the therapist's) responsibility, then the patient will not learn to take responsibility for his feelings and behavior. Whenever the patient becomes upset with something, the therapist may "jump in" and try to modify the negative feeling. Since narcissists often have intolerance for negative feelings, this too rapid intervention will reinforce the belief that negative feelings are bad and cannot be tolerated.

If the therapist believes that he must meet the patient's needs, the patient will escalate demands to test the therapist's willingness to gratify him. This further reinforces the patient's sense of entitlement and hinders the development of insight. As boundaries become blurred, the patient attempts to absorb or incorporate the therapist: the patient expects more time for sessions, the right to come late, the right to pay bills late or not at all, and freedom to make frequent calls between sessions.

Similar to the therapist who tries to gratify the patient, the self-sacrificing therapist puts his needs second to the patient's demands. This therapist believes that the only thing that counts is that the patient gets what he wants. For example, one self-sacrificing therapist would extend 45-minute sessions to 80 minutes because the "patient needed my time." The therapist would respond to between-session calls with long discussions with the patient about material that could be discussed in the next session. Moreover, the therapist did not send the patient a bill for 6 months; when the patient did not pay the bill, the therapist did not press collection. Some self-sacrificing therapists use the patient as a replacement for the friends that are missing in their own lives. Consequently, for the therapist who has blurred the boundary between professional and personal relationships, it often seems difficult to set limits on people who have become "friends in need." The patient will normalize his demandingness and wonder, "Why aren't other people as giving to me as my therapist is?" Rather than develop insight into his entitlement, the patient feels further vindicated in his demands.

Challenging Automatic Thoughts and Assumptions in the Countertransference

First, you should examine your own thinking if you are having any strong emotional response to a patient in therapy—that is, are you angry, anxious, sad, frightened, frustrated, or bored during your interactions with the patient? Second, you should ask yourself, Is this treatment getting stuck? Is the patient not changing? Third, are you finding that you are reluctant to refer this patient for a different modality, such as medication or marital therapy? Are you becoming too attached to your role in the process?

We should keep several points in mind in treating a patient. First, the goal of therapy is to help the patient, not to help the therapist. Second, no therapy works for everyone. Third, therapy requires the collaboration of both patient and therapist—the therapist cannot do it entirely on her own. Keeping these points in mind, let us examine some of the typical cognitive distortions of therapists doing cognitive-behavioral therapy (see Table 12.1).

In examining the cognitive distortions and maladaptive assumptions that you, as a therapist, have, you can use all the techniques that are useful in challenging your patient's thinking. For example, consider the typical assumption of demanding standards, or perfectionism: "I should be able to help [cure] all my patients." You might try the following challenges to this assumption:

- How would you define "cure" or "help"?
- What are the advantages and disadvantages of demanding perfection?
- Do you think that other therapists should cure or help all their patients?
- Is there a good reason why you hold yourself to a higher standard?
- Is there anyone beside you that thinks that you should be perfect?
- What if you don't cure all your patients? What would that imply? (*vertical descent*)
- How likely is it that these outcomes will come true?
- Who established the rule that you have to cure all your patients?
- Are you discounting the positives—that is, all the patients you have helped? How many patients have you helped that other therapists have not helped?
- Even if you are not a perfect therapist, what are some things that you can still do to help other patients? What are some things that you can still do in your personal life?
- What advice would you give a colleague who thought she should be a perfect therapist?

Activation of Therapist Schemas

The therapist's frustration is a natural reaction to the narcissist's behavior. But why does the narcissist elicit such a range of different responses

TABLE 12.1. Countertransference Cognitive Distortions

Distortion	Example	Rational response
Personalizing	"The patient isn't getting better because I'm not that good a therapist."	Patients do not get better for a lot of reasons. The patient had this problem before therapy began. You have helped a lot of other patients.
Catastrophizing	"It's awful that the patient is thinking of suicide."	Thinking about suicide is very common with depressed patients. You are here to help people think through their problems. There is no advantage in your getting catastrophic. Nothing terrible has happened yet. There are a lot of things that you can do to help: you can counsel the patient on alternatives, examine short-term and long-term goals, help the patient challenge his negative and hopeless thinking, modify the medication, get assurance with a suicide contract, and arrange for hospitalization during this time of crisis.
Labeling (of patient)	"This patient is just a pain to deal with."	The patient is a human being who is suffering. He doesn't want to suffer and the difficulty and resistance that the patient expresses is probably causing him more discomfort than it is causing you. Try to see life through his eyes and develop a shared curiosity with the patient about the current problems.
Labeling (of self)	"I must be a lousy therapist."	There are some people you work well with and others that you don't. Even the "famous" therapists make mistakes. Consider the range of patients that you have worked with—Aren't there some who have been helped? No therapist is perfect.
Mind reading	"The patient thinks I'm incompetent."	That's unlikely if the patient keeps coming for help. Even if the patient did think you were incompetent, it doesn't follow that you are. You probably don't know what the patient is really thinking. If the patient thinks you are incompetent, it may be that this is the way that the patient responds to support in his life.
Fortune telling	"This patient will never get better."	You don't know that this is true. In reality, many people improve a little bit and have good times and bad times. Look back at the mood fluctuations of this patient over time and you will discover some better times. There are a variety of techniques and interventions that you have yet to try.
All-or-nothing thinking	"Nothing seems to work."	Again, there may be some fluctuation in functioning for this patient. Have the patient keep a mood log and you will find that his mood varies with time of day, activities, and thoughts.

(continued)

TABLE 12.1. (*continued*)

Distortion	Example	Rational response
Emotional reasoning	"I feel lousy seeing this patient, so the therapy must be going poorly."	Your feelings are no guide as to whether the patient is getting anything out of treatment. However, you might examine if the way you are feeling may be similar to the way other people feel in trying to help this person.
Discounting the positives	"Anyone could have helped that patient."	You don't know if that's true, but even if it were, you helped someone. That's what counts.
Overgeneralizing	"I didn't help this patient. I can't help any patients."	You don't really know that you did not help this patient. But even if you did not help him, you still have helped others and you still can help new patients.

in different people? The answer to this question—and one of the methods of helping the narcissist—is to first examine the therapist's schemas. For example, consider the therapist who focuses on the narcissist's lack of "fairness." The therapist's automatic thoughts were: "He should be fair," "People should do the right thing," and "If they don't, then I don't want to have anything to do with them." Another therapist with the fairness schema thought: "She should be punished." Obviously, the therapist who is responding to his "justice schema" will have difficulty empathizing with the patient and may lose the patient because of punitive or distancing retaliation against the patient.

The therapist's own narcissistic view of being a "special person" may be activated when the narcissist idealizes her. The therapist may be emotionally seduced by the narcissist's flattery of the patient's social and economic status. This "mutual admiration society" between patient and therapist during the idealization phase of treatment may have both positive and negative consequences. First, both patient and therapist may feel "good" about the treatment and there may be an initial mutual commitment to working on problems. But, second, the negative consequences of the mutual idealization may result in both parties failing to live up to the expectations of the other, perception of special privileges on the part of the patient, the inability of the therapist to perceive significant pathology in the patient, and the patient's belief that there is nothing really wrong with him.

The therapist who is dependent may initially be impressed and pleased with the narcissist. The patient may represent to her the kind of person she is looking for in her personal life: someone who is confident and successful, someone with poise and charm, someone who can take care of her. The patient may recognize his impact on the therapist and attempt emotional and sexual seduction. The therapist's dependency may result in her inability to challenge the patient's thinking or to see the pathology in the patient's character structure. Further, the dependent therapist, guided by fears of abandonment, may feel that "keeping" the patient in therapy is essential, since rejection by such a "superior" person would be true evidence of the therapist's failure. Consequently, the therapist may fail to collect payments due, extend sessions beyond the allotted time, call the patient repeatedly when the patient misses a session, and otherwise demonstrate to the patient that the therapist needs the patient more than the patient needs the therapist.

The therapist's schemas of personal inadequacy and fears of abandonment may result in significant anxiety in dealing with the narcissist. The patient's condescending, distancing, and devaluing maneuvers may be interpreted by the therapist as less an indication of the patient's pathology and more as proof of the therapist's inferiority. The therapist may feel that she is not meeting the narcissist's needs and believe that the patient's frustration is evidence that the rules need to be modified: that sessions need to be extended, that payments do not need to be collected, that limits do not need to be set, and that anything must be done to calm the narcissist.

Therapist schemas about fairness, specialness, abandonment, responsibility, humiliation, persecution, and inadequacy are easily activated by the narcissist. Therapists may attempt to compensate when their schemas are activated by punishing (fairness schema), mutual admiration (specialness schema), relinquishing limits (abandonment schema), self-criticism (responsibility schema), retaliation and humiliation of the patient (humiliation schema), withdrawing or retaliating (persecution schema), and self-criticism or nonassertion (inadequacy schema).

What is the consequence for the narcissist when the therapist responds in this manner? Consider the following as responses to the therapist's countertransference:

Therapist	*Patient*
• Punishment	Retaliation, withdrawal
• Mutual admiration	Seduction, denial of problems
• Relinquishing limits	Increased demandingness, devaluation of therapist
• Self-criticism	Sense of superiority, devaluation of therapist, threats
• Retaliation/humiliation	Retaliation, withdrawal

- Withdrawal   Withdrawal
- Nonassertion   Increased demandingness,
                      devaluation of therapist

What assumptions of the patient are confirmed by the therapist's countertransference response?

Therapist	*Patient's belief that is confirmed*
• Punishment	"People can't be trusted."
• Mutual admiration	"I really am special and unique. I don't have problems."
• Relinquishing limits	"I'm entitled to have what I want. Rules don't apply to me."
• Self-criticism	"Others are inferior to me. No one can help me."
• Retaliation/humiliation	"If I trust people, they'll hurt me."
• Withdrawal	"No one cares about me. No one is there for me."
• Nonassertion	"People are weaker than I am. I can take advantage."

How Does the Countertransference Reflect How Others React to the Patient?

We have seen how the therapist may respond with feelings of inadequacy, humiliation, fears of abandonment, mutual admiration and idealization, or schemas of fairness. The therapist may respond with punishment, adulation, indulgence, self-criticism, withdrawal, or nonassertion. But the therapist is not alone. Others in the patient's life are responding this way too. The therapist who feels devalued and responds with retaliation may ask, "Do the patient's friends retaliate?" If the therapist finds that she is functioning as a "need gratifier" for the patient—by sacrificing limits—she may recognize that the patient's wife is in a similar role with the patient.

Patients do not live in a world that is isolated from their own behavior. They have an impact on others. If the therapist is nonassertive with the narcissistic patient, then the patient may conclude that the therapist approves of the patient's behavior or that the therapist is weak. Narcissists may selectively socialize with people who indulge their pathology. I have referred to this as the "interactive reality" (Leahy, 1991, 1992): individuals selectively pursue relationships that allow them to maintain their disorder. Thus narcissists may select either dependent personalities who will defer to the narcissist or they may select other narcissists with whom they can share a sense of being special and superior.

The consequence of this complimentarity is that the narcissist's schemas are continually reinforced. When he looks for evidence that he is superior, he can point to the dependent personalities who look up to him or to the other narcissists who flatter his ego in mutual gratification contracts. For example, a successful business executive complained that his wife was "boring" because she had few interests of her own. He recalled that his mother was domineering and cold and that he never wanted to have a partner similar to his mother. When he examined his choices of women during his life, each of them was deferent, dependent, and needed him financially. Consequently, he kept choosing women who would not dominate him and who would service his expanding ego, but because of their dependency they would not satisfy his needs for companionship and interest.

Did Others Make the Patient Feel This Way?

The patient's behavior toward the therapist often reflects how others treated the patient. *What the therapist feels may be similar to how the patient has felt in other relationships.* For example, a successful executive who alternated between idealizing the therapist, giving lip service to agreeing with the therapist, and then ignoring the therapist's recommendations, described how he always felt inferior to his father, whom he idealized, but against whom he rebelled. He felt that his father was condescending and never listened to him. This was exactly the feeling the therapist had: that the patient was condescending and did not really listen to him.

Another patient, who alternated between idealizing and devaluing the therapist, indicated that his father gave him conflicting messages: "We expect great things from you" and "You can't do anything right." These were the same conflicting messages that he was giving the therapist. This patient indicated that he believed that the therapist would be like everyone else and would eventually reject him. Therefore, his strategy would be to reject the therapist first.

DYSFUNCTIONAL COMMUNICATION PATTERNS
AND COUNTERTRANSFERENCE

Many patients will display communication patterns that make it difficult for the therapist to "stay on task." Sociolinguist Deborah Tannen (1990) has described these varying "conversational" styles and indicated how disparity between speakers can lead to mutual frustration. For example, some patients expect validation and empathy and simply want to share their feelings, whereas the therapist may appear too "task oriented," thereby invalidating the patient. Consequently, the patient complains more and the therapist, attempting problem solving, continues to demand change.

A therapist inclined toward demanding problem solving and who cringed from complaining patients noted that his own mother often nagged and complained—much to his dismay. He indicated that, as a child, he often felt oppressed by this emotional ventilation. He often appeared to be a "taskmaster" as a therapist. The therapist's demanding, problem-solving style of communication was often dysfunctional for the patient who needed validation. Finally, recognizing the source of his countertransference assisted the therapist in working with patients who complained.

The therapist may become frustrated when the patient repeatedly interrupts, changes the topic, does not acknowledge what the therapist has just said, repeats apparently trivial details, complains and whines, or simply remains silent. Countertransference responses may include anger, frustration, and boredom. These therapist responses may lead the therapist to criticize the patient, give up on him, or talk over the patient's statements or silence. The angry therapist is thinking, "All he wants to do is complain. He's not doing what he's supposed to do"; the frustrated therapist is thinking, "I can't stand this. He's keeping me from getting my work done"; and the bored therapist is thinking, "This is going nowhere. I may as well give up. I can't wait for this session to end."

The patient's conversational style activates the therapist's schema. If the therapist's schema is "demanding standards" and "competence," then the patient's complaining or silence will frustrate the therapist, perhaps leading the therapist to "demand" that the patient conform with her standards of what a patient "should" be. These demands on the part of the therapist may take the form of criticism, further confirming the patient's belief that "no one cares about me anyway."

The patient's conversational style and the therapist's frustration may be used to help both better understand the patient's predicament and coping style. One patient initially presented with numerous complaints about her husband, continually punctuating these complaints with "Do I make sense?" and "Do you understand?" Ironically, everything she said made sense, but her constant reassurance seeking began to frustrate the therapist's "demanding standards." Rather than criticize the patient for not complying with the implicit rules of the "ideal conversational style," the therapist pointed out that the patient was constantly seeking out reassurance that she was not being misunderstood.

THERAPIST: You seem to wonder if I am understanding what you are feeling. Why do you doubt that I can understand you?

PATIENT: Sometimes I can't put my feelings into words. I don't know if I make sense.

THERAPIST: Do you have this feeling with other people?

PATIENT: Yes. My husband, Bill, is always telling me how stupid I am—that I don't make any sense. And, when I was a kid, my mother only wanted to talk about her feelings.

THERAPIST: So the people who are important in your life don't seem to give you credit for your feelings. Let's take some of the angry feelings that you have toward Bill. What does he say that makes you angry?

PATIENT: He calls me an "idiot."

THERAPIST: How do you think other wives would feel if their husband called them an "idiot"?

PATIENT: I think they'd be angry too.

THERAPIST: So, why would I not be able to understand that you feel the same way that other people would feel? Maybe your feelings make sense. But maybe Bill wants to blame you for your feelings and you believe him when he says that you don't make sense.

DEPENDENCY DEMANDS
AND COUNTERTRANSFERENCE

Another patient behavior that may seem problematic for the therapist is frequent phone calls between sessions. Therapists respond with a variety of assumptions and schemas of their own: "She shouldn't call between sessions," "I'm being controlled. I'll lose my private life," "She's narcissistic [borderline, demanding, etc.]," "I can't stand this. This is awful," or "I've got to put a stop to this at once." Alternatively, some therapists respond with self-sacrificing schemas and assumptions: "This means that she needs me," "I have to meet her needs right now," "She must trust me to be calling me now," "She can't handle her problems on her own," "This is an emergency," or "This is my job. I have to be available all the time."

Making distinctions between true emergencies, demandingness, and dependency is not always simple. The therapist does have an obligation to respond to the patient. If the patient is suicidal or extremely upset, the therapist should be willing to include some phone consultation between sessions. But therapists often respond with their countertransference: either they arbitrarily set limits or they indulge the patient unnecessarily. For example, one therapist would wait until the next day to respond to the patient. He assumed the patient was being unreasonable "once again" and that he had to set limits on the patient. Consequently, the therapist responded in a passive–aggressive manner by waiting a whole day to respond to calls. This led the patient to believe the therapist did not care about her feelings and could not be counted on for professional services. In contrast, another therapist would return the patient's calls even when she, the therapist, was on vacation (and even though appropriate backup was available). Moreover, the therapist would spend over an hour on the phone with the patient, trying to calm her down, and would not charge for her services. This led the patient to believe the therapist had no rights, needed the patient, and that she, the patient, was totally unable to handle any problems on her own.

The first step in dealing with frequent phone contact is to address the assumptions of the countertransference. Let us begin with the therapist who distances and devalues. What are the costs and benefits of labeling the patient as a narcissist or borderline, and then dismissing the patient's concerns? The costs are that the patient will feel demeaned and rejected, will probably quit therapy, will confirm his negative belief about others as untrustworthy and selfish, and will justify his own tendency to distance and devalue others. In addition, the therapist will be less likely to show empathy in the future (further rupturing the therapeutic alliance) and will not examine, with the patient, beliefs about seeking and needing help. The therapist may believe there are benefits for labeling the patient and distancing himself. He may believe this keeps him from taking things personally, it does not reinforce the patient's demandingness, and it protects the therapist's boundaries. There is some truth for both costs and benefits. The question arises as to whether the therapist can accomplish these goals without distancing or devaluing the patient.

Consider the therapist's automatic thoughts: "She shouldn't call between sessions," "I'm being controlled. I'll lose my private life." The therapist may use the following rational responses: "Why shouldn't the patient call between sessions? Why shouldn't the patient respond in a needy, dependent way? After all, that's why he's in therapy. He has problems solving his problems. He feels overwhelmed. What may seem minor to me, feels like a life-and-death emergency to him." To challenge the idea that he'll lose his private life, the therapist might use these responses: "How much of an interference is a few minutes on the phone? Am I jumping to conclusions? Do I really believe that *every* patient *every* minute of the day and night will be calling me? What if I were to build into my expectations that some patients will make calls in between sessions and that I have to learn how to handle that?"

To challenge the labeling of the patient as "narcissistic" (or "borderline") so that the patient can be dismissed, the therapist might consider the following responses: "Just because someone calls me doesn't mean that he is narcissistic. Labeling a patient so that I can distance myself from him is countertherapeutic. It's like saying, 'The reasons he's acting like he's depressed is that he's depressed.' Using tautologies or labels only keeps me from thinking creatively about how to help this person. Not everything about this patient is narcissistic. If I label the patient and dismiss him I'll never learn how he sees things and how I can help him." To challenge the idea that "I can't stand this. It's awful," the therapist can say to himself: "There's nothing awful about a 10-minute inconvenience. I can still do everything else that I want to do. I can use the patient's perception of emergency to understand the patient better. I can think of a million things worse than a phone call. I can't imagine if I told someone else about this that she would think it's awful." And, finally, to challenge the idea that "I have to put a stop to this at once," the therapist might think: "There's no emergency here. I can try to learn more about why the patient thinks that he cannot tolerate negative feelings or help himself. One or two phone calls does not mean that I'm sliding down a slippery slope. I can help the patient develop some guidelines for phone contact."

The therapist who directly addresses his countertransference may find it easier to address the patient who makes frequent phone calls. The following guidelines are useful.

Observe the Phenomenon

The therapist can directly say, "I've noticed that you have felt the need to call me between sessions. I wonder if we can talk about what is going on for you in between sessions so that we can work on some ways that you can help yourself?"

Elicit Automatic Thoughts about Feelings and Problems

The therapist can inquire about how the patient relates to his negative feelings. For example, does the patient immediately assume that when he has a negative feeling it cannot be tolerated, that he has to get rid of the feeling immediately, that he believes the negative feeling will spin out of control, that he needs validation or he needs to be cared about, or that he has no ability to moderate his feelings?

Examine the Patient's Negative Thoughts about Contacting the Therapist

The therapist can ask if the patient has any feelings about calling the therapist. Responses might include, "I need you to be there for me.

You'll get angry with me and reject me. I am angry at you for not being there [returning my call immediately]. I'm all alone in the world. I know that when I'm upset I can always call on you."

Examine Past Transference Relationships

The therapist can ask, "When you've needed other people to be there for you, what has happened?" Patients have answered that "My other therapist was always there" or "My mother never listened to me—she was too wrapped up in her own problems" or "I was always made to feel that I didn't have a right to my feelings." The therapist might ask, "How are these feelings the same when you seek help from me?"

Use Collaborative Problem Solving to Negotiate Contact

It is important that the patient believes that in true emergencies he can contact the therapist, but it is equally important that there be limits set on this contact. The therapist can present this as a problem for the two of them to solve: "Let's try to figure out a way that I can be responsive to true emergencies, but that you can learn to use self-help to deal with some of the feelings that you are having."

Increase Self-Help Assignments

The therapist can suggest homework for moderating negative feelings, challenging negative thoughts, and problem solving. Difficulties between sessions can be used as opportunities for the patient to test the belief that she is helpless and always needs someone else to change her feelings. For example, the therapist and patient can identify which techniques in session seem to work and examine how these techniques can be used outside sessions. I have found that patients find it useful to ask themselves, "What would my therapist tell me to do? What questions would he ask me if I were talking to him?" Patient's can tape-record sessions and then use these tapes between sessions or during difficult times to activate their ability to challenge their thinking.

Review Self-Help

As therapists, we often focus on the negative. For example, we might ask the patient about a problem that she needs help with now. But it is often useful to ask patients how they have helped themselves during the previous week. For patients who have called the therapist in between sessions, it is important to follow up on *when they did not need the therapist to solve their problems*. Given the importance of self-help assignments, we can ask the patient, "Is there any time during the past week when you had some difficulty but you solved the problem yourself?" This reinforces the patient's belief that the therapist will recognize and appreciate self-help.

Troubleshoot Problems

Giving patients direction on how to handle problems is seldom enough. The therapist can help the patient anticipate when problems will arise and explain how the patient may feel discouraged in handling these problems. For example, the patient who has been requesting reassurance from the therapist via frequent phone calls can be told, "There have been times that you felt that you could not rely on your own decision making and that you needed me to make decisions for you. At these times you have felt the need to call me for reassurance. Let's look at how you can handle some of this in between sessions." The therapist can suggest:

> "What are the costs and benefits or needing reassurance from me and
>   others?"
> "Let's think of a decision that you might have to make and how you
>   can use costs and benefits to make that decision."
> "Is there any evidence that you have made decisions that have
>   worked out?"
> "Would you be willing to spend at least 1 hour doing some written
>   cognitive therapy homework before calling me? That way you
>   can test out your own skills in making decisions."
> "I cannot make your decisions. Are you trying to shift the responsi-
>   bility to others, so that if the decision is wrong you will regret it
>   less?"
> "Let's do a role play. I'll try to convince you that you cannot make
>   decisions and you try to challenge me."

The patient can either tape-record the "troubleshooting" therapy session or write out extensive notes to be used as flashcards. The therapist should ask the patient for feedback on this discussion. Does the patient think that the therapist is annoyed and trying to get rid of the patient? The therapist can point out that cognitive therapy is a self-help therapy. How would the patient feel if she went to a personal trainer who suggested exercising in between training sessions?

Allow Slipups

None of us is perfect. The therapist and patient can try to anticipate that slipups will occur. The patient may not do the things that the therapist recommends. The therapist can indicate that slipups will be opportunities to learn. During a slipup the most significant automatic thoughts and schemas are activated. What will these be? For example, the therapist and patient, while troubleshooting, might recognize that the patient may have a slipup because she believes that she cannot tolerate any negative affect and has to contact the therapist immediately. This sense of urgency can then be examined using cognitive-behavioral techniques.

It is essential that the patient recognize that slipups are part of developing as a human being. The patient may look at a slipup as "proof" that she can never change, that she is hopeless, or that she has failed the therapist. Or slipups may be viewed as evidence that the therapy does not work and that the therapist is incompetent. Even these thoughts can be examined and challenged: "Slipups are inevitable in all development. We go off diets, decide not to exercise, put off doing our work. Are you saying that you have to be perfect to make progress? How can we use a slipup as a way of testing whether the therapy works? For example, if you decide not to do the self-help, can we test out how you feel after doing nothing? Can we compare that to how you feel when you do the self-help?" This is similar to the classic A–B–A–B experimental design, in which an intervention is introduced, removed, and then reintroduced. Feeling worse during a slipup may be taken as a "natural experiment" through which we learn that the therapy actually works when it is utilized.

THE VERBALLY ABUSIVE PATIENT

Therapy is difficult work, but it can become intolerable for many therapists when the patient becomes verbally abusive. Our contract with the patient is to provide therapy, not to be a whipping post for his rage. It may be unavoidable that some patients will ventilate their frustration and anger, but it is not essential that patients be allowed to intimidate and verbally abuse the therapist.

Verbally abusive behavior includes demeaning and insulting comments about the therapist's competence, gender, ethnicity, family, or values. Telling the therapist that he or she is "an idiot," "a chump," "a goddamn Jew," "a mick," or "an asshole"—or making inappropriate comments about the therapist's husband or wife—is not to be tolerated. Therapists who routinely tolerate verbally abusive behavior indulge the patient with the idea that this behavior is acceptable. It is likely that it is this abusive behavior that has resulted in the patient's continual problems with intimate and work relationships. If this behavior is not tolerated (or is even illegal) outside of therapy, then it is not to be tolerated inside therapy.

Therapy should have as its goal preparing the patient for the "real" world. Acting out aggression handicaps the patient for other relationships. The patient who is allowed to continue his abusive behavior in therapy comes to view the therapist as weak, incompetent, and deserving of abuse.

I have taken the following assertive position regarding being a therapist (which I generalize to all the therapists who work within our institute): *The therapist's welfare comes first.* My belief is that the patient always has the option of quitting treatment to find another therapist of his choosing. I do not have the option of finding another self. This is what I do every day. If therapy becomes so unpleasant that I hate seeing my patients, then none of my patients will be helped. Furthermore, regarding my staff, I would rather a patient drop out of treatment than continue his abusive behavior toward a valued staff member, who might leave our group because of this abuse. Furthermore, employment law may require me to set limits to any abusive patient behavior directed toward my staff.

The therapist does have the legal and ethical right to terminate a patient unilaterally. The patient should be provided with advanced notice that a transfer will be made in the treatment. In the few cases in which I have indicated that I would unilaterally end the treatment unless a patient's behavior changed, the patient was surprised to learn that I had this right. However, the therapist is not "abandoning" the patient if he gives the patient advanced notice and makes another referral. Notifying patients of the consequences of their behavior, coupled with a willingness to examine the causes and pursue mutual solutions, has generally had a palliative effect. In some cases, the therapeutic relationship has been dramatically improved.

Inappropriate behavior within the session—such as screaming, throwing things, making threats, or making sexual overtures—is sufficient to terminate the session immediately. For example, the therapist can say, "It seems like today is not a good day for us to work. You are too upset. I find that I cannot do my work when someone is screaming [throwing things]. So I will have to end our meeting now." If the patient makes sexually inappropriate remarks, the therapist can be assertive and say, "These comments are not appropriate. This behavior cannot be tolerated in our meetings. If it continues, I will have to end the session and, if necessary, terminate treatment."

The therapist should ask herself, "If a colleague made these sexually inappropriate comments to me, what would I say?" Asserting oneself in the face of sexual harassment does not change simply because the

278 COGNITIVE THERAPY AND COUNTERTRANSFERENCE

harasser is a patient. In cases in which the abusive behavior or inappropriate behavior is extremely disturbing, the therapist should tell the patient that the therapy needs to be terminated.

Identify Abusive Behavior

It may be difficult to distinguish "at the boundary" what is abusive and what is simply angry ventilation. One guideline to use would be to ask, "What would be the most unpleasant behavior that would be tolerated in a work setting without being considered harassment?" For example, it is legal (but, perhaps, not socially skilled) in a work setting to say, "I think you did a terrible job" or "You annoy me." It is not legal to say, "You're an asshole," or "I want to have sex with you." It is legal to sit and remain silent, but it is not legal to lunge forward in a threatening manner or to engage in unwanted touching of the other person (the latter two constitute assault and battery). It is legal to make a phone call to ask for help, but it is not legal to make repeated phone calls to another party, yell at them, and hang up. All of these behaviors constitute harassment in the real world—some are misdemeanors, some are felonies. There is no reason why a patient should be allowed to abuse a therapist, just as there is no reason why one employee should be allowed to abuse another employee.

Identify Your Right Not to Be Abused

Consistent with the observation that therapists have a right to protect their own welfare and that they certainly have a right not to be abused, the clinician should keep in mind that helping people is not equivalent to indulging their sadism. Therapists are committed to a professional role of helping patients. However, patients who make it impossible for the therapist to act like a professional and to be treated with the respect due their position sacrifice their right to be a patient with that therapist. The therapist may need to examine his or her self-sacrificing schemas—or schemas of perfectionism, abandonment, and approval seeking. The double-standard technique is a useful intervention for the countertransference: "Would I encourage a friend to stay in a professional relationship where he or she was being abused?"

Tolerating Abuse Reinforces Abuse

We know that spouses who "tolerate" abuse (i.e., who do not have their spouse arrested) are more likely to be abused in the future. Setting limits on abusive behavior conveys an important message to the patient: *This behavior is not tolerated.* Continuing to see a patient who is abusive or inappropriate enables the patient to maintain a highly dysfunctional pattern of behavior. Providing a rationale for the therapist's authority to terminate an abusive relationship is more likely to evoke higher functioning from the patient than permissiveness or authoritarian hostility—just as it does with childrearing (see Baumrind, 1971).

Establish Guidelines Early

At the first sign of potentially abusive or acting-out behavior (such as yelling or throwing things), the therapist should establish limits: "I find that it is very difficult for me to work with people who yell [throw things, etc.]. I know that you are upset, but this behavior is not acceptable in my office. We can talk about why you are upset, but if this behavior reoccurs, the session will be ended and I will have to consider whether I will be able to continue working with you."

Limit setting is, in a sense, respectful of the patient. The therapist is indicating that she expects that the patient will be able to abide by standard rules of conduct. Lowering the bar by tolerating abusive behavior implies that the patient is unable to conform to standard rules—suggesting that the patient is incompetent. The therapist may make this point by saying, "I know that you will be able to act in a way that shows that you are able to control your behavior even when you are upset. Perhaps I will be helpful to you in this regard."

Other assertive statements that may interfere with abusive behavior include: "That is not acceptable," "That comment is inappropriate," "This is not therapy when you make comments like that," or "These comments will have to stop if we are to continue with this meeting." Some patients may be encouraged to use "time-out" within a session. Therapist and patient can agree to 5 minutes of silent reflection and relaxation, while both consider what is going on and how to make it better. In some cases, the patient may find it very helpful to announce, "I need a few minutes of time-out, so I am going to the bathroom [or waiting room], and I'll be back in a few minutes." Needless to say, the therapist should never be the one to leave the room.

Discuss the Abusive Behavior with the Patient

Quite often, in coercive family systems (Patterson, 1982), both parties in a dyad are so relieved that the conflict has abated that they do not want to discuss it later. I have found it useful to put the abusive behavior on the agenda as the first item of the next meeting. Consistent with Linehan's (1993) recommendations, I indicate to the patient that the therapy has to work for "both of us." For example, the therapist can say: "In our working together, I will try the best I can to help you meet your needs. I will try to do a good job in taking care of you. But I want you to take care of my needs too. What I mean by this is that I have a need to be treated with respect, to be treated like a human being. You and I both have that need. So I want you to treat me with respect if you want me to treat you with respect."

Some patients may reply, "I don't have to meet your needs. I pay you." I indicate that it is true that they pay me, but the payment is not sufficient for me to work with them. "In all working relationships, I expect both the other person and I will treat each other with respect—regardless of who is paying whom. I am being paid to do therapy, not to be treated disrespectfully." After the therapist has discussed the issue of abusive behavior in the session, the therapist can say, "It is time for us to talk about how we can work together to solve these problems. So, the first thing for us to discuss is, 'What would be some good guidelines for you and me in working together?' "

Make "Respect" a Mutual Goal

Respect cannot be viewed as a unilateral right of the therapist. The therapist can say, "Just as it is important that I ask you to show respect for me, I want you to tell me how I can show respect for you. Can you tell me some specific things that I can do so that you will feel more cared about and respected by me?" Patients have found that this is very helpful to them because it encourages them to express themselves directly about their needs, rather than "requires" that they act out their frustration. One patient indicated, "You could show more respect for me if you gave me more credit for the things that I have done." Another patient indicated, "You could respect me more if you went over my homework every time."

Be Assertive about Your Feelings

In contrast to the view that the therapist should be neutral, I believe that it is helpful to the patient to get good reality testing about the effects of his behavior. For example, the patient who insults the therapist, calls him incompetent, and tells him the therapy is idiotic can be told by the therapist: "You know, when you say those things, it annoys me. It makes me feel like we are wasting our time in this kind of discussion. Now, I want to work with you, but this kind of behavior is going to get in the way. Is this how you want to spend the session—insulting me?"

Or the therapist can say to the patient who is physically intimidating, "I find that it is not possible for me to work with people who try to be physically intimidating [or who scream, etc.]. I can't concentrate and I feel uncomfortable with that behavior. So, either you will have to stop this behavior, or we will have to terminate our meeting today."

Validation, Validation, Validation

The patient may agree to the guidelines for mutual respect and the guidelines for limit setting, but she may still believe that the therapist does not care about her feelings and needs. The therapist can elicit feedback about the discussion about "mutual respect": "How do you feel about our discussion today about how we can work together?" (Actually, I have found that patients usually begin these discussions in a defensive and angry state, but feel relieved, understood, and, indeed, protected. Several patients, who had been very angry with me, indicated at the end of the discussion of mutual respect that it was the only time that they had been able to talk about their feelings with someone whom they were angry toward.)

The patient can be told, "It may be that you have found that you needed to resort to this intense, angry behavior, because no one would listen to you if you spoke more quietly." Patients who engage in abusive behavior are often able to identify how parents invalidate them. "How did it make you feel when your mother would not listen to you?" or "How did it make you feel when your father told you that you should not feel that way?" Typical responses include, "That my feelings were not important" and "I felt angry." The therapist can reply, "Perhaps you were getting angry with me because you had those same thoughts and feelings."

Establish Mutual Guidelines and Evaluate Progress

Newman (1994, 1997) has suggested that the therapist and the patient can effectively address their impasse by establishing some mutual guidelines. The therapist and patient can negotiate a style and plan of working together, preferably writing down the specific guidelines. For example, the therapist confronted a patient whose mania was interfering with therapy: "Right now you are going through a difficult time. I get the sense that you are displeased with some things that I am doing. I also think that we need to examine some changes that can be made in your behavior. Let's write down some changes that we want the other person to make." This led to a set of practical rules. The patient requested that the therapist stick to the agenda, not "argue" with him, and be available for one phone call in between sessions. The therapist requested that the patient not insult him, not extend sessions, and not make repeated phone calls.

Subsequent sessions involved a short review of how each was following the guidelines. This mutually respectful "behavioral contracting" was of considerable value in maintaining the therapeutic relationship. The patient indicated that no one ever seemed to take the time or effort to discuss these problems. The therapist felt relieved because he did not have to feel frustrated about his autonomy and demanding standards.

SUMMARY

The issue of countertransference could take up at least an entire volume. Cognitive and behavioral therapists have been remiss in addressing this important issue. I view the countertransference as a unique "projective technique"—that is, the patient can project his problems onto the therapeutic relationship. In the therapeutic relationship, the therapist has direct access to how someone can experience the patient. However, the therapist must recognize that she, the therapist, brings to the relationship her own schematic issues. In the relationship, the therapist can engage in "corrective" work, whereby interpersonal issues with the patient can be addressed in a direct fashion. The therapist, aware of her countertransference, can see it as a source of information about the patient and as a potential sabotaging factor in the treatment. I have examined several schematic dimensions in the countertransference, but I leave it to the reader to consider the various permutations that are available involving different countertransference and patient schemas. Identifying the significance of his or her countertransference allows the therapist to provide more meaningful, deeper, more conceptual therapy. Most importantly, the therapist who is effective in understanding his or her own countertransference responses can provide the patient with a unique opportunity in therapy sessions to correct interpersonal impasses.

13

Conclusions

In this volume I have attempted to outline a multidimensional model of resistance. Although I have described seven dimensions of resistance in therapy, it is clear to me that this model is not fully comprehensive. Other significant processes of resistance—including emotional dysregulation, attachment processes, family or dyadic systems, characterological explanations, reliance on cognitive defenses, and fixation resulting from traumatic experiences—each deserve mention and review. My decision not to include these processes is not because I view these and other processes of resistance as less important, but rather because such coverage would be beyond the scope of one book. Moreover, the emphasis I wish to place on the *cognitive* model of resistance is better suited to the dimensions I have covered. It may be true that many of the themes of resistance mentioned above are relevant to the cognitive dimensions I have discussed and that a further exploration of these other themes of resistance could be enhanced by a cognitive formulation. I do not mean the cognitive formulation is primary, thereby subsuming issues such as attachment processes or traumatic effects. I simply mean that an "integrative" theoretical–clinical model might enhance all approaches.

In Table 13.1, I have summarized the main features of each of the seven modalities of resistance. One can see that the resistant individual may utilize more than one of these modalities—in some cases, the patient may utilize all seven. Furthermore, as I have attempted to demonstrate, certain of these dimensions may be more likely to trigger a countertransference response in some therapists. This is the consequence of therapist–patient schema mismatch. The therapist who is overly focused on productivity and rationality will find the validation resistance to be quite problematic, whereas the therapist concerned with rejection will

TABLE 13.1. Dimensions of Resistance

Dimension	Example
Validation	Emphasis on empathy and validation of emotions and thoughts, mirroring, being understood means being "cared for" or "protected." Self-invalidation, inhibition or suppression of affect, dissociation, distraction from emotion, avoidance, escape.
Self-consistency	Cognitive dissonance, self-verification, and self-perception processes. Emphasis on heuristics. Commitment to prior behavior, identity, and sunk-costs.
Schematic resistance	Schematic processing: selective attention, recall, and recognition of information. Avoidance, compensation, and maintenance of schemas. Specific vulnerabilities to events dependent on schema.
Moral resistance	Emphasis on personal causality, imperatives, obligations, and guilt. Obsessive beliefs in personal responsibility.
Victim resistance	Emphasis on deflecting responsibility—blaming, victim and martyr roles. Moral self-righteousness, persecutor–defendant–judge scripts, and help rejection.
Risk aversion	Search for danger or loss potential, perception of unpredictability and uncontrollability, rules for "quitting" early, minimization of loss versus maximization of gain.
Self-handicapping	Attempts to obscure self-evaluation, disattribution, excuse generation, judgment focus, and self-limitation.

find the narcissistic schema of superiority and devaluation of others to be troublesome.

Although "cognitive-behavioral purists" may cringe at the use of the term "resistance," I do hope that new insights and interventions become apparent from the multidimensional model I have outlined here. Perhaps some would have preferred a substitute for "resistance," such as "treatment noncompliance," "challenging patients or issues," "nonresponsive to treatment" or "not motivated for treatment." I have no quarrel with such terminology. But my choice of "resistance" is based on my clinical observation that many patients in therapy actually struggle as much with themselves as with the therapist in maintaining a losing position.

Resistance to therapy, at first, seemed to me to be a paradox. Why would a patient voluntarily pursue treatment, disclose painful information, with the apparent intention to modify dysfunctional patterns, and then reject the treatment offered? Why would someone hold onto pain if a possible solution were available? We could claim, with psychoanalysis, that the patient "has a need to suffer," and then feel confident that the patient's masochism has sabotaged therapy. Or we could even attribute almost everything that the patient does outside of therapy to convoluted transferential processes—as if the patient came into therapy simply to manifest his pathology and punish the therapist.

I have eschewed such explanations of resistance. Indeed, I argue that the patient's resistance in therapy is based on processes that the patient believes protect him from further loss or harm. For example, even validation resistance—which seems such a fundamental aspect of human nature—is partly related to the patient's fear that people who are invalidating are not to be trusted. Moral resistance is also self-protective: the patient resists change lest he relinquish his moral values. Resistance, as I have conceptualized it throughout this book, is not a consequence of masochism, but rather a process whereby the individual protects valued aspects of self-functioning.

The multidimensional model proposes that there are (at least) seven important processes affecting resistance. These include validation, self-consistency, schematic resistance, moral resistance, victim roles, risk aversion, and self-handicapping. Validation resistance may appear to be the "least cognitive," since we generally view validation as part of an attachment process. Yet, as fundamental to human nature as validation is, I have attempted to identify some cognitive and behavioral implications of this issue. Some patients may have unique, demanding rules for validation, expecting that only "mirroring" will suffice. Others may believe that their feelings, or aspects of themselves, are so repugnant that they could never share them with anyone. Furthermore, the cognitive model, especially its emphasis on "testing" or "challenging" negative thoughts, may be experienced as especially invalidating to some individuals. My discussion of validation, then, attempted to examine some of the "meanings" or "rules" related to validation and invalidation and to incorporate these insights into a range of interventions.

Self-consistency is, perhaps, the hallmark of what we mean by "self." Some may argue that the "self" is simply a fiction, a reification of an illusion that we have traits (see Mischel, 1968). Even though we can question the validity of the existence of traits, individuals do believe that they have a "self"—that is, that they do have some consistent ways of thinking, believing, and relating (see Harter, 1999). My discussion of self-consistency processes is neutral regarding the existence of a consistent self. This will, of course, seem odd to anyone who thinks about a model of self-consistency that does not address whether there is *actual consistency*. Again, my emphasis in this book has been on the phenomenology of resistance, not on the accuracy of the traits that may or may not characterize individuals. I have simply suggested that people seek consistency. Whether they achieve it is an entirely different question.

My discussion of self-consistency focused on the issue of "sunk-costs." (I extend the discussion of self-consistency to "schematic resistance" which seemed to me to deserve a separate chapter—if not a separate book.) I have found that almost anyone can understand the idea of sunk-costs, since all of us have "thrown good money after bad." Individuals, fearing regret, anticipating further mistakes, and trying to redeem their past mistakes, may resist change because they are less interested in future benefits than in justifying past decisions. These people are "backward looking" rather than "forward looking" in making decisions. They believe "I can't just walk away from it," even though it may be apparent to everyone else that this is precisely what they "should" do. If there ever were a "cognitive trap," it is the "sunk-cost."

Individuals trapped by a sunk-cost often claim that "you just don't understand." This is actually true. Because the therapist is not submerged like the patient is in the sunk-cost, she is not burdened by the necessity to justify the past and save face. Furthermore, many sunk-cost traps are related to the patient's schematic vulnerabilities. The woman who fears that she is undesirable and unlovable is likely to get trapped in the sunk-cost of a losing relationship, but is not so likely to get trapped by sunk-costs in her business relationships. Perhaps we can think of these as "schematic sunk-costs." In any case, I have identified a number of cognitive interventions that may help patients understand this process and assist them in extricating themselves.

The third aspect of resistance, schematic resistance, has been the focus of considerable attention (Beck et al., 1990; Guidano & Liotti, 1983; Leahy, 1985, 1996a; Needleman, 1999; Young, 1990). According to this model, many patients are prevented from making progress because of the persisting effects of their early maladaptive schemas. These early maladaptive schemas may be more resistant to modification for several reasons. First, their onset may be associated with emotionally compelling events that occurred at an early age prior to the use of language and cognitive skills that might allow higher level processing. Second, the individual may have developed schematic adaptations that result in avoidance, compensation, or schema maintenance, thereby conserving the schema. Third, therapy may activate the schema, leading to "protective" maneuvers, which interferes with current change. Finally, the schematic theme may be so familiar to the patient that it does not occur to him that there is a different way of functioning.

Whenever one develops a model, there seems to be some temptation to propose a sequential-causal model, such that certain processes are "prior" to other processes. The model that I have proposed is too preliminary to merit such a definitive proposal. I can certainly see that there are reciprocal influences. For example, a rejection schema may result in risk-aversion and risk-aversion may lead to self-handicapping. But one can argue that risk-aversion may lead to a rejection schema. Perhaps the chicken-and-egg problem can be left for another day. My clinical experience suggests that several modalities of resistance operate simultaneously.

Finally, I have found that developing a curiosity—and sharing this curiosity with the patient—allows resistance to become a dynamic and meaningful part of the collaborative experience of therapy. If we can set aside the tendency to personalize resistance—that is, if we can avoid thinking that the patient is "out to get us"—we can help others escape from the barriers of their resistant self-protection. By getting into their shoes, we can help them find the pathway out.

References

Abramson, L. Y., Metalsky, G. I., & Alloy, L. (1989). Hopelessness depression: A theory-based subtype of depression. *Psychological Review, 96,* 358–372.

Abramson, L. Y., Seligman, M. E. P., & Teasdale, J. D. (1978). Learned helplessness in humans: Critique and reformulation. *Journal of Abnormal Psychology, 87,* 102–109.

Adler, A. (1964). *Social interest: A challenge to mankind.* New York: Capricorn Books. (Original work published 1926)

Alford, B., & Beck, A. T. (1997). *The integrative power of cognitive therapy.* New York: Guilford Press.

Alloy, L., Abramson, L. Y., Metalsky, G. I., & Hartledge, S. (1988). The hopelessness theory of depression. *British Journal of Clinical Psychology, 27,* 5–12.

Arkes, H. R. (1991). The costs and benefits of judgment errors: Implications for debiasing. *Psychological Bulletin, 110,* 486–498.

Arkes, H. R. (1996). The psychology of waste. *Journal of Behavioral Decision Making, 9,* 213–224.

Arkes, H. R., & Ayton, P. (1999). The sunk cost and concorde effects: Are humans less rational than lower animals? *Psychological Bulletin, 125,* 591–600.

Arkes, H. R., & Blumer, C. (1985). The psychology of sunk cost. *Organizational Behavior and Human Decision Processes, 35,* 124–140.

Arkin, R. M., & Oleson, K. C. (1998). Self-handicapping. In J. M. Darley and J. Cooper (Eds.), *Attribution in social interaction: The legacy of Edward E. Jones* (pp. 313–347). Washington, DC: American Psychological Association Press.

Aronson, E. (1995). *The social animal.* New York: Freeman.

Barlow, D. (1988). *Anxiety and its disorders: The nature and treatment of anxiety and panic.* New York: Guilford Press.

Barlow, F. D., & Craske, M. G. (1988). The phenomenology of panic. In S.

Rachman & J. D. Maser (Eds.), *Panic: psychological perspectives* (pp. 11–35). Hillsdale, NJ: Erlbaum.

Baron, J. (1994). *Thinking and deciding* (2nd ed.). Cambridge, UK: Cambridge University Press.

Baucom, D. H. (1987). Attributions in distressed relations: How can we explain them? In S. Duck & D. Perlman (Eds.), *Heterosexual relations, marriage, and divorce* (pp. 177–206). London: Sage.

Baucom, D. H., & Epstein, N. (1990) *Cognitive-behavioral marital therapy.* New York: Brunner/Mazel.

Baumrind, D. (1971). Current patterns of parental authority. *Developmental Psychology Monographs, 4*(Part 1, 2).

Beck, A. T. (1967). *Depression: Causes and treatment.* Philadelphia: University of Pennsylvania Press.

Beck, A. T. (1976). *Cognitive therapy and the emotional disorders.* New York: International Universities Press.

Beck, A. T. (1997). Beyond belief: A theory of modes, personality, and psychotherapy. In P. M. Salkovskis (Ed.), *Frontiers of cognitive therapy* (pp. 1–25). New York: Guilford Press.

Beck, A. T., Emery, G., & Greenberg, R. L. (1985). *Anxiety disorders and phobias: A cognitive perspective.* New York: Basic Books.

Beck, A. T., Freeman, A., & Associates. (1990). *Cognitive therapy of personality disorders.* New York: Guilford Press.

Beck, A. T., Rush, A. J., Shaw, B. F., & Emery, G. (1979). *Cognitive therapy of depression.* New York: Guilford Press.

Beck, J. (1996). *Cognitive therapy: Basics and beyond.* New York: Guilford Press.

Becker, G. S. (1976). *The economic approach to human behavior.* Chicago: University of Chicago Press.

Becker, G. S. (1991). *A treatise on the family.* Cambridge, MA: Harvard University Press.

Becker, G. S., Grossman, M., & Murphy, K. M. (1991). Rational addiction and the effect of price on consumption. *American Economic Review, 81,* 237–241.

Belli, R. F., & Loftus, E. F. (1997). The plausibility of autobiographical memory. In D. C. Rubin (Ed.), *Remembering our past: Studies in autobiographical memory* (pp. 157–179). New York: Cambridge University Press.

Berglas, S., & Jones, E. E. (1978). Drug choice as a self-handicapping strategy in response to noncontingent success. *Journal of Personality and Social Psychology, 36,* 405–417.

Berlyne, D. (1978). Curiosity and learning. *Motivation and Emotion, 2,* 97–175.

Bornstein, B. H., & Chapman, G. B. (1995). Learning lessons from sunk costs. *Journal of Experimental Psychology: Applied, 1,* 251–269.

Bornstein, M., & Arterberry, M. (1999). Perceptual development. In M. Bornstein & M. Lamb (Eds.), *Developmental psychology: An advanced textbook* (pp. 231–276). Hillsdale, NJ: Erlbaum.

Bornstein, M., Kessen, W., & Weiskopf, S. (1976). The categories of hue in infancy. *Science, 191,* 201–202.

Bower, G. (1981). Mood and memory. *American Psychologist, 36,* 129–148.

Bowlby, J. (1969). *Attachment and loss: Vol. 1. Attachment.* New York: Basic Books.

Bowlby, J. (1973). *Attachment and loss: Vol. 2. Separation: Anxiety and anger.* New York: Basic Books.

Bowlby, J. (1980). *Attachment and loss: Vol. 3. Loss: Sadness and depression.* London: Hogarth Press.

Brecht, B. (1991). *Mother Courage and her children* (Eric Bentley, Trans.) New York: Grove Press. (Original work published 1941)

Brehm, S. S., & Brehm, J. W. (1970). *A theory of psychological reactence.* New York: Academic Press.

Breuer, J., & Freud, S. (1955). Studies on hysteria. In J. Strachey (Ed. and Trans.), *The standard edition of the complete psychological works of Sigmund Freud* (Vol. 2). London: Hogarth Press. (Original work published 1895)

Brown, G. W. & Harris, T. (1978). Social origins of depression. New York: Free Press.

Bruner, J. (1992). Another look at New Look 1. *American Psychologist, 47,* 780–783.

Burns, D. D. (1980). *Feeling good: The new mood therapy.* New York: New American Library.

Burns, D. D. (1989). *The feeling good handbook: Using the new mood therapy in everyday life.* New York: Morrow.

Burns, D. D. (1990). *The feeling good handbook.* New York: Plume.

Clark, D. A., Beck, A. T., & Alford, B. (1999). *The scientific foundations of cognitive theory and therapy of depression.* New York: Wiley.

Conway, M. A., & Rubin, D. C. (1993). The structure of autobiographical memory. In A. E. Collins, S. E. Gathercole, M. A. Conway, & P. E. M. Morris (Eds.), *Theories of memory* (pp. 103–137). Hove, Sussex, UK: Erlbaum.

Coyne, J. C., & Pepper, C. M. (1998). The therapeutic alliance in brief strategic therapy. In J. D. Safran & J. C. Muran (Eds.), *The therapeutic alliance in brief psychotherapy* (pp. 147–169). Washington, DC: American Psychological Association Press.

Daniel, K. (1995). The marriage premium. In M. Tommasi & K. Ierulli (Eds.), *The new economics of human behavior* (pp. 113–128). Cambridge, UK: Cambridge University Press.

Dawes, R. M. (1987). *Rational choice in an uncertain world.* New York: Harcourt.

DeRubeis, R., & Feeley, M. (1990). Determinants of change in cognitive therapy. *Cognitive Therapy and Research, 14,* 469–482.

Dowd, E. T. (1999). *Cognitive hypnotherapy.* Northvale, NJ: Jason Aronson.

Dweck, C. S. (1975). The role of expectations and attributions in the alleviation of learned helplessness. *Journal of Personality and Social Psychology, 31,* 674–685.

Dweck, C. S., & Goetz, T. E. (1978). Attributions and learned helplessness. In J. H. Harvey, W. J. Ickes, & R. F. Kidd (Eds.), *New directions in attribution research* (Vol. 2). Hillsdale, NJ: Erlbaum.

D'Zurilla, T. J. (1988). Problem-solving therapies. In K. Dobson (Ed.), *Handbook of cognitive-behavioral therapies* (pp. 85–135). New York: Guilford Press.

Eisenberger, R. (1992). Learned industriousness. *Psychological Review, 99,* 248–267.

Eisenberger, R., Carlson, J., Guile, M., & Shapiro, N. (1979). Transfer of effort across behaviors. *Learning and Motivation, 10,* 178–197.

Ellis, A. (1985). *Overcoming resistance: Rational-emotive therapy with difficult clients.* New York: Springer.

Ellis, A., & Grieger, R. (Eds.). (1977). *Handbook of rational-emotive therapy.* New York: Springer.

Festinger, L. (1957). *A theory of cognitive dissonance.* Stanford, CA: Stanford University Press.

Fisher, R., & Ury, W. (1981). *Getting to yes: Negotiating agreement without giving in.* Boston: Houghton Mifflin.

Foa, E. B., & Kozak, M. J. (1991). Emotional processing: Theory, research, and clinical implications for anxiety disorders. In J. D. Safran & L. S. Greenberg (Eds.), *Emotion, psychotherapy, and change* (pp. 21–49). New York: Guilford Press.

Foa, E. B., & Rothbaum, B. O. (1998). *Treating the trauma of rape: Cognitive-behavioral therapy for PTSD.* New York: Guilford Press.

Frankl, V. (1959). *From death camp to existentialism.* Boston: Beacon Press.

Freud, A. (1946). *The ego and the mechanisms of defence.* New York: International Universities Press.

Freud, S. (1958). The dynamics of transference. In J. Strachey (Ed. and Trans.), *The standard edition of the complete psychological works of Sigmund Freud* (Vol. 12, pp. 97–108). London: Hogarth Press. (Original work published 1912)

Freud, S. (1961). The ego and the id. In J. Strachey (Ed. and Trans.), *The standard edition of the complete psychological works of Sigmund Freud* (Vol. 19, pp. 1–66). London: Hogarth Press. (Original work published 1923)

Freud, S. (1963). Mourning and melancholia. In J. Strachey (Ed. and Trans.), *The standard edition of the complete psychological works of Sigmund Freud* (Vol. 14, pp. 237–260). London: Hogarth Press. (Original work published 1917)

Freud, S. (1964). Analysis terminable and interminable. In J. Strachey (Ed. and Trans.), *The standard edition of the complete psychological works of Sigmund Freud* (Vol. 23, pp. 209–253). London: Hogarth Press. (Original work published 1937)

Fromm, E. (1941). *Escape from freedom.* New York: Rinehart.

Fuller, L. (1967). *Legal fictions.* Stanford, CA: Stanford University Press. (Original work published 1931)

Garland, H. (1990). Throwing good money after bad: The effect of sunk costs on the decision to escalate commitment to an ongoing project. *Journal of Applied Psychology, 75,* 728–731.

Garland, H., & Newport, S. (1991). Effects of absolute and relative sunk costs on the decision to persist with a course of action. *Organizational Behavior and Human Decision Processes, 48,* 55–69.

Geer, J. H., Davison, G. C., & Gatchel, R. I. (1970). Reduction of stress in humans through nonveridical perceived control of aversive stimulation. *Journal of Personality and Social Psychology, 16,* 731–738.

Geer, J. H., & Maisel, E. (1972). Evaluating the effects of the prediction-control confound. *Journal of Personality and Social Psychology, 23,* 314–319.

Gilovich, T., Medvec,V. H., & Chen, S. (1995). Commission, omission, and dissonance reduction: Coping with regret in the "Monty Hall" problem. *Personality and Social Psychology Bulletin, 21,* 182–189.

Greenberg, L., & Paivio, S. (1997). *Working with emotions in psychotherapy.* New York: Guilford Press.

Grossman, M. (1995). The economic approach to addictive behavior. In M. Tommasi & K. Ierulli (Eds.), *The new economics of human behavior* (pp. 157–171). Cambridge, UK: Cambridge University Press.

Guidano, V. F. (1987). *The complexity of the self.* New York: Guilford Press.

Guidano, V., & Liotti, G. (1983). *Cognitive processes and the emotional disorders.* New York: Guilford Press.

Hare, R. M. (1981). *Moral thinking: Its levels, method, and point.* Oxford, UK: Oxford University Press.

Hart, H. L. A. (1968). *Punishment and responsibility.* Oxford, UK: Oxford University Press.

Hart, H. L. A., & Honore, T. (1985). *Causation in the law.* Oxford, UK: Clarendon Press.

Harter, S. (1999). *The construction of the self: A developmental perspective.* New York: Guilford Press.

Hastie, R. (1981). Schematic principles in human memory. In E. T. Higgins, C. P. Herman, & M. P. Zanna (Eds.). *Social cognition: The Ontario Symposium* (Vol. 1, pp. 39–88). Hillsdale, NJ: Erlbaum.

Heider, F. (1958). *The psychology of interpersonal relations.* New York: Wiley.

Heschel, A. J. (Ed.). (1997). *Between God and man: An interpretation of Judaism from the writings of Abraham Joshua Heschel* (F. A. Rothschild, Ed.). Tampa, FL: Free Press.

Ingram, R. E., Miranda, J., & Segal, Z. V. (1998). *Cognitive vulnerability to depression.* New York: Guilford Press.

Jacobson, E. (1938). *Progressive relaxation.* Chicago: University of Chicago Press.

Jones, E. E., & Davis, K. E. (1966). From acts to dispositions: The attribution process in person perception. In L. Berkowitz (Ed.), *Advances in experimental social psychology* (Vol. 2, pp. 219–266). San Diego, CA: Academic Press.

Jones, E. E., & Rhodewalt, F. (1982). *The Self-Handicapping Scale.* (Available from F. Rhodewalt, Department of Psychology, University of Utah.)

Kahneman, D., & Tversky, A. (1979). Prospect theory: An analysis of decision under risk. *Econometrica, 47,* 263–291.

Kegan, R. (1982). *The evolving self: Problem and process in human development.* Cambridge, MA: Harvard University Press.

Kelley, H. H. (1971). *Attribution in social interaction.* Morristown, NJ: General Learning Press.

Kelly, G. A. (1955). *The psychology of personal constructs*. New York: Norton.

Kennedy-Moore, E., & Watson, J. C. (1999). *Expressing emotions: Myths, realities, and therapeutic strategies*. New York: Guilford Press.

Kernberg, O. (1975). *Borderline conditions and pathological narcissism*. New York: Jason Aronson.

Kernberg, O. (1978). *Object relations theory and clinical psychoanalysis*. New York: Jason Aronson.

Kierkegaard, S. (1954a). *Fear and trembling: A dialectical lyric*. Princeton, NJ: Princeton University Press. (Original work published 1843)

Kierkegaard, S. (1954b). *Either/or*. Princeton, NJ: Princeton University Press. (Original work published 1843)

Kiesler, C. A. (1969). *The psychology of commitment*. New York: Academic Press.

Koffka, K. (1963). *The principles of gestalt psychology*. New York: Harcourt-Brace. (Original work published 1935)

Kohler, W. (1929). *Gestalt psychology*. New York: Liveright.

Kohut, H. (1971). *The analysis of the self*. New York: International Universities Press.

Kohut, H. (1977). *The restoration of the self*. New York: International Universities Press.

Langer, E. (1990). *Mindfulness*. New York: Perseus Press.

Leahy, R. L. (1978). *Children's judgments of excuses*. Paper delivered at the Southeastern Conference on Human Development, Atlanta, GA.

Leahy, R. L. (1983). Development of self and the problems of social cognition: Identity formation and depression. In L. Wheeler & P. Shaver (Eds.), *Review of personality and social psychology* (pp. 206–236). Beverly Hills, CA: Sage.

Leahy, R. L. (1985). The costs of development: Clinical implications. In R. L. Leahy (Ed.), *The development of the self* (pp. 267–294). San Diego, CA: Academic Press.

Leahy, R. L. (1991). Scripts in cognitive therapy: The systemic perspective. *Journal of Cognitive Psychotherapy, 5*, 291–304.

Leahy, R. L. (1992). Cognitive therapy on Wall Street: Schemas and scripts of invulnerability. *Journal of Cognitive Psychotherapy, 6*, 1–14.

Leahy, R. L. (1995). Cognitive development and cognitive therapy. *Journal of Cognitive Psychotherapy, 9*, 173–184.

Leahy, R. L. (1996a). *Cognitive therapy: Basic principles and applications*. Northvale, NJ: Jason Aronson.

Leahy, R. L. (1996b). *An investment model of resistance*. Paper presented at the meeting of the Association for the Advancement of Behavior Therapy, New York City.

Leahy, R. L. (1997a). An investment model of depressive resistance. *Journal of Cognitive Psychotherapy, 11*, 3–19.

Leahy, R. L. (1997b). Depression and resistance: An investment model of decision making. *Behavior Therapist, 20*, 3–6.

Leahy, R. L. (1997c). Resistance and self-limitation. In R. L. Leahy (Ed.), *Practicing cognitive therapy: A guide to interventions* (pp. 61–86). Northvale, NJ: Jason Aronson.

Leahy, R. L. (Ed.). (1997d). *Practicing cognitive therapy: A guide to interventions*. Northvale, NJ: Jason Aronson.

Leahy, R. L. (1997e). Cognitive therapy interventions. In R. L. Leahy (Ed.), *Practicing cognitive therapy: A guide to interventions*. Northvale, NJ: Jason Aronson.

Leahy, R. L. (1997f). Reflections on cognitive therapy. In R. L. Leahy (Ed.), *Practicing cognitive therapy: A guide to interventions*. Northvale, NJ: Jason Aronson.

Leahy, R. L. (1999a). Strategic self-limitation. *Journal of Cognitive Psychotherapy, 13,* 275–293.

Leahy, R. L. (1999b). Decision-making and mania. *Journal of Cognitive Psychotherapy, 13,* 1–23.

Leahy, R. L. (1999c). *A cognitive model of manic decision-making*. Paper presented at the meeting of the Association for Advancement of Behavior Therapy, Toronto.

Leahy, R. L. (1999d). *Depressive decision-making*. Paper presented at the meeting of the Association for Advancement of Behavior Therapy, Toronto.

Leahy, R. L. (1999e). *Self-limitation*. Paper presented at the meeting of the Association for Advancement of Behavior Therapy, Toronto.

Leahy, R. L. (2000a). Mood and decisions: Implications for bipolar disorder. *Behavior Therapist, 62*–63.

Leahy, R. L. (2000b). Sunk-costs and resistance to change. *Journal of Cognitive Psychotherapy, 14,* 355–371.

Leahy, R. L. (2000c). *Some implications of a Piagetian-developmental constructivist approach to cognitive therapy*. Paper presented at the International Congress on Constructivism in Psychotherapy, Geneva.

Leahy, R. L. (2000d). *Constructing risk and resistance in psychotherapy*. Paper presented at the International Congress on Constructivism in Psychotherapy, Geneva.

Leahy, R. L., & Beck, A. T. (1988). Cognitive therapy of depression and mania. In A. Georgotas & R. Cancro (Eds.), *Depression and mania* (pp. 517–537). New York: Elsevier.

Leahy, R. L., & Holland, S. (2000). *Treatment plans and interventions for depression and anxiety disorders*. New York: Guilford Press.

Leahy, R. L., & Shirk, S. (1984). The development of social cognition: Conceptions of personality. In L. Wheeler (Ed.), *Annals of child development* (Vol. 1, pp. 175–200). Greenwich, CT: JAI Press.

Lerner, M. J., & Miller, D. T. (1978). Just world research and the attribution process: Looking back and ahead. *Psychological Bulletin, 85,* 1030–1051.

Lewinsohn, P. M., Breckenridge, J. S., Antonuccio, D. O., & Teri, L. (1987). Group therapy for depression: The coping with depression course. In P. Keller & S. R. Heyman (Eds.), *Innovations in clinical practice: A sourcebook* (Vol. 6, pp. 361–375). Sarasota, FL: Professional Resource Exchange.

Light, D. (1970). *Becoming psychiatrists*. New York: Norton.

Linehan, M. (1993). *Cognitive-behavioral treatment of borderline personality disorder*. New York: Guilford Press.

Loftus, E., & Ketcham, K. (1994). *The myth of repressed memory*. New York: St. Martin's Press.

Mahoney, M. (1991). *Human change processes: The scientific foundations of psychotherapy*. New York: Basic Books.

Marks, I. M. (1987). *Fears, phobia, and rituals: Panic, anxiety and their disorders*. New York: Oxford University Press.

Masterson, J. F. (1976). *Psychotherapy of the borderline adult*. New York: Brunner/Mazel.

Masterson, J. F. (1981). *The narcissistic and borderline disorders*. New York: Brunner/Mazel

McClelland, D. C. (1951). *Personality*. New York: Sloane, Dryden, Holt.

Miller, W. R., & Rollnick, S. (1991). *Motivational interviewing: Preparing people to change addictive behavior*. New York: Guilford Press.

Millon, T., Davis, R., Millon, C., Escovar, L., & Meagher, S. (2000). *Personality disorders in modern life*. New York: Wiley.

Mischel, W. (1968). *Personality and assessment*. New York: Wiley.

Murray, H. (1938). *Explorations in personality*. New York: Oxford University Press.

Needleman, L. D. (1999). *Cognitive case conceptualization: A guidebook for practitioners*. Mahway, NJ: Erlbaum.

Newman, C. (1994). Understanding client resistance: Methods for enhancing motivation to change. *Cognitive and Behavioral Practice, 1*, 47–69.

Newman, C. (1997). Maintaining professionalism in the face of emotional abuse from clients. *Cognitive and Behavioral Practice, 4*, 1–29.

Newman, C., Leahy, R. L., Beck, A. T., Reilly-Harrington, N., & Gyulai, L. (2001). *Bipolar disorder: A cognitive therapy approach*. Washington, DC: American Psychological Association Press.

Nezu, A., & Nezu, C. (1989). Unipolar depression. In A. Nezu & C. Nezu (Eds.), *Clinical decision making in behavior therapy: A problem-solving perspective* (pp. 117–156). Champaign, IL: Research Press.

Otto, R. (1950). *The idea of the holy* (J. W. Harvey, Trans.). Oxford, UK: Oxford University Press. (Original work published 1923)

Padesky, C. (1996) Developing cognitive therapist competency: Teaching and supervision models. In P. M. Salkovskis (Ed.), *Frontiers of cognitive therapy* (pp. 226–292). New York: Guilford Press.

Patterson, G. R. (1982). *Coercive family process*. Eugene, OR: Castalia.

Pelikan, J. (1999). *Jesus through the centuries: His place in the history of culture*. New Haven: Yale University Press.

Pennebaker, J. W. (1995). *Emotion, disclosure, and health*. Washington, DC: American Psychological Association Press.

Persons, J. (1989). *Cognitive therapy in practice: A case formulation approach*. New York: Norton.

Peterson, C., Maier, S., & Seligman, M. E. P. (1993) *Learned helplessness: A theory for the age of personal control*. New York: Oxford University Press.

Piaget, J. (1934). *The moral judgment of the child*. New York: Free Press.

Piaget, J. (1970a). *Genetic epistemology*. New York: Norton.

Piaget, J. (1970b). *Structuralism*. New York: Harper.

Pope, K. S., & Vasquez, M. J. T. (1998). *Ethics in psychotherapy and counseling: A practical guide.* New York: Jossey-Bass.

Premack, D. (1965). Reinforcement theory. In D. Levine (Ed.), *Nebraska Symposium on Motivation* (Vol. 13, pp. 123–180). Lincoln: University of Nebraska Press.

Rachman, S. J. (1993). Obsessions, responsibility, and guilt. *Behavior Research and Therapy, 31,* 149–154.

Rehm, L. P. (1977). A self-control model of depression. *Behavior Therapy, 8,* 787–804.

Rehm, L. P. (1990). Cognitive and behavioral theories. In B. B. Wolman & G. Stricker (Eds.), *Depressive disorders: Facts, theories, and treatment methods* (pp. 64–91). New York: Wiley.

Riskind, J., Sarampote, C., & Mercier, M. A. (1996). For every malady a sovereign cure: Optimism training. *Journal of Cognitive Psychotherapy, 10,* 105–117.

Rogers, C. R. (1950). A theory of therapy, personality, and interpersonal relationships as developed in the client-centered framework. In S. Koch (Ed.), *Psychology: The study of a science* (Vol. 3). New York: McGraw-Hill.

Rogers, C. R. (1965). *Client-centered therapy: Its current practice, implications, and theory.* Boston: Houghton Mifflin.

Safran, J. D. (1998). *Widening the scope of cognitive therapy: The therapeutic relationship, emotion and the process of change.* Northvale, NJ: Jason Aronson.

Safran, J. D., & Muran, C. (2000). *Negotiating the therapeutic alliance.* New York: Guilford Press.

Safran, J. D., & Segal, Z. V. (1990). *Interpersonal process in cognitive therapy.* New York: Basic Books.

Salkovskis, P. M. (1989). Cognitive-behavioral factors and the persistence of intrusive thoughts in obsessive problems. *Behaviour Research and Therapy, 23,* 571–583.

Salkovskis, P. M. (1996). The cognitive approach to anxiety: Threat beliefs, safety-seeking behavior, and the special case of health anxiety and obsessions. In P. M. Salkovksis (Ed.), *Frontiers of cognitive therapy* (pp. 48–74). New York: Guilford Press.

Salkovskis, P. M., & Kirk, J. (1989). Obsessional disorders. In K. Hawton, P. M. Salkovskis, J. Kirk, & D. M. Clark (Eds.), *Cognitive behaviour therapy for psychiatric problems: A practical guide* (pp. 179–208). Oxford, UK: Oxford University Press.

Salkovskis, P. M., & Kirk, J. (1997). Obsessive–compulsive disorder. In D. M. Clark & C. G. Fairburn (Eds.). *Science and practice of cognitive behaviour therapy* (pp. 179–208). Oxford, UK: Oxford University Press.

Sartre, J. P. (1964). *Being and nothingness: An essay in phenomenological ontology.* New York: Citadel Press. (Original work published 1956)

Schafer, R. (1954). *Psychoanalytic interpretation in Rorschach testing: Theory and application.* New York: Grune & Stratton.

Schwartz, B. (1986). *The battle for human nature: Science, morality and modern life.* New York: Norton.

Schwartz, B., & Lacey, H. (1982). *Behaviorism, science and human nature*. New York: Norton.

Seligman, M. E. P. (1990). *Learned optimism*. New York: Knopf.

Shapiro, D. (1965). *Neurotic styles*. New York: Norton.

Shorter, E. (1997). *A history of psychiatry: From the age of the asylum to the age of prozac*. New York: Wiley.

Simon, H. A. (1979). Rational decision making in business organizations. *American Economic Review, 79*, 293–304.

Smucker, M., & Dancu, C. V. (1999). *Cognitive-behavioral treatment for adult survivors of childhood trauma*. Northvale, NJ: Jason Aronson.

Snyder, C. R., Higgins, R. L., & Stucky, R. J. (1983). *Excuses: Masquerades in search of grace*. New York: Wiley.

Staw, B. M. (1976). Knee-deep in the Big Muddy: A study of escalating commitment to a chosen course of action. *Organizational Behavior and Human Performance, 16*, 27–44.

Staw, B. M. (1981). The escalation of commitment to a course of action. *Academy of Management Review, 6*, 577–587.

Staw, B. M., & Ross, J. (1987). Behavior in escalation situations: Antecedents, prototypes, and solutions. In L. L. Cummings & B. M. Staw (Eds.), *Research in organizational behavior* (Vol. 9, pp. 39–78). Greenwich, CT: JAI Press.

Steiner, R. (1980). *The death of tragedy*. New York: Oxford University Press.

Strean, H. S. (1990). *Resolving resistances in psychotherapy*. New York: Brunner/Mazel.

Stuart, R. B. (1980). *Helping couples change: A social-learning approach to marital therapy*. New York: Guilford Press.

Swann, W. B. (1983). Self-verification: Bringing social reality into harmony with the self. In J. Suls & A. G. Greenwald (Eds.), *Psychological perspectives on the self* (Vol. 2, pp. 33–66). Hillsdale NJ: Erlbaum.

Swann, W. B., Stein-Seroussi, A., & Giesler, R. B. (1992). Why people self-verify. *Journal of Personality and Social Psychology, 62*, 392–401.

Tannen, D. (1990). *You just don't understand: Women and men in conversations*. New York: Morrow.

Taylor, S. (1990). *Positive illusions: Creative self-deception and the healthy mind*. New York: Basic Books.

Temoshak, L., & Dreher, H. (1992). *The Type C connection: The behavioral links to cancer and your health*. New York: Random House.

Thaler, R. (1980). Toward a positive theory of consumer choice. *Journal of Economic Behavior and Organization, 1*, 39–60.

Thaler, R. (1992). *The winner's curse: Paradoxes and anomalies of economic life*. Princeton, NJ: Princeton University Press.

Tommasi, M., & Ierulli, K. (Eds.). (1995). *The new economics of human behavior*. Cambridge, UK: Cambridge University Press.

Tompkins, M. (1999). Using a case formulation to manage treatment nonresponse. *Journal of Cognitive Psychotherapy: An International Quarterly, 13*, 317–330.

Traue, H. C., & Pennebaker, J. W. (1993). *Emotion, inhibition, and health*. Kirkland, WA: Hogrefe & Huber.

Unamuno, M. de (1990). *The tragic sense of life* (J. E. C. Flitch, Trans.). North Hampton, NH: Dover Publications. (Original work published 1921)

Waddington, C. H. (1957). *The strategy of the genes: A discussion of some aspects of theoretical biology*. London: Allen and Unwin.

Wegner, D. M. (1989). *White bears and other unwanted thoughts: Suppression, obsession, and the psychology of mental control*. New York: Guilford Press.

Weiner, B. (1974). Achievement motivation as conceptualized by an attribution theorist. In B. Weiner (Ed.), *Achievement motivation and attribution theory*. Morristown, NJ: General Learning Press.

Weiner, B. (1985). An attribution theory of achievement motivation and emotion. *Psychological Review, 92,* 548–573.

Weiner, B. (1995). *Judgments of responsibility: A foundation of a theory of social conduct*. New York: Guilford Press.

Wells, A. (1997). *Cognitive therapy of anxiety disorders: A practice manual and conceptual guide*. Chichester, UK: Wiley.

Westen, D. (1998). The scientific legacy of Sigmund Freud: Toward a psychodynamically informed psychological science. *Psychological Bulletin, 124,* 333–371.

Whyte, G. (1993). Escalating commitment in individual and group decision making: A prospect theory approach. *Organizational Behavior and Human Decision Processes, 54,* 430–455.

Wilson, E. O. (1975). *Sociobiology: The new synthesis*. Cambridge, MA: Harvard University Press.

Wilson, J. Q. (1993). *The moral sense*. New York: Free Press.

Winnicott, D. W. (1986). *Holding and interpretation*. New York: Grove Press.

Young, J. E. (1990). *Cognitive therapy for personality disorders: A schema-focused approach*. Sarasota, FL: Professional Resource Exchange.

Index

("f" indicates a figure, "t" indicates a table)